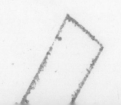

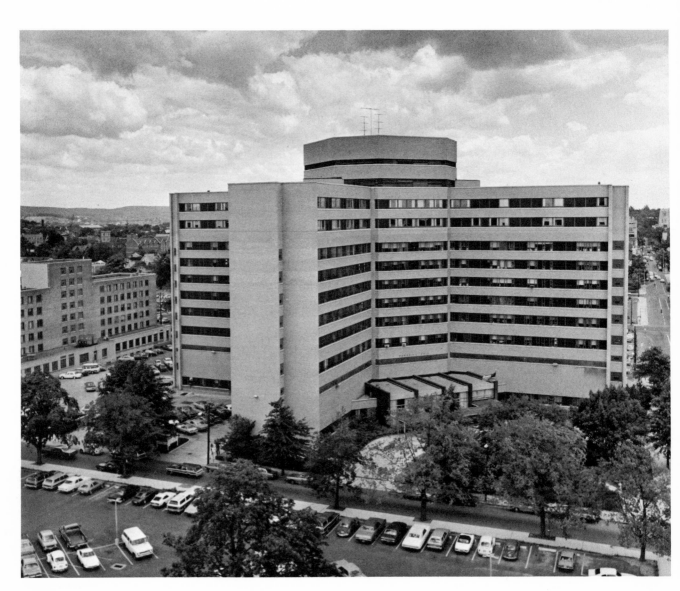

Frontispiece. Memorial Unit, Yale–New Haven Hospital, New Haven, Connecticut, 1974, as completed with the addition of two new stories.

THE HOSPITAL: A Social and Architectural History

THE HOSPITAL: A SOCIAL AND ARCHITECTURAL HISTORY

John D. Thompson and Grace Goldin

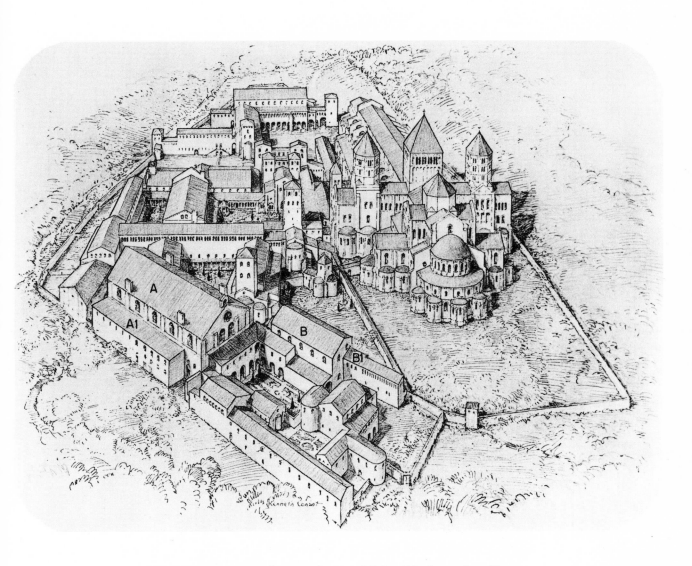

New Haven and London   Yale University Press

1975

Published with assistance from
the Louis Stern Memorial Fund.

Library of Congress catalog card number: 74-19574
International standard book number: 0-300-0 1829-0

Designed by John O. C. McCrillis
and set in Garamond type.
Printed in the United States of America by
The Murray Printing Co., Forge Village, Mass.

Published in Great Britain, Europe, and Africa by
Yale University Press, Ltd., London.
Distributed in Latin America by Kaiman & Polon,
Inc., New York City; in India by UBS Publishers' Distributors Pvt.,
Ltd., Delhi; in Japan by John Weatherhill, Inc., Tokyo.

for E. M. Bluestone, M.D.,
who never lost sight of the
patient in the plan

Contents

List of Illustrations

Frontispiece. Memorial Unit, Yale–New Haven Hospital, 1974. Photo by Stuart Langer; courtesy Yale–New Haven Hospital.

1. Hall for dreamer–patients, Asklepieion of Epidauros, fifth century B.C. From Alfonse Defrasse and Henri Lechat, *Épidaure*. Paris: May and Motteroz, 1895, p. 131.

2. Latrines, North Market Hall, Miletus. From Arnin von Gerkan, "Der Nordmarkt und der Hafen an der Löwenbucht" in Theodor Weigand, ed., *Milet, Ergebnisse der Ausgrabungen und Untersuchungen seit den jahre 1899*, Berlin and Leipzig, 1922, 1: figs 20–21; courtesy Walter Horn.

3. Model of the Asklepieion of Pergamon by H. Schleif. From Erich Boehringer, "Pergamon," *Neue Deutsche Ausgrabungen in Mittelmeergebiet und im Vorderen Orient*, Berlin: Gebr. Mann, 1959, fig. 25.

4. Floor plan and reconstruction of Roman military hospital (*valetudinarium*) of Vindonissa (Windisch, Switzerland, first century A.D.). From Mario Tabanelli, "Gli ospedale delle legioni Romane, lungo 'Limes' Germanico ed Orientale," *Atti del Primo Congresso di Storia Ospitaliera*, Reggio Emilia (1960): 1264.

5. A nursing brother kissing the wounds of a patient. Photo courtesy George Kubler, of a painting in Peru (probably Lima).

6. Site plan, monastery of Turmanin, about 475 A.D. From Georges Tchalenko, *Villages antiques de la Syrie du Nord,* Institut français d'archéologie de Beyrouth, B.A.H. tome L, Paris, Geuthner, 1953–58, 2, pl. 16.

7. The convent building of Turmanin as it looked about 1865. From Charles Jean Melchior de Vogüé, *Syrie centrale,* Paris: J. Baudry, 1865–77, 1: pl. 131.

8. Plan of St. Gall monastery, Switzerland, about 820. Courtesy Walter Horn.

9. Elevation and plan of the cattle barn of Ezinge, province Groningen, The Netherlands, third century B.C. Walter Horn's reconstruction, drawn by Walter Schwartz; courtesy Walter Horn.

10. Three building types of the St. Gall plan as reconstructed by Walter Horn and drawn by William Hill; courtesy Walter Horn.

11. Model of the St. Gall plan by Walter Horn and Ernest Born. Photo by Schmolz and Ullrich, Köln; courtesy Walter Horn.

12. View of Cluny monastery and infirmary about 1043, as restored by Kenneth J. Conant. Courtesy Medieval Academy of America. Photo Ufford and Nedzweski.

13. Ground plan of the monastery of Cluny about 1050, as restored by Kenneth J. Conant. Courtesy Medieval Academy of America. Photo Ufford and Nedzweski.

14. Ground plan of Cluny monastery about 1157, as restored by Kenneth J. Conant. Courtesy Medieval Academy of America. Photo Ufford and Nedzweski.

15. Elevations and bird's eye view of Cluny monastery about 1157, as restored by Kenneth J. Conant. Courtesy Medieval Academy of America. Photos Ufford and Nedzweski.

16. Drain of dormitory necessarium, Kirkstall Abbey, England. Courtesy Charles H. Talbot. Photo by A. W. Haggis.

17. Plan of buildings and drains of Christ Church priory, Canterbury, by Robert Willis after a Norman drawing of 1165. From Willis, *The Conventual Buildings of Christ Church in Canterbury,* London: Kent Architectural Society, 1869, pl. 2.

18. Plan of Ourscamp infirmary by Viollet-le-Duc. From *Dictionnaire raisonné de l'architecture française,* Paris: Morel, 1875, 6: 106.

19. Ourscamp infirmary in 1967, exterior and interior views. Photos by Grace Goldin.

20. Interior of the Hôtel-Dieu of St. Jean in Angers in the nineteenth century. From A. Ver-

List of Tables

Acknowledgments

The first thanks go to the readers of the history, whose criticisms and suggestions were incorporated in it to the best of our ability: Professor Dieter Jetter of the University of Köln, who carefully reviewed all of Part 1 twice; Dr. Egill Snorrason of the Rigshospital, Copenhagen; Professor George Rosen of Yale University; and Dr. Charles H. Talbot of the Wellcome Library, London, who read the section dealing with medieval hospitals. Mr. Miles C. Hardie, then Director of the King's Fund Centre, London, plied us with materials for chapter 9, on contemporary British hospital design, and painstakingly excised mistakes in it. We thank for special encouragement during the preparation of Parts 1 and 2 the late Dr. Richard H. Shryock, Dr. Kenneth J. Conant, Professor Derek de Solla Price of Yale University, and Professor Erna Lesky of the University of Vienna. The generosity and patient helpfulness of Professor Walter Horn of the University of California, Berkeley, and his unfailing interest in Part 1 entitle him to be its patron. Errors remaining in the pages dealing with the past and contemporary history of the hospital are of our own unaided making.

To the staffs of the medical museums, and especially of European and American hospitals visited in the course of gathering historical materials, sincere thanks for a friendly welcome and freedom to photograph and photocopy. Some individual obligations are footnoted under the specific hospitals discussed.

Warm thanks are owing to Miss Madeline Stanton, Mr. Ferenc Gyorgyey, Mr. Stanley Truelson, and the staff of the Medical-Historical Library of Yale University for a decade of eager assistance; to Miss Lydia Wentworth and Mrs. Sonja Bay of the Art Library of Yale University; and to Mrs. Lisabeth M. Holloway of the Library of the College of Physicians, Philadelphia.

As for the studies on the modern hospital whose results are reported here, it is impossible to list all the faculty and staff who contributed to them. Mr. Robert Pelletier and Dr. Robert B. Fetter were the principal coinvestigators; their collaboration in specific chapters is indicated. Special mention should be made of the late Mrs. Nancy Lincoln, who worked on the investigation into the modern hospital for many years, adding to it, as she did to everything, the touch of humanity. Other staff making major contributions were Mrs. Catherine Calder, Mrs. Liliane McClenning, Dr. Joel Kavet, Mr. John F. O'Connor, and Mr. Hugh Maher. The advice of Dr. Charles Flagle was constantly sought while contending with problems involved in certain phases of this research.

No book was luckier in those who joined to produce it. Miss Bev Pope was responsible for the labeling of plans and pictures, for the charts and graphs, and the best of the photographic printing. The uniform excellence of her work enhances many pages. An expert team at the Yale University Press, under the directorship of Chester Kerr, was involved with this volume: Mr. Alexander Metro, Mrs. Anne Wilde, Mrs. Tina Weiner, Ms. Jill Danzig. The superb design of the book and disposition of illustrations on the pages are the work of Mr. John McCrillis. Our wonderful editor, Mrs. Jane Isay, conducted the complex production with her customary verve and wit, and with know-how and understanding of a rare order. To all, the authors' profound thanks.

John D. Thompson initiated this book and formulated the elements of ward design on which the whole is based. He directed and wrote the Yale Studies in Hospital Function and Design and the concluding chapters analyzing the modern hospital. Grace Goldin wrote the history of hospitals and chose its accompanying illustrations.

Some of the historical research was supported by grants from the American Philosophical Society and The Wellcome Institute, London. The research as a whole was supported for 6 years by U.S. Public Health Grants #5ROI H5-10063 and #HM 00543, and the cost of reproducing the illustrations was covered by U.S. Public Health Grant #1ROI LM-01952-1.

Introduction

This book is about the hospital ward, also called the *nursing unit* or *inpatient unit.* It is called inpatient unit because hospital patients stay overnight, as well as to distinguish it from the outpatient departments, where they come and go. It is called nursing unit to differentiate it from areas of the hospital not directly given over to patient care: the space for administrative offices, teaching, research, mechanical services, and the housing of staff.

We have collected, examined, illustrated, and evaluated many ward plans, past and present. Part 1 gives a history of nursing unit floor plans since Roman times in some European countries and the United States (chapters 1–6). Part 2 reviews contemporary planning problems in the United States and Great Britain (chapters 7 and 9). Part 3 contains the Yale Studies in Hospital Function and Design, which were concerned with hospital problems of today and particularly with the evaluation of a scientifically above-average contemporary ward plan, that of the Memorial Unit of the Yale–New Haven Hospital (chapters 10–17). Part 4 (chapters 18 and 19) considers the structure and possible future applications of the concept of progressive patient care.

In the historical section no attempt was made to trace the origin of the hospital as an institution or to describe hospital care earlier than the first century or in any part of Asia, Africa, Australia, South America, Mexico, Canada, and so forth at any date. A glance at the table of contents will show that the range undertaken was vast enough. Hospitals chosen for discussion were often, but not necessarily, "important" ones. Each ward we examine in some detail does represent the way people were thinking about group housing for the sick at that time and place. (Up to a century ago, they were thinking mainly in terms of the pauper sick or those without kin or friends to care for them; most patients were nursed at home.) In many instances, other examples from different countries might serve as well but we chose the ones we did because reliable information about them was relatively easy to come by, because we were intrigued by certain aspects of them, or because they were wards we were given the opportunity to visit. A year's residence in Copenhagen by one of the authors during the preparation of the book resulted in a disproportionate concern with Danish hospitals, particularly so since no other part of Scandinavia is mentioned. Great Britain is amply represented because there was no language difficulty with the sources. An arbitrary principle of choice was unavoidable.

The distinction is drawn between what we have termed *designed* and *derived* historic hospital plans. Designed hospitals were those in which an attempt was made to plan for the function of nursing care. In derived hospitals, the buildings were actually borrowed from monasteries, palaces, estates, prisons, barracks, or they were consciously constructed in current architectural forms for any one of them—in a spirit of public-mindedness, to be sure, but also with the hope of adorning the community and providing a lasting monument to the beneficence of the charitable founders. The success (if one may call it that) of a ward design depended until relatively recently on how well the building form chosen adapted to nursing purposes. For example, the barracks form seemed to make for a better nursing unit than did a monastery or palace.

About a hundred years ago, planning for function took the upper hand. Today the hospital is thought of as a functional machine. In our second section we review recent American and English literature having to do with planning for increased privacy or better supervision. This affords a closer and more detailed look at the actual forms assumed by wards in our time and at the agitated controversy over how to build them, in which many interested parties join: architects, hospital administrators, physicians, nurses, patients, and the community or governmental agency that must finance each hospital project.

In our third section we present the Yale Studies in Hospital Function and Design. It was the intention of the research team to examine, as carefully and objectively as possible, building axioms of our time as embodied in a ward complex of recent date and above-average construction standards: the Memorial Unit of the Yale–New Haven Hospital. Many aspects of the actual working wards were tested by questionnaires, simple comparisons with other ward units, and the more sophisticated technique of comparison with conceptual, mathematical, and computer models. A detailed description of the methodology employed will be found in chapter 10. A valid methodology should be like a yardstick that is able to measure not only the object immediately at hand but any similar object as well. Once we had arrived at a workable evaluation technique for the Yale–New Haven Hospital, we could offer that methodology to any administrator for application to his own hospital to determine his own needs. For example, the Yale Traffic Index, a formula evolved in one of the studies in this book (chapter 15), can be applied to a ward unit of any shape or size to determine its efficiency in terms of nursing steps.

In the fourth section we treat the concept of progressive patient care, first as presently operating within the hospital, where separate areas may be assigned to intensive, intermediate, self-, and long-term care. After that, the concept is applied to a progressive patient care system of hospitals that we call progressive patient care writ large—a pattern for the future.

The design of any nursing unit is composed of four ingredients: the *healthful environment* it provides for patients, the amount of *privacy* it allows patients, the extent to which it exercises *supervision and control* over patients, and the *efficiency* with which it can be operated. These we call the four elements of ward design. This book is an elaboration of the four elements since all our research has been an attempt to examine aspects of one element or another.

But at the outset we must make one point clear: neither privacy, nor supervision and control, nor economy and efficiency, nor a sanitary environment may be treated separately and pursued as an end in itself. In no unit do all four elements appear in their pure, distilled states. It would be a physical impossibility. As the air about us is a combination of oxygen, hydrogen, and nitrogen, so the nursing unit atmosphere is a combination of privacy and supervision, efficiency and sanitation. One cannot say of any one element in the nursing unit, any more than of one element in the air, the more the merrier. The well-run unit is not a concentrate but a judicious mixture of all four elements.

Efficiency, or its by-product economy—a preoccupation of our times—may demand less than the optimum in the way of supervision and control. With too much emphasis on efficiency and economy, sanitary provisions may be found imperfect. Intensive supervision and control necessarily impinge upon the patient's privacy. The administrator, architect, and nurse must determine in advance how much of each ingredient should be provided to achieve the perfect

mix for their particular nursing unit. They will soon realize that emphasis on one ingredient means giving up another, and they must be clear about the true cost of each element in the design. Like the administrator who has to balance 100 percent availability of labor rooms against their cost and the reasonable utilization of each one, hospital personnel who want optimum privacy for their nursing unit must figure out what it is going to cost them in terms of efficiency, economy, supervision, and control.

It is assumed in the third section that one ward, designed as a careful mixture of the four design components, will meet the needs of all patients. Our efforts in Part 3 were limited to describing what went on in such a ward. We assumed that what went on should have gone on. The studies in Part 4, on progressive patient care, go beyond this assumption to deal with problems of a completely different order. They extend the inquiry to the question of whether the patient should have been in that particular ward at all. The functional pressures of modern scientific medicine have burst the one-unit system wide open and have resulted in a need for three or four different inpatient units where patients might be housed within the hospital in the course of a single illness.

In the separate units the four design components cannot be judiciously mixed; one element must predominate at the expense of the others. For example, intensive-treatment requirements of the acutely ill coronary patient may result in a nursing unit design primarily concerned with supervision and in which privacy is eliminated, overall efficiency sacrificed, and selected sanitary facilities eliminated. When the patient improves, it will be better to treat him in a completely different unit with optimal privacy and efficiency and to surround him with the usual amenities that make his return home easier.

The studies of Part 3 are already history. In Part 4, ward planning takes one more step. It is typical of today's thinking that solutions arrived at in our final chapter are open ended because the work is unfinished; we call for reactions from those who decide on plans for tomorrow's hospitals. Solutions are still in the making. Like other aspects of contemporary life, they will be vastly complicated.

PART 1

A History of Ward Design in Europe and the United States

CHAPTER 1

Early Forms

Greek Asklepieia

Nursing wards are not meant to be living areas. Normally, group housing is planned for occupants who sometimes stand, sometimes sit down, and sometimes lie down, but the chief occupants of a nursing area—those for whom it was designed—are horizontal most of the time. Because the patients are bedridden, the central and most important part of a nursing ward is the bed area.

However, a ward unit also consists of service rooms for helpers, which have to allow primarily for the first two postures. The helpers stand or sit to prepare medication or food, to keep records, or to take a rest, and only for nightwatchers is there need for a bed in the service rooms. Another area that must allow for the sitting posture is that of the patients' privies, whose number and size depend upon how ambulatory the patients are expected to be.

The central area is a bed area. In this respect, historical and modern nursing units are similar. In addition to it there must be service rooms for the nurses and for cooking, medical preparation, and treatment. In this volume we are not concerned with operation rooms, emergency rooms, or outpatient areas for the sick who do not sleep over in the hospital. We limit ourselves to the *inpatient unit,* the bed area and service rooms directly attendant upon it.

The subject of ward planning is a vast one. In reviewing it historically, we further limit ourselves with very few exceptions to Western Europe and the United States. Wherever possible we have tried to treat historical examples whose actual floor plans have come down to us. We cannot attempt to recreate origins in Egypt, India, or even Greece. The Greek material presents a dilemma. What shall one say about the open halls of Greco-Roman Asklepieia, where attendant priests converted patients' dreams into a therapeutic regimen? They undeniably were places for inpatient nursing, including bed rest, treatments, medication, baths, diet, and exercise, and we do possess a number of floor plans of the large halls in which patients gathered to dream their dreams. Figure 1 shows the double hall for dreamer–patients at the Asklepieion of Athens, founded fifth century B.C. The rooms were 24 feet deep by 108 and 96 feet long and completely closed on three sides and opening to the south with a row of pillars—the typical form of a Greek stoa (portico)—oriented to the sun.

However, the whole approach to hospitalization was foreign to our own. Some "patients" were simply stand-ins for others at home too ill to undertake the pilgrimage. Whatever a patient dreamed that the god Asklepios told him to do was then carried out in the form of treatment, although it went dead against the medical convictions of the time. For example, in the second century A.D. a sufferer from tumor of the groin was sent on a long horseback ride. In carrying out the god's prescription presented to him in a dream, the patient satisfied certain masochistic longings; and, by the way, he recovered.[1]

The architectural forms of a gathering place for the

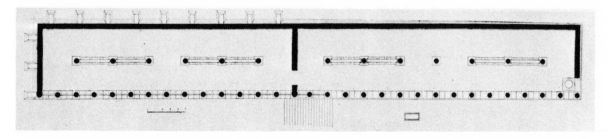

Fig. 1. Double hall for dreamer–patients at the Asklepieion of Epidauros, fifth century B.C., as restored along the lines of a branch building, the Asklepieion of Athens. The left-hand hall was built directly on the ground. The right-hand hall, flush with it, rested upon a full basement. The circle (extreme right) was a well. Patients could see the temple through the portico from their beds.

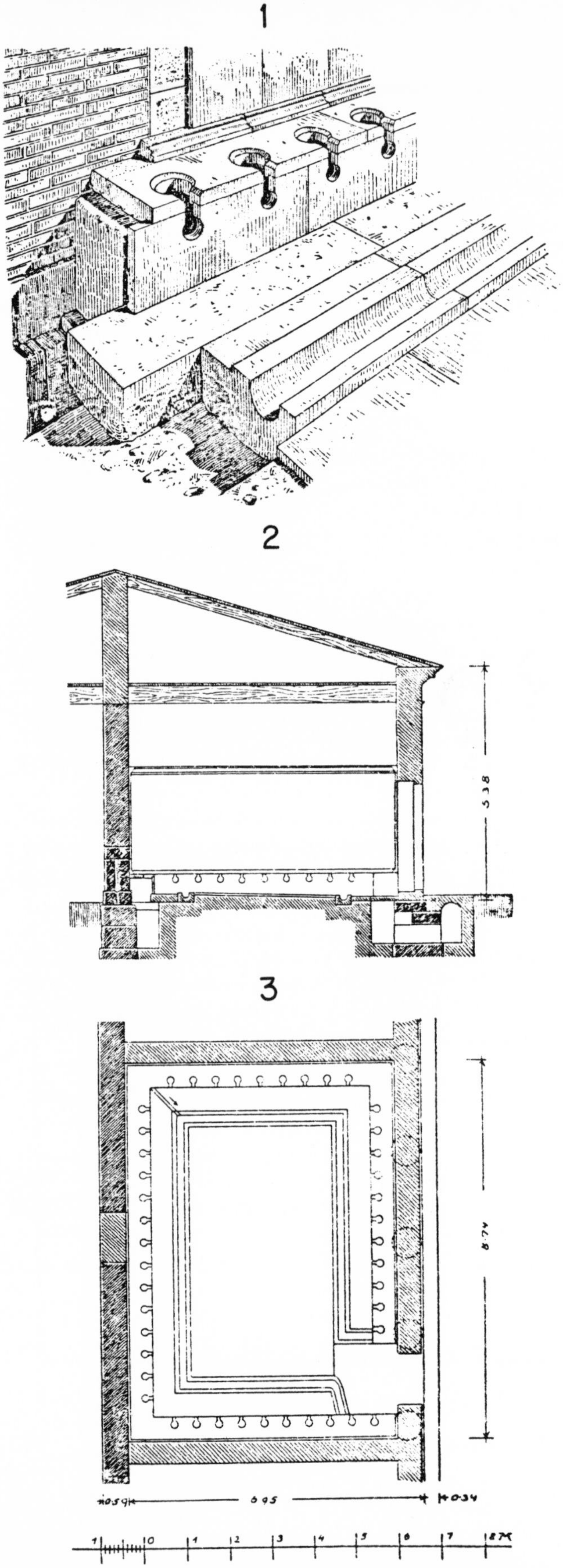

Fig. 2. Latrines, said by Walter Horn to be virtually identical in form and placement with those at the Asklepieion of Pergamon; these are from the North Market Hall of Miletus. 1, Elevation; 2, transverse section of latrines; 3, plan.

sick may influence later building although the medical theory behind them is questionable, and in this sense the halls of the Asklepieia may have played their part in determining the layout of large medieval wards, but the ways in which that influence was transmitted and the intermediate forms it took during a very dark half-millennium are so unclear that we content ourselves with the simple statement that dreamer–patients at the Asklepieia were nursed in large open halls.

Asklepieia naturally did not lack latrines, or *necessaria* as they were aptly called in the Middle Ages. Figure 2 shows one of two latrines (for the two sexes) at the Asklepieion of Pergamon in what is now Turkey (Hellenistic, second century A.D.). Pergamon seems also to have had fairly extensive bathing facilities for patients, both tubs and mud baths, with radioactive waters from a sacred spring.[2]

How complicated a site might become is seen in a model of the sacred enclosure at Pergamon (fig. 3) where in addition to a rectangular incubation hall for dreamers (A) and latrines (B1 and B2), a temple is found (C) in the form of a small replica of the Pantheon, (built some twenty years earlier) as well as a room for the emperor also serving as a library (D), a large stadium (E), and an interesting, outstanding two-storied circular structure (F) with six apses on the second floor connected to the ground floor by stairs outside and inside the building. Six round bath basins were found upstairs and other such tubs in the lower story with arrangements for drawing up water. Toward the south was an outer walk with a row of windows. The circular opening in the roof might be covered by awnings. This structure has been and perhaps can only be interpreted as a treatment hall.[3]

Roman Military Hospitals: Vindonissa

The first plan to be presented here of what people in our time might consider a real hospital is one designed by the Roman state for its soldiers in the field, the military hospital of Vindonissa (the modern Windisch) in Switzerland (first century A.D.; figs. 4a and 4b). Similar buildings seem to have been provided by the state for gladiators and by large plantation owners for their slaves. In all three instances, the patients had no homes to go to and were thought too valuable to be cast out to die, which, by and large, was what happened to paupers in distress in Roman times.

Roman army camps were established at intervals along the borders of the empire. They were square in plan, and the streets were laid out on a grid with the town center at the point where the principal north–south and east–west streets crossed. Hospitals were deliberately placed far from that busy center, near an outer wall, and can sometimes be distinguished from other barracks buildings only by writings or surgi-

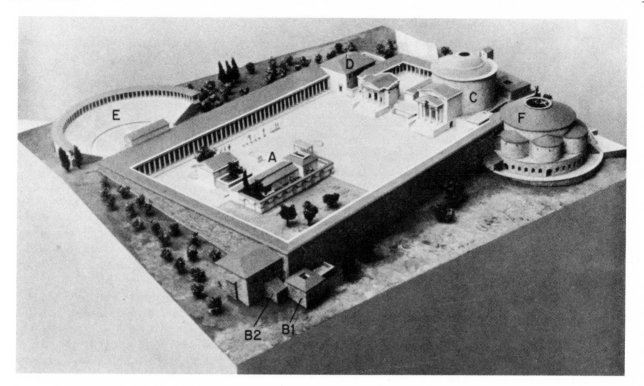

Fig. 3. A model of the Asklepieion of Pergamon by H. Schleif. A, Hall for dreamers; B1 and B2, latrines; C, temple; D, emperor's room; E, stadium; F, treatment hall.

cal instruments discovered in the foundations when they were excavated.[4]

As the Greek Asklepieion was simply a stoa, or ordinary business arcade, put to nursing use, so the Roman *valetudinarium,* or military hospital, was a regular barracks adapted for sick and wounded soldiers. In general, early hospitals used what we would call *derived plans,* plans originally evolved for other purposes and adapted to nursing. Very much later, functional hospital forms were deliberately created in response to medical or nursing needs. These we call *designed plans.* Also possible are transitional forms, in which some elements of deliberate design may be seen to modify a recognizably derived plan.

The plan of the barracks at Vindonissa is completely symmetrical. There is one large hall at the entrance (A) and another in the courtyard (B). The large hall might have been used as a meeting or dining room, the small rooms behind the portico (C . . . C) for nurses and administrators. If it was indeed a nursing building and not simply a barracks—doubts have been expressed on the subject[5]—the patient rooms (D . . . D) ran around both sides of a corridor (E . . . E) about as wide as they were deep.[6]

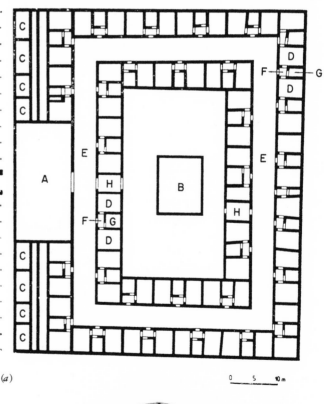

(a)

Fig. 4. (a) Floor plan and (b) reconstruction of the Roman military hospital (*valetudinarium*) of Vindonissa (Windisch, Switzerland, first century A.D.). A, Entrance hall; B, courtyard hall; C, small rooms behind the portico for nurses and administrators; D, typical patient rooms; E, corridor; F, vestibules; G, back rooms; H, passageways.

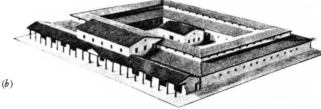

(b)

In the reconstructed elevation, a clerestory was given the corridor since there would be no other way to light it. The plan does not show privy arrangements but we must assume them because Roman plumbing was both excellent and ubiquitous. A latrine with a brick floor was found in the valetudinarium of Novaesium (first century A.D.) with a sewer originating there that ran out of the building. At Vindonissa there must also have been a kitchen, perhaps the separate house in the courtyard. A plan of the second valetudinarium at Carnuntum (second century A.D.) shows a probable kitchen with hearth in one of the small rooms off the corridor and in many others, presumably for patients, signs of hypocaust heating (that is, heat rising within the walls from some subterranean furnace).

One design peculiarity, the pattern of the patient rooms, is found in particularly striking form at Vindonissa. They are not entered directly from the corridor but from a little vestibule between every two rooms (F), which means that dust and noise from the corridor must have been considerably reduced. The vestibule has doors in all four walls: to the corridor, to the rooms on either side, and to a little room in back (G) whose purpose is anybody's guess. Was it used for stores, for linens, for a watcher?

The room pattern is extremely regular, broken only by two passageways (H . . . H) for making a shortcut across the court. Into each of these 60 patient rooms, approximately 11 by 15 feet, no more than three beds could fit—either three with the foot of the beds toward the door or two corner beds with their heads against the window wall and one with its foot toward the door. Space was customarily calculated for the valetudinarium at 200 men[7] and we have accounted for 180; a question arises whether beds were laid along that enormous corridor.

These rooms are remarkable for the degree of privacy they offer. Dr. Egill Snorrason suggests to us that a floor plan emphasizing privacy had been worked out for Roman houses, because the owners would not sleep with their considerable staff of slaves, and that it was carried over here.

An Early Christian Monastic Hospice: Turmanin in Syria

With the hospice of Turmanin (A.D. 475) we move into a totally different world, that of early Christian monasticism. The question immediately arises whether one should even consider hospices, essentially inns for pilgrims, in a history of the design of nursing wards for the sick. Our answer is that from the very beginning of the Christian era distinctions between "acts of mercy" became so blurred that one could no longer think of one of them without the others, and the resultant institutions for performing acts of mercy had

to be designed for multiple functions. All were founded upon one text: "For I was an hungred, and ye gave me meat: I was thirsty, and ye gave me drink: I was a stranger, and ye took me in: Naked, and ye clothed me: I was sick, and ye visited me: I was in prison, and ye came unto me" (Matt. 25: 35–36).

To these six works of mercy a seventh, burying the dead, was absorbed in the thirteenth century from a passage in Tobit (1: 16–17).[8] For a thousand years Christian charitable institutions (the term includes not only what we would call hospitals for the sick but also many other arrangements for social relief) were shaped by the Seven Works of Mercy. An admirable number of nurses and administrators took literally the text, "Inasmuch as ye have done it unto one of the least of my brethren, ye have done it unto me." Many laymen volunteered financial support or remembered the charity in their wills. Motives were not disinterested: St. Chrysostom had said, "If there were no poor, the greater part of your sins would not be removed; they are the healers of your wounds."

Since in the guiding text all categories of social assistance were jumbled together, Christian charitable foundations might cater to one, some, or all of the victims of wretchedness: aged, infirm, dying, diseased, wounded, blind, crippled, idiot, insane; orphans, paupers, wanderers, pilgrims. This is very different from hospitalizing slaves or soldiers as valuable assets. Assistance was directed toward the social classes held most in contempt by the classical world. The victim's degree of misery enhanced his value and the merit of the attendant. Fabiola, a fourth-century Roman matron, turned her own home into a refuge for the sick and collaborated in founding a hospice in the port of Rome for pilgrims from Africa.[9] St. Jerome eulogizes her: "How often did she carry on her own shoulders poor filthy wretches tortured by epilepsy! How often did she wash away the purulent matter from wounds which others could not even endure to look upon!"[10] Eight hundred years later St. Elizabeth of Hungary, while gathering the afflicted on her estates together and putting them to bed in her own castle, exclaimed to her servants, "How well it is for us, that thus we bathe and cover our Lord!"[11] (fig. 5).

In the same spirit, hospitality was proffered to the wanderer. Thus wrote St. Theodore, Abbot of Stude, in the sixth century:

> Come, draw near to this hospitable roof, O you travellers overcome by fatigue! Accept the offerings of hospitality, the bread that will nourish your hearts, the good drink flowing freely, clothing to protect you from the cold. These, my friends, are the blessings I, Theognoste, have received from my master Christ, giver of all riches.

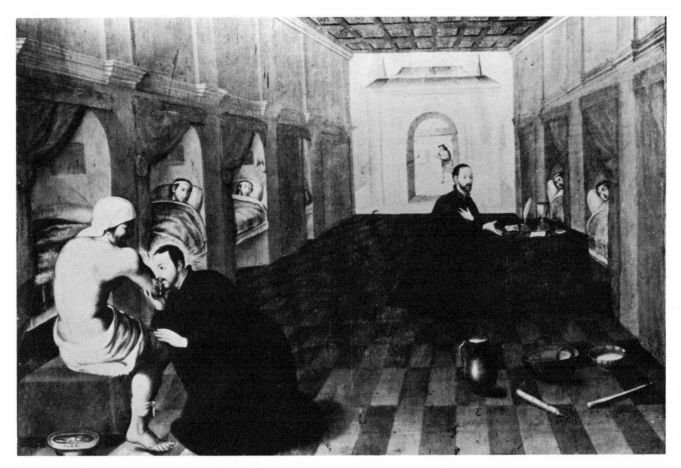

Thank him, for it is he who nourishes the world; for me utter only the prayer that in exchange for this hospitality I shall be fortunate enough to be taken into the bosom of Abraham.[12]

The text, although it dates from the following century, might have been mounted above the portal of the hospice that was a part of the monastery at Turmanin. The building group (fig. 6) comprises a church, a convent building, a house for the priest–administrator, and a tomb, together with a couple of quarries, one of them an open-air cistern. The convent building has been thought to be a *pandochaeion,* an inn for dispensing hospitality to pilgrims.[13]

Turmanin was on the main road from Antioch to Qalat-Siman, the great cross-shaped church (cf. figs. 31a and 31b) built over the pillar to which St. Simeon Stylites confined himself for nearly forty years in prayer and meditation, preaching twice a day, reconciling and counseling individuals, and attracting vast throngs of pilgrims—to himself during his lifetime, to the pillar and church after his death. In the convent building of Turmanin (fig. 7) these travelers would receive the monks' hospitality overnight or for as long as they required. It must be remembered that almost by definition a pilgrim is more or less sick, he or she having undertaken a long journey as a form of penance. Travel on foot over primitive roads may itself be quite painful, aside from illnesses contracted along the way, strange and insufficient food, and the sackcloth shirts

Fig. 5. A nursing brother (probably St. John of God) kissing the wounds of a patient.

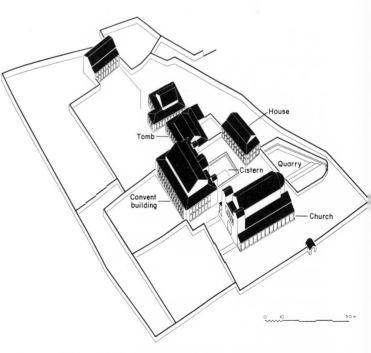

Fig. 6. Site plan of the monastery of Turmanin, Syria, about 475 A.D.

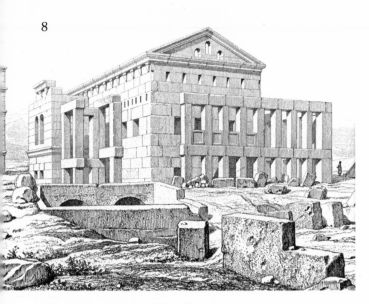

Fig. 7. The convent building of Turmanin as it looked about 1865.

may have housed the monastic community as well. One knows that such buildings were used as inns but it seems to be hard even for experts to say exactly which ones were. Another more frequent inn form is oblong with porticoes along only one side—particularly suitable for temporary summer guests. Tchalenko (*1*, 209) tells us that such buildings came in two sizes, "one of small dimensions, doubtless the ground and first floor were rented to travelers in easy circumstances; the other much larger, *without interior divisions* [our italics], containing stables and lodgings" for the poorer classes.[17] A principle is established in the fifth and sixth centuries that may then have been centuries or millenia old: *One can always purchase privacy with money.*

It is easy to imagine the porticoes at Turmanin populated by weary, half-sick or convalescent pilgrims, but they were not necessarily designed for the purpose, since the administrator's house and even the collective tomb had such porticoes on two or more sides. At one point the portico of the convent building of Turmanin is broken by a small jutting annex added later. This structure is identified as an oratory, probably because there are two tall arched windows on the upper story (compared with squared windows elsewhere) and because it has been inserted in the middle of the long eastern wall, that is, oriented in the manner of chapels and churches—including the basilica of Turmanin.

Limestone for the building was hewn from a quarry immediately in front of it; afterward the quarry was beautifully finished as an open-air reservoir with a balustrade like that in the chancel of churches. An underground cistern was discovered alongside it. Cisterns were and are terribly important in northern Syria. In a dry land of few wells, water must be saved from the winter rains for use throughout the year in tanks either open to the sky or underground. Those underground were constructed in the shape of a truncated cone, 12 to 15 feet in inner diameter and the same height. The top, closed over by flagstones, had a little opening covered by a wooden lid.[17] Two towers to either side of the oratory, wrongly identified by de Vogüé as stairwells, were actually for drawing the water up, one from such a cistern, the other from the open reservoir.[18] Some years the rains failed utterly.

or pebbled shoes some felt obliged to wear. For this reason the convent shelter must be more than an inn, nursing care would necessarily be included in hospitality, and a hospice had to be part hospital.[14] Provision was also made for those who died of their illness. Shallow graves in the churchyard are out of the question in limestone terrain, but a two-story common tomb, one among many in that neighborhood, was found there half hollowed out of, half built up with, the rock. There is now no trace of where the monks of the monastery lived, aside from the one house for the monk–administrator; Tchalenko imagines their scattered huts, long since destroyed, somewhere within the walls.[15]

The convent building was a large, open, two-storied rectangle approximately 90 by 47 feet, surrounded on all four sides of both stories by porticos of monumental square limestone pillars 2 feet across and 15 feet tall, with 6-foot-tall square stone blocks between them.[16] In size and construction it resembles a pandochaeion of the North-West Monastery in the town of Deir-Siman, one of three monasteries in that town alone that took in the overflowing crowds at the church of Qalat-Siman. At any rate, it is assumed that this building and others like it were pandochaeia. The building type is common and undifferentiated and

Fig. 8. The plan of St. Gall monastery, Switzerland, about 820. 1. Church, 2. annex for preparation of holy bread and oil, 3. Dormitory of the monks above, warming room below, 4. monks' privy, 5. monks' laundry and bathhouse, 6. refectory of the monks below, vestiary above, 7. cellar of the monks below, larder above, 8. monks' kitchen, 9. monks' bake-and-brewhouse, 10. kitchen, bake-and-brewhouse for distinguished guests, 11. House for Distinguished Guests, 12. outer school, 13. abbot's house, 14. kitchen, cellar, and bathhouse of abbot, 15. house for bloodletting, 16. House of the Physicians, 17. novitiate and infirmary, 18. kitchen and bath for the sick, 19. kitchen and bath for the novices, 20. gardener's house, 21. henhouse, 22. house of the fowlkeepers, 23. goosehouse, 24. granary, 25. Great Collective Workshop, 26. annex of Great Collective Workshop, 27. mill, 28. mortar, 29. drying kiln, 30. house of coopers and wheelwrights, and brewers' granary, 31. Hospice for Pilgrims and Paupers, 32. kitchen, bake-and-brewhouse for pilgrims and paupers, 33. house for horses and oxen and their keepers, 34. house for emperor's following (identification not certain), 35. house for sheep and shepherds, 36. house for goats and goatherds, 37. house for cows and cowherds, 38. house for servants of outlying estates and for servants traveling with the emperor's court (not certain, cf. no. 34), 39. house for swine and swineherds, 40. house for brood mares and foals and their keepers, W. monks' cloister yard, X. monks' vegetable garden, Y. cemetery and orchard, Z. medicinal herb garden.

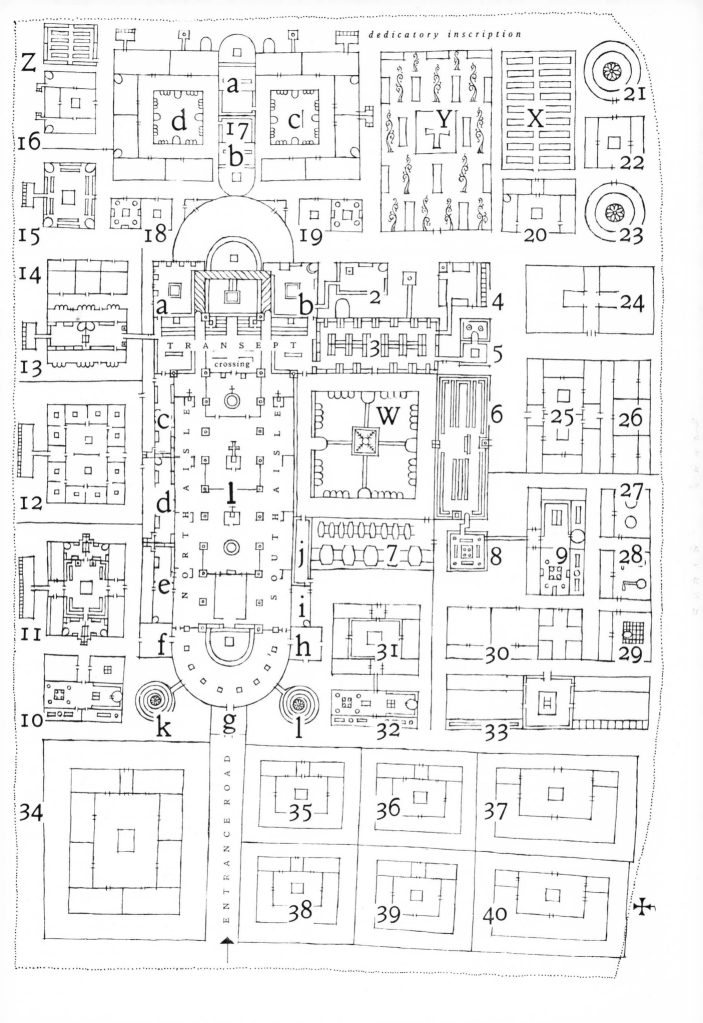

dedicatory inscription

In this hospice one can imagine the feet of pilgrims being washed as a ritual act, but the rare luxury of a full bath would have been beyond the reach of pilgrim or monk, however much they may have longed for it.

The Plan of St. Gall Monastery, Switzerland

The plan of Turmanin is a rather good introduction to the layout of a monastery, which appears here in a simple and rudimentary form. But because of its very simplicity it is a wretched representative of Christian charitable institutions in the Eastern Empire. At an extraordinarily early date they were so specialized as to deserve the name of hospitals. In A.D. 370, St. Basil opened at Caesarea (Syria) a famous group of institutions that included a hospital and a leprosarium. Four maternity hospitals were endowed in Alexandria in 610.[19] A list has been compiled of 40 medieval hospitals or hostels in Constantinople alone.[20] Texts inform us of the most minute details of administration at the twelfth- to fifteenth-century Hospital of the Pantocrator in Constantinople: its 50 beds in 5 sections, one section each for surgical patients, medical patients, and women, two for patients with less serious illnesses. Each section had one extra bed for an emergency patient. Two latrines; all outbuildings lit at night; pharmacy, kitchen, butchery, laundry; a menu for the daily diet, an inventory of bedclothes and housekeeping utensils; a list of surgical implements, and a schedule for the numerous personnel[21]—everything concerning the Pantocrator seems to have come down to us but its floor plan. We have floor plans too for the elaborate Moslem hospitals, which attained a refinement and medical sophistication unknown in Western Europe for centuries, but the subject is too vast and difficult to tackle here, and most of the sites involved lie beyond our designated area. Therefore we enter upon the discussion of the subject of medieval Christian hospitals by its usual front door: the plan of the monastery of St. Gall in Switzerland (fig. 8).

The hospitality and infirmary divisions of the monastery of St. Gall exist only on paper, or rather on the parchment of what Walter Horn defined for us in a letter as

> a masterplan for a monastic settlement worked out during two ecclesiastical reform synods held at Aachen in 816 and 817. The original is not preserved, but is known to us through a copy made in the Scriptorium of the Abbey of Reichenau upon the request of Abbot Gozbert (816–836) of St. Gall, who used it as a guide for the reconstruction of the monastery of St. Gall.

Even more than the inns of Deir-Siman, the plan of St. Gall speaks eloquently of distinctions among persons, the first being that between monks and laymen, masters and servants. Saint Benedict recommended that monks themselves perform all tasks required for a self-supporting community. But, under the feudal system of the north, villeins and workmen were part of the original estate given to a monastery, and as an integral human complement of these possessions they had to give their services to it. Thus specialized crafts and menial jobs passed into the hands of laymen.[22] It has been estimated that at St. Gall, for a population of 110 monks there were 130 to 150 servants performing the work of the monastery and living within its walls.[23] Their sleeping quarters were outside the cloister for the monks, yet still within the monastery walls, in the various workshops (fig. 8, nos. 25, 26, 30), the houses for monastic livestock and their keepers (nos. 33, 35, 36, 37, 39, and 40), the mill and mortar houses (nos. 27, 28), and the bake-and-brewhouses (nos. 10 and 32).

A second distinction documented by this plan is that between rich and poor pilgrims. The latter, arriving on foot at the western gate, would walk past the barnyard area (there was no monumental approach to a monastery, its important areas being turned inward toward the cloister) to present himself at the semicircular portico of the central, cross-shaped church. There he would be welcomed by the monk porter and directed through a vestibule on his right to the Hospice for Pilgrims and Paupers (fig. 8, no. 31), where he would find not only other pilgrims but also a group of paupers maintained by the monastery.[24] A visiting nobleman or king, who always arrived by horse and with a retinue of vassals and servants, would be shown through an identical vestibule on his left to the House for Distinguished Guests (fig. 8, no. 11). The nobleman was also received free and might or might not leave rich gifts upon departure. The Hospice for Pilgrims and the House for Distinguished Guests were roughly the same size (one pictures the Hospice as considerably more crowded). Each had its own bake-and-brewhouse, and each had rooms for servants. But there the likeness ends. The House for Distinguished Guests shows tables and benches in the main hall, whereas in the Hospice for Pilgrims there were only benches around the walls. The poor were given, basically, bread and beer to eat; thus the Hospice for Pilgrims and Paupers had no separate kitchen although its bakery had a kitchen stove. The kitchen installed in an annex to the House for Distinguished Guests (fig. 8, no. 10) was equipped to prepare richer and more varied food than the monks' strict vegetarian fare. The poor of the Hospice might sleep on the benches or in rows on the floor of the two dormitories. But in the House for Distinguished

Guests (fig. 8, no. 11), four smaller rooms were placed at the service of the noble rich, each with only four beds, a corner fireplace (corner fireplaces in this plan are indicated by ovals and imply an outer wall of something other than wood), and its own necessarium (privy). To either side of the entrance were rooms for the servants accompanying the wealthy visitors. At the rear were stables, and beyond the stables a necessarium with no fewer than eighteen toilet seats. There were no privies at the hospice, none attached to the sleeping quarters for craftsmen, workmen, herdsmen. Barnyards must have been thought adequate sanitary facilities; richer odors were superimposed upon those of the pigpen. On the other hand, the monks' dormitory was decently provided with a necessarium of nine seats, lit all night by a lamp at the corner nearest the dormitory that threw its light both ways (to ensure moral demeanor during a monk's most private moments).[25]

Novices, both those vowed to the cloister in childhood by their parents and those seeking admittance as adults, must according to the Rule live elsewhere than the monks, another distinction seen in the St. Gall plan. The novices' cloister lies east of the apse of the big church (fig. 8, no. 17); it is a mirror image of the monks' infirmary, sharing with it a small double-ended church on the same axis as the large one. Close examination reveals that there is absolutely no way to cross from the novices' to the infirmary cloister and that the common church has neatly been divided in half with two entrances, one into the novitiate, the other into the dormitory. The kitchens for preparing the special foods are under one roof with the baths for the novices and the sick (fig. 8, nos. 18 and 19).

The monks' infirmary was closed to laymen. It catered to three types of the infirm: the superannuated, who slept in the dormitory; the sick, for whom a special room was set apart "for dangerous illnesses," meaning perhaps also contagious diseases that could be isolated here; and those who had let blood and shared for a few days the relaxed discipline and richer fare of the infirmary. Meat was not served in the monks' refectory but it was served here, and recuperating from bloodletting might come to seem a kind of vacation from the monotonous, rigorous routine.

The bloodletting house (fig. 8, no. 15), directly across from the monks' infirmary, speaks eloquently of those bled and purged there at stated intervals for every ill of the body or mind—there are four corner stoves in the open hall and seven toilet seats in that necessarium alone. Four round wooden bathtubs for an estimated 12 to 20 sick or superannuated monks in the infirmary,[26] compared to two bathtubs for 77 well monks in the cloister dormitory (fig. 8, no. 4), very well illustrate the dictum of St. Benedict, "Let the use

of baths be afforded to the sick as often as may be expedient, but to the healthy, and especially to the young, let them be granted seldom."[27] This is not to say the 77 never washed themselves. They kept themselves reasonably clean by cold sponge baths; the hot tub was a luxury.

Another distinction observed in this plan is that between inpatients and outpatients, the terms meaning, respectively, those inside and those outside the cloistered area of the monastery. By this definition, inpatients would include monks sent to the infirmary to be treated for acute illnesses, to recover from being bled, or to end their days there, plus the sick novices in their own infirmary. Outpatients would be the exhausted, half-sick transients and the resident poor in the Hospice for Pilgrims and Paupers, and, above all, those for whom a room for "patients very ill" was set aside in the House of the Physicians behind the infirmary. For where else could the "patients very ill" have come from? Dangerously ill monks and novices had their own infirmaries with fireplace and privies attached.[28] It makes sense to assume with Walter Horn that those who lay in the House of the Physicians (fig. 8 no. 16) were sorely stricken members of the monastery's lay community with nowhere else to go: servants, workers, craftsmen.[29] They too had their own privies, the chief physician slept opposite, medicine for them and the entire community was stored under a lean-to at the rear of the house, and medicinal herbs grew outside the physician's windows (fig. 8, Z). The names of the herbs in the garden are given on the plan. The physician, who was sometimes a layman, also treated the sick of the monks' infirmary, but there was no shortcut between one intensive care group and another. The entrance to the infirmary cloister lay beside the western apse of the infirmary church.

Thus the entire northeastern corner of the monastery was given over to medical purposes, which leads to yet another distinction of the plan—that between the sick and the well. This was a matter of location, and the abbot was the link between the two areas. It was his religious duty to live in close conjunction with the sick, as the Rule of St. Benedict advised him to do:

> Before all things and above all things care must be taken of the sick, so that they may be served in very deed as Christ himself; for he said: 'I was sick and ye visited me.' . . . Therefore let the abbot take the greatest care that they suffer no neglect. For these sick brethren let there be assigned a special room and an attendant who is God-fearing, diligent, and careful. . . . Let the abbot take the greatest care that the sick not be neglected

by the cellarers and attendants; for he must answer for all the misdeeds of his disciples.[30]

On the other hand, the abbot was in charge of hospitality as well as of the hospital, and hospitality must be proffered outside the cloister. Although any guest, rich or poor, sick or well, must be received "like Christ," if all those rich or poor layfolk were admitted into the cloister they would disrupt its reason for being.[31] The abbot therefore entertained the rich in his own quarters, for there was literally no other spot within the monastery where he was permitted to join the nobility at meals. As laymen, noble folk were interdicted from eating with the monks in their refectory (only visiting monks were allowed to do that), and no monk was allowed to eat at the House for Distinguished Guests. The abbot alone was permitted to serve in his house and partake there of food fit for a king.

One last distinction to be observed in this plan is that between classic and vernacular architecture. Scholars have long agreed that the huge church, main cloister, and twin cloisters east of the apse were planned to be executed in stone, the church in Early Romanesque style and the cloisters in a form derived from the classic Roman atrium court. The abbot's house, two stories tall, must also be thought of as at least partly a stone construction. Arcades are given at the ground floor here as well as in the main cloister.

But it is now believed that the out-buildings—31 structures of a total of 40—were planned to be built in wood. They are all variants of one basic floor plan, whether used for pigs, paupers, or prominent guests. The plan shows a square central hall with a smaller square in the middle, which represents an open hearth and the hole in the roof above it to let out the smoke. This hole must have been covered or the fire would have been doused by rain. Around the hall are rooms

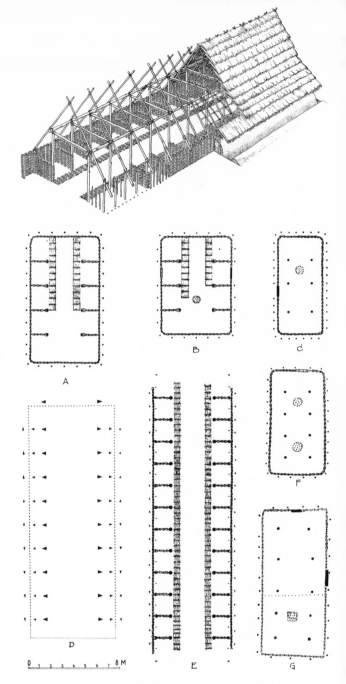

Fig. 9. (*a*) Elevation and (*b*) plan showing the basic structure of a barn, The Netherlands, third century B.C.

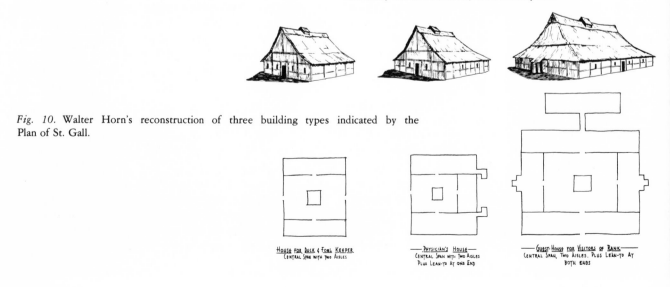

Fig. 10. Walter Horn's reconstruction of three building types indicated by the Plan of St. Gall.

House for Duck & Fowl Keeper
Central Span with Two Aisles

—Physician's House—
Central Span with Two Aisles
Plus Lean-to At one End

—Guest-House for Visitors of Rank—
Central Span, Two Aisles, Plus Lean-to At Both Ends

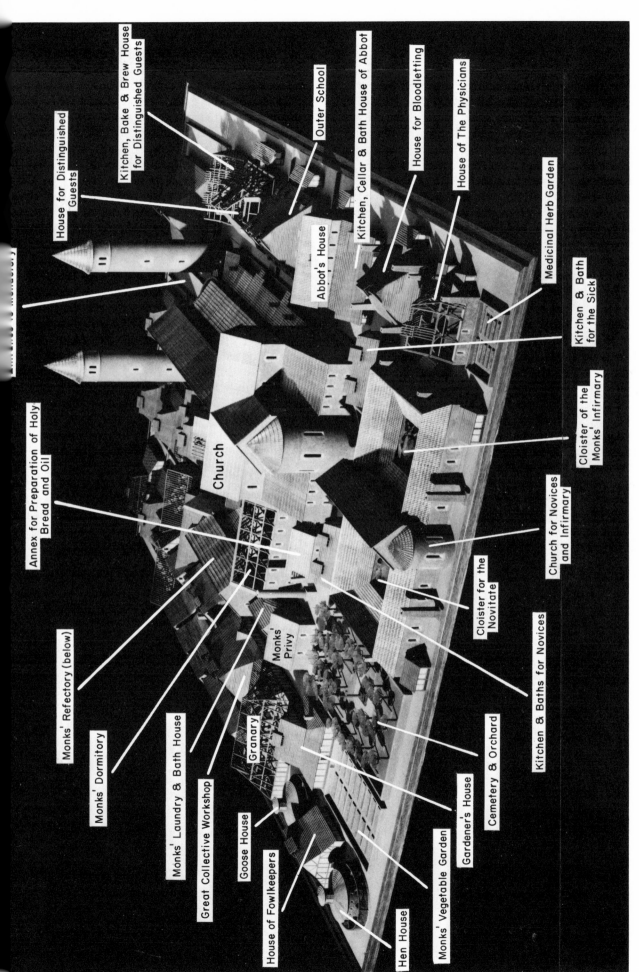

House for Distinguished Guests

Kitchen, Bake & Brew House for Distinguished Guests

Outer School

Kitchen, Cellar & Bath House of Abbot

House for Bloodletting

House of The Physicians

Abbot's House

Medicinal Herb Garden

Kitchen & Bath for the Sick

Cloister of the Monks' Infirmary

Church for Novices and Infirmary

Annex for Preparation of Holy Bread and Oil

Church

Cloister for the Novitiate

Monks' Refectory (below)

Monks' Dormitory

Monks' Laundry & Bath House

Great Collective Workshop

Goose House

Granary

Monks' Privy

Kitchen & Baths for Novices

House of Fowlkeepers

Hen House

Monks' Vegetable Garden

Gardener's House

Cemetery & Orchard

Fig. 11. A model of the reconstruction of the St. Gall plan by Walter Horn and Ernest Born, looking west. In the foreground are the medical installations that appear at the top of the plan. Some buildings were left unfinished to show their construction.

on one (the cooper's house), two (the poultry keeper's), three (the gardener's, the physicians') or four sides (the Hospice for Pilgrims and Paupers, the House for Distinguished Guests, and others). In the nineteenth century an attempt was made to concoct an elevation in stone with a square clerestory and lantern surmounting it, which had the defect of looking like nothing ever built in the whole history of architecture.[32] In 1958 Walter Horn suggested a much more plausible form. His basic unit is the wooden barn, a structure omnipresent on American farms even today and dating back at least to the twelfth or perhaps the fourteenth century B.C.[33]

By its timber frame a barn is naturally divided lengthwise into central hall and two side aisles, which are in turn subdivided as cubicles by the procession of supporting posts (fig. 9). Barn houses have survived almost unchanged for 2500 years because they are simply and logically built and because they are infinitely adaptable. They can be used for storage or for animals as we use barns today. (Our barns are topped by a ventilator very similar to that devised so long ago to keep the rain off the fire.) They could be used from the very beginning for any combination of animals and people, the animals stalled in the side aisles, the people occupying the central living space. They could be used only for people who worked and ate in the central hall and slept in the aisles, either cubicled or open; all this "without entailing even the slightest changes in . . . basic structural dispositions."[34]

Such service structures must have been the ones implied in the St. Gall plan. The only sources of light for the hall were the front door and the covered smoke vent. Simpler buildings such as sheepfolds and sties would have been built of wood with partitions just high enough to keep the animals out of the servants' areas. Elegant buildings such as the House for Distinguished Guests could have had stone walls clear to the steep-pitched timber roof, both on the outside and along the aisles.[35] These walls rendered the private bedrooms really private but in so doing cut off the sole source of heat (the fire) and of light, such as it was, from the hole in the roof. Hence corner fireplaces were added and we must imagine windows in the outer walls. The two rooms for the dangerously ill in the House of the Physicians show stoves and probably had such windows. Sometimes aisle rooms under the eaves are indicated on three or even four sides of the plan. Their ceilings would be low while in the center an open hall rose to the rooftree (fig. 10). Even the elegant House for Distinguished Guests had but one front door, meaning that horses would have to be led right across the central hall to the stable—which pretty well defines the Carolingian notion of elegance.

Forms of classical and vernacular origin are seen in a photograph of the reconstruction model of the plan of St. Gall by Walter Horn and Ernest Born, taken from its northeastern corner and showing the infirmary cloister and House of the Physicians (fig. 11).

CHAPTER 2

The Open Ward

Monastic Hospitals

Whether and to what extent what we call the Plan of St. Gall was actually realized when Abbot Gozbert in the year 830 began to rebuild the monastery of St. Gall, is not known and could only be ascertained through excavations. But the plan itself was of course a conceptual reality—and a paradigm—and for that reason it is fascinating to compare it with what was actually built two centuries later at the monastery of Cluny.

At Cluny we can watch the infirmary evolve from a long building subdivided into four rooms into a large open hall, a dominant form of ward construction under both religious and lay auspices until the eighteenth century. Increased size of important rooms reflects a growing security and prosperity after the chaos and destruction of the Dark Ages. Even the temporary consolidation of warring territories under Charlemagne had been half-barbarous in character. But the rise of towns, the Crusades, and consequent opening of new trade routes led to a prosperity reflected in religious architecture first of all. The open ward, which falls into this category, is yet another derived plan, so resembling that of contemporary churches that it is sometimes difficult to assign a specimen to one category or the other.

The nucleus of the medieval conventual buildings of Cluny, which included the infirmaries, was replaced in the current style after 1750; the third and final church of Cluny was almost entirely dismantled after the French Revolution and sold off as building material. However, a fairly dependable plan (now lost) was made in 1622, and copies of this plan, with the results of excavation (1928–50), make it possible to identify the elements of the medieval plan and to work out their chronological sequence. In describing the successive infirmaries of the monastery, we depend upon reconstructions by Kenneth J. Conant, who spent the better part of his life in the investigation of this extraordinary site. Figure 12 shows how the infirmary may have looked around 1043 (no. 1), and its relationship to the monks' dormitory (2), St. Mary's Chapel (3), and the important Second Church of Cluny (4). It resembled a basilica, with a high central section lit by clerestory; a one-story veranda, open

from end to end, facing the church; and a corresponding side aisle on the far side with divisions for the latrines. The Horn and Born model of St. Gall has privies in approximately the outhouse form familiar to us today; on the plan they are connected with the buildings they serve by a narrow corridor. At Cluny the lean-to has been made part of a substantial stone building. Conant's restored ground plan (fig. 13) clearly shows the inner structure of this infirmary: the latrines, the four rooms (23' × 27'), and the mandatum, or kitchen for special foods, which had been in a separate building at St. Gall. Comparison between the two plans makes still clearer how scattered functions have been brought together under one roof.

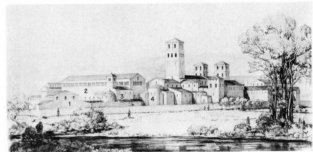

Fig. 12. A view of the monastery and infirmary of Cluny about 1043, as restored by Kenneth J. Conant. 1, Infirmary; 2, monks' dormitory; 3, St. Mary's Chapel; 4, Second Church of Cluny.

Hospitality areas at Cluny monastery were similar to those of St. Gall: a large guest house for travelers, both men and women, to the left of the church; a hospice for the poor near the entrance gate; a tiny almonry for the abbey's poor pensioners—12 or 18 paupers symbolic of the thousands of passersby receiving alms.[1] As the monastery grew, a vast church, Cluny III, was projected and other structures were enlarged proportionately. Comparison between the plans of 1050 and 1157 (fig. 14) is particularly interesting because we can see the abbot facing the problems hospital administrators do today when they have to expand architecturally around an irreducible patient population. The program began with a necessary enlargement of St. Mary's Chapel. The new chapel would extend right through the old infirmary, so before it could be started another infirmary, St. Hugh's (no. 2),

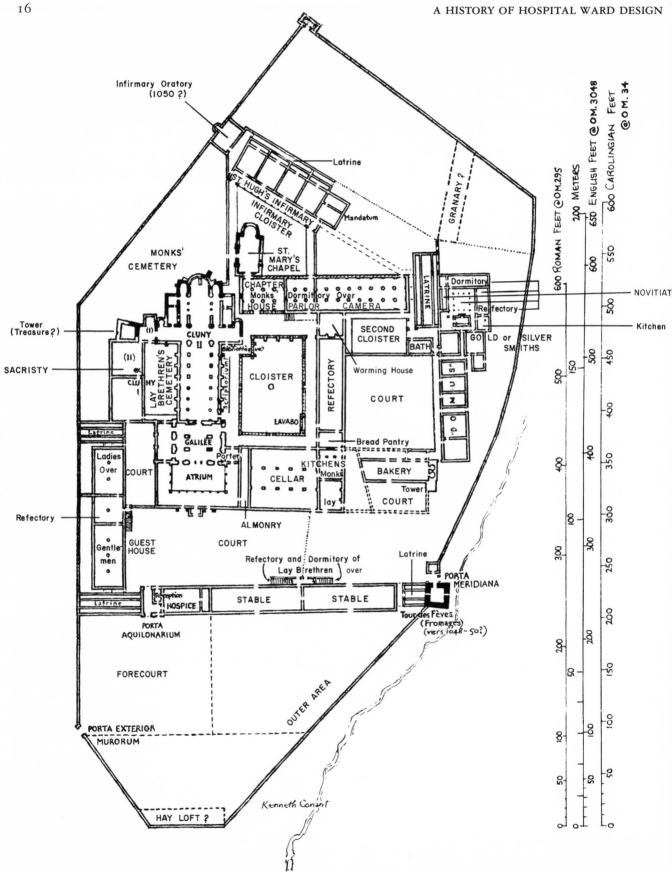

Fig. 13. Ground plan of the monastery of Cluny about 1050, as restored by Kenneth J. Conant.

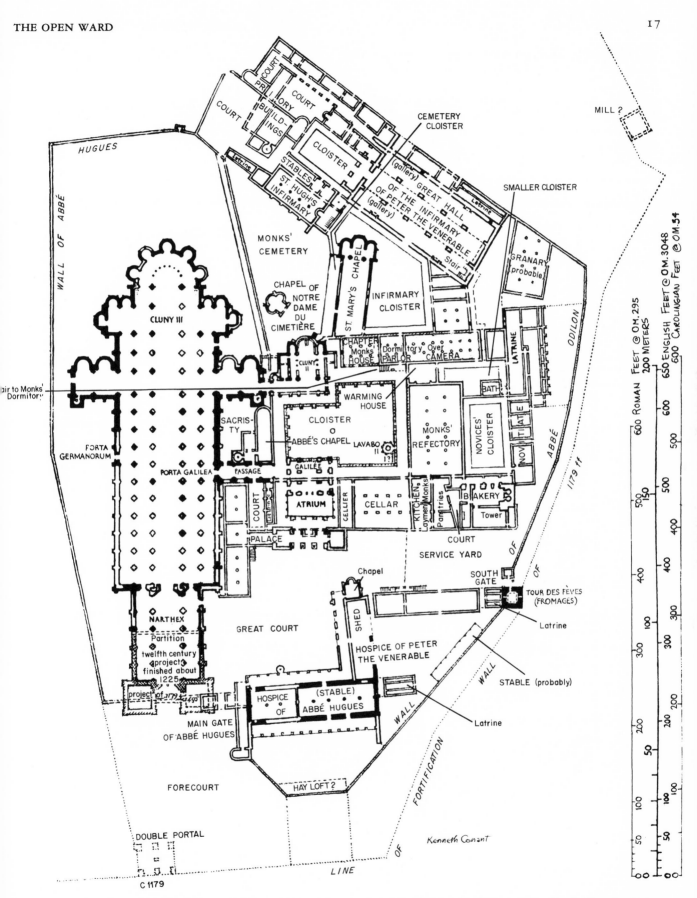

Fig. 14. Ground plan of the monastery of Cluny about 1157, as restored by Kenneth J. Conant. 1, St. Mary's Chapel, which had been much enlarged; 2, St. Hugh's infirmary, built 1082; 3, the great infirmary of Peter the Venerable, built about 1135.

was built (1082) incorporating as its vestibule a small apsed oratory east of the old infirmary. It broke away from the pattern of medium-sized rooms; it was a two-story open hall, 40 by 80 feet, that accommodated about 24 sick monks. Because of the dampness of the neighborhood, patients were kept only on the upper story.[2] Privy seats of the attached necessarium would have been on the same level, for a time at least in the extension at the north.

About 1135, when the monks numbered 460 (an all-time high), a huge infirmary hall, two-thirds the height of the church of Cluny III, was added. Conant's restorations of this infirmary (fig. 15a) show a three-aisled hall about 212 feet long through the eastern porch, 112 feet wide including the attached privies, and 87 feet high to the central rooftree. The center aisle may have been open clear to the roof or to a high, rounded ceiling.[3] The infirmary could accommodate 80–100 patients. Conant writes us that he cannot resist imagining the open downstairs area with its two rows of pillars and four jolly fireplaces as a kind of club for ambulatory patients.[4]

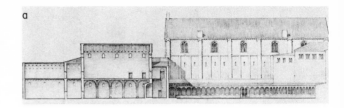

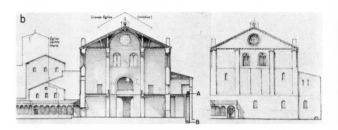

Fig. 15. Cluny monastery around 1157, as restored by Kenneth J. Conant. (*a*) Infirmaries of St. Hugh (longitudinal section) and Peter the Venerable (long side); (*b*) infirmary of Peter the Venerable: left, cross section with (A) privy seat and (B) drain; right, western elevation; (*c*) bird's eye view of the entire monastery with (A) infirmary of Peter the Venerable; (A1) its necessarium; (B) infirmary of St. Hugh; (B1) its necessarium.

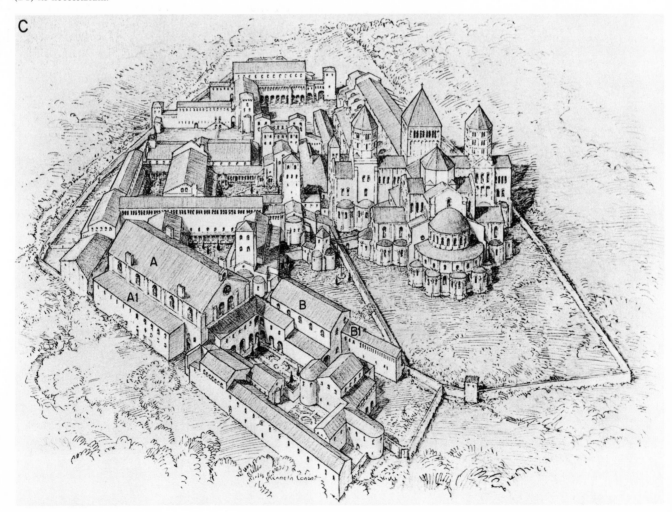

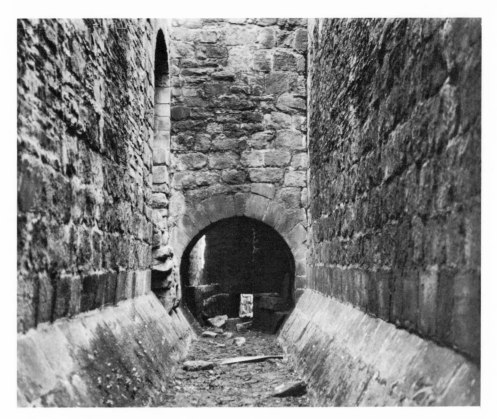

Fig. 16. Drain of the dormitory necessarium of Kirkstall Abbey, England. Entrance door to the seats that were above it is on the left.

Monasteries were built near water, and streams were diverted to feed the fountains and flush the sewers. The relationship between privy seat (A) and sewer (B) shows particularly well in Conant's cross section of the Infirmary of Peter the Venerable (fig. 15b). The external relationship of the buildings is shown in figure 15c. The scale of the drain of a monastery necessarium is seen in a photograph of the one at Kirkstall Abbey (1155; fig. 16). The door from the monks' dormitory is at left and one must of course imagine this sewer roofed over at the level of the doorsill.

A drawing of 1165 describes the complete water system of the Priory of Christ Church, Canterbury. Its complicated perspectives were reduced to a diagram by Robert Willis (fig. 17). From a source at the bottom (north) of the plan the water was piped through five settling tanks, over the city moat (i.e., dump) on a trestle, under the city wall, and into the monastery grounds. It was conveyed beneath a corner of the infirmary without being tapped there to a series of tanks, each one on lower ground than the last. It emerged in the Great Cloister to feed the laver, where the monks washed their hands in their own individual jets of water before eating. At that point the pipes divide. One branch serves the needs of kitchen, brewhouse, bakehouse, and the hall on the site of the almonry; a subbranch takes off for the bathhouse and the prior's own bathtub. Another branch running east from the Great Cloister surfaces in a laver at the door of the infirmary, which also used a well

in the same courtyard. (The infirmaries of both Cluny and Canterbury, as of most monasteries, had their own cloisters.[5]) After further wanderings, used water, augmented by rainwater collected in gutters from the roofs of the Great Cloister, was directed to flush the infirmary necessarium and the dormitory necessarium (55 seats, each one 3 inches wider than the choir stalls)[6] and was then carried by sewer to the city moat.

The infirmary looked rather like the first one at Cluny, a basilica with clerestory, but here the lower side-aisles were open to the nave and used for floor space. An attached kitchen (A) was seemingly decided upon, but the privies (B) were put in a separate structure. Infirmary hall and chapel formed one building, yet the hall—that is, the ward—was entirely separated from the chapel by a wall to the ceiling with a single central door. An interesting and significant differentiation was discovered in the shape of the piers that survive from the actual building. In the ward they were plain cylindrical columns with scalloped capitals, in the chapel they were compound columns with capitals richly carved.[7]

The Great Hall

For building big there are two prerequisites—comparative peace and enough money. In Western Europe during the Dark and very early Middle Ages more of both commodities was available in the monasteries then in the world at large. In them the open ward of

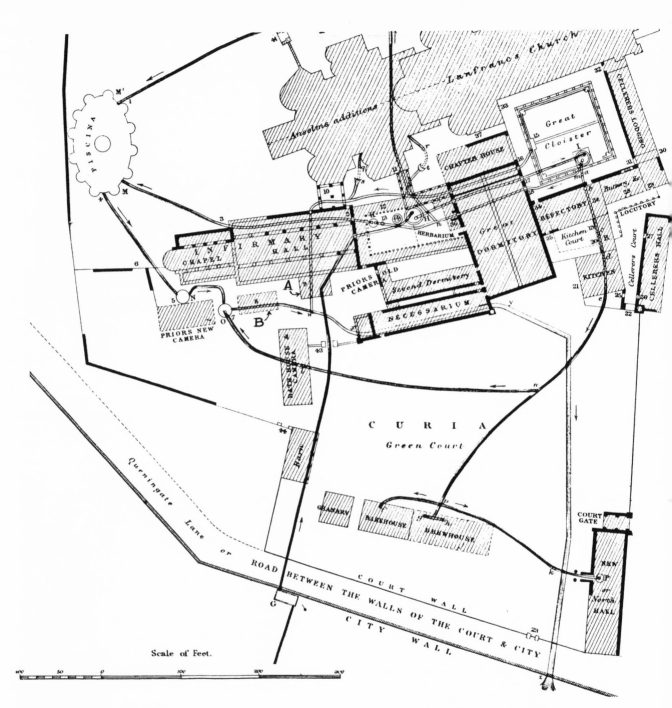

Fig. 17. Plan of the buildings and drains of Christ Church priory, Canterbury, by Robert Willis, after a Norman drawing of 1165. A, Attached kitchen; B, detached necessarium.

considerable dimensions developed, and during the twelfth century, when towns were formed, trade again flourished, and the towns became wealthy, the form was copied outside the cloister. Works of charity grew very numerous. A small foundation might be small indeed, merely an almshouse for twelve aged paupers, in which case an ordinary house could be taken over unchanged. Many a large foundation began in such quarters and expanded later. For certain patients special enclosures that revealed their function might be designed: leprosaria, plague houses. But the solution generally adopted for the hospice–hospital—that catchall for the poor and for assorted cases of illness and decrepitude—was the open ward, taken

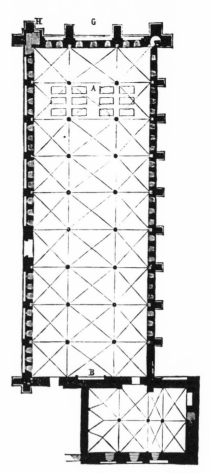

over from the monasteries, adapted, enlarged, refined,
and eventually mass-produced.

Regardless of sponsor, this was the dominant hospital
idiom. The bishop who erected a hospital across from
or alongside his cathedral, as the Council of Aachen
bade him do; the Order of the Holy Ghost, sanctioned
by the Pope himself, which built a string of hospitals
clear across Europe; a military order, such as the
Knights of St. John of Jerusalem (the Hospitalers),
which founded hospitals at key points along the Cru-
sader routes; the prince of a city, who proved his
Christian piety to his subjects by endowing a work
of charity; guilds and fraternities that established
hospitals for their own sick or impoverished members
as well as for the poor; a group of rich burghers who
designed the grandest monument they could afford
to the glory of God but still more to the glory of their
town; or a pious donor who remembered a hospital
in his will for the good of his own soul—all built open
wards. The form prevailed for nearly four centuries.

Whatever else the open ward was provided with by
way of appendages, bed space, altar, kitchen, and
privies were a must. In surviving structures we cannot always identify all four areas: the infirmary of the
Abbey of Ourscamp, France (1210), which escaped
destruction only because it was used as a parish church,
understandably shows no sign of the original privies.
It also shows no sign of an altar. On Viollet-le-Duc's
plan (fig. 18) the kitchen is at the rear, an open fireplace at B, and his guess about the bed placement
is superimposed. According to this arrangement,
leaving the two end bays free for circulation of air
and staff, an open area 160 by 52 feet would take 84
beds. And the nursing staff would work in relatively
clean air near the windows, which at Ourscamp are
quite remarkable (figs. 19a and 19b). The rose window
and two tall windows below it did not open and were

Fig. 19. Ourscamp infirmary in 1967. (a) The entrance in relation
to the apse of the abbey church; (b) rear view; (c) interior showing the three types of windows: the bottom row for air, and the
two top rows for light.

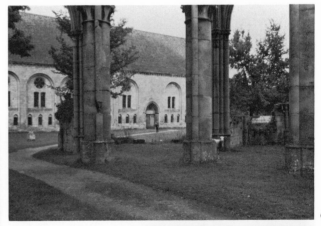

(a)

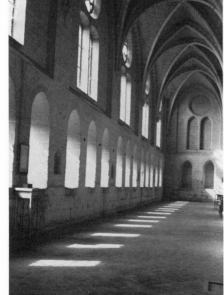

(c)

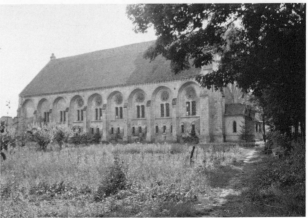

(b)

intended to flood the room with light as though it were a church. The three small windows near the ground, which are the size and height of a person, opened and could be used for ventilation (fig. 19c). These "sacred" and "secular" windows express the double function of a hospital ward.[8] Sick and very human beings, feeding and eliminating and being bandaged and vomiting and screaming with pain, were at the same time potential candidates for salvation, on their way to heaven—and in the near future too. The infirmary at Ourscamp came to be known as the *salle des morts*.

It was too cold in the great stone halls to lie in an open bed. Such was not the custom even in homes. With inadequate heating, a person in bed was safer from drafts behind curtains, where he could warm up his cube of air with his own breath if nothing better offered. Thus the interior of the salle des morts may have looked something like that of a similar ward at the Hôtel-Dieu of St. Jean in Angers (fig. 20). The hospital at Angers, founded by a layman in 1153, is shown here in operation in the middle of the nineteenth century. Well-built stone hospitals, if properly maintained, survive as long as cathedrals. After the ward was built (1184), the chapel was attached to the rear of it in a position similar to that of the kitchen at Ourscamp, but there is no direct door through; the entrance is from the cloister. Behind that cloister today may be found privy sewers of unspecified date, and they still smell.

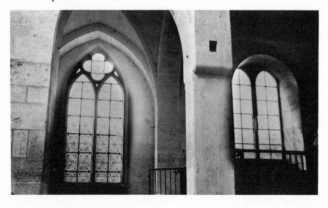

Fig. 21. Left, a sacred and right, a secular window, lighting, respectively, the chapel and the ward of the Hôpital Notre Dame des Fontenilles, Tonnerre, France (founded 1293). Note vaulted ceiling over the chapel area; the ward is barrel roofed (see fig. 22). Photo taken in 1971.

Probably the most striking example still standing of a ward opening into its own chapel is the Hôpital Notre Dame des Fontenilles of Tonnerre, France (1293). The sacred windows are separated from the profane. The ward is surrounded by large arched windows for air, while around the apse that contains the chapel are far larger windows absolutely like those

of churches (fig. 21). Today the ward seems rather dark by comparison with the dazzling chapel (fig. 22). Dieter Jetter reminds us that whereas the window glass of the ward would have been colorless, as it is today, the altar was surrounded by stained glass as in a cathedral and thus the quantity of light would be more evenly distributed. The contrast in *quality* of light between ward and altar would have been immense, for over the altar would abide a light like that to be expected in heaven. Such a differentiation at Canterbury was suggested by the finding of simple piers in the ward and ornate piers in the chapel.[9] At the Hospital del Rey of Burgos, Spain (eighteenth century) one sees today a far more elaborated ceiling over the chapel area. In any ward–chapel combination the chapel was built in an architectural mode as distinct from that of the ward as heaven is from earth. "All was completely different," Dr. Jetter sums it up. "The chapel material—stone and never wood, if possible; the size and shape of the windows; the height of the room; the level of the floor; the vaulting. *This* is the meaning of sacred and profane architecture!"

The hall at Tonnerre measures 288 by 61 feet. Its wooden barrel vault, the largest still standing in Europe, is perforated by a pattern of clover-shaped ventilation holes, which draw upon the cubage of the attic clear to the rooftree to supplement the not inconsiderable air supply of the hall itself (fig. 23). The relationship between ward and service area is particularly relevant because the hospital was founded for the sick poor by the widow queen Marguerite de Bourgogne, sister-in-law of Louis IX, to atone for her sins during her married life and, as she put it, "with a desire to merit that reward the Evangelist has promised us."[10] Following the classic Christian pattern, she nursed patients with her own hands and intelligently administered the affairs and personnel of the hospital for the remainder of her life. In a plan by Viollet-le-Duc (fig. 24), her house (L) is shown beside the hospital and connected to it by a little bridge at second-story level leading into a tower with a winding staircase, just at the juncture of chapel and ward. Overlooking the chapel are two windows through which the queen may have witnessed Mass, afterward descending the winding stair to tend the patients, whose beds were in cubicles along the two long walls. She could also look down into their cubicles from a balcony that ran below the level of the windowsills, from which it would be possible to mount the two stone steps to each window in order to manipulate the shutters and moderate the light.

The plan shows quarters for the nursing brethren (K) just below the queen's house on either side of a kitchen (M). In their front yard was that useful appendage, a cemetery (P). The laundry (R) is down

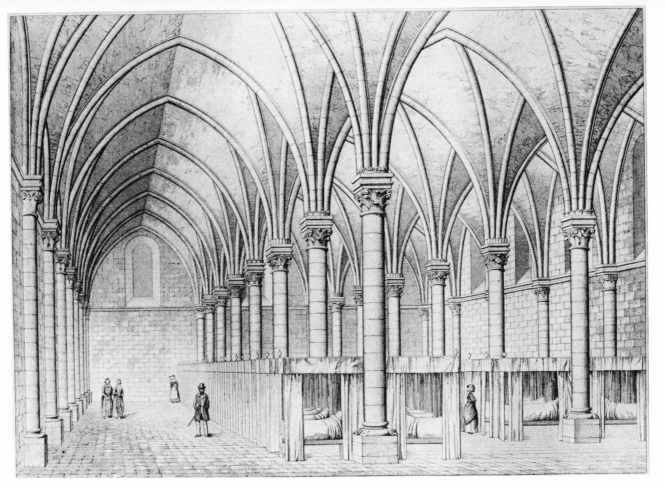

Fig. 20. Interior of the Hôtel-Dieu of St. Jean in Angers, France (founded 1153) in the nineteenth century.

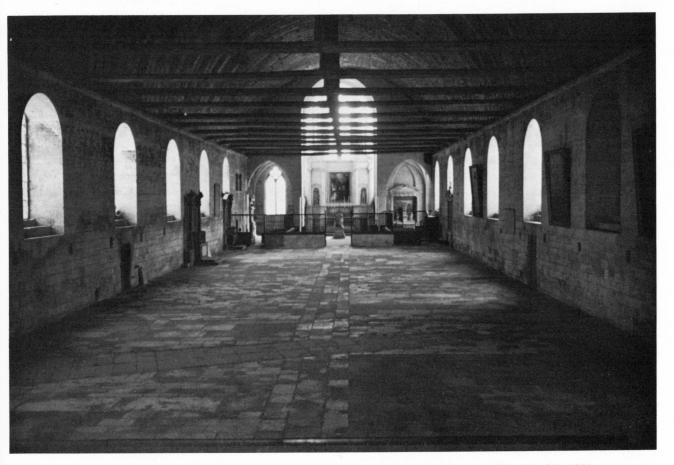

Fig. 22. Interior of the thirteenth-century barrel-vaulted hospital in Tonnerre, looking toward the chapel, in 1971.

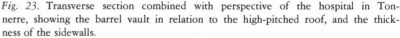

Fig. 23. Transverse section combined with perspective of the hospital in Tonnerre, showing the barrel vault in relation to the high-pitched roof, and the thickness of the sidewalls.

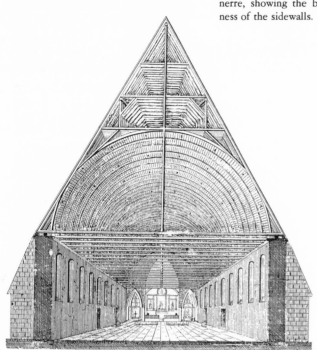

by the river, which, surrounding the hospital on two sides, served a very practical purpose. The two sewers that ran riverward past the long sides of the ward were flushed by a diverted arm of the river and also by a spring and brook.[11] Along the main street was a public well (X).[12] The hospital lay outside the city wall, its grounds enclosed by a wall of its own. At night, when the city gates were shut, a poor sick person or wanderer could still find shelter. (Perhaps the authorities gave a thought to contagion too.)

The many open ward and chapel arrangements all over Christendom can be sorted out according to the relationship of ward to chapel. Was the chapel closed off or at a distance from the ward with an indirect entrance as at Angers, or could patients see the altar from their beds? A clear view was of especial importance in the twelfth century. Sacramental communion had become rare; we are told that St. Louis, who every day attended one or more masses, only communicated six times a year. A feast for the eyes was all the more passionately desired. "Bishops . . . in about 1210, ordered the host to be held only breast high and to be raised higher only after the words of consecration, lest the people should adore it too soon." It was therefore a "regulation of . . . a gesture already in use, the emphasis being provoked by the especial religious value attached in those days to seeing the host."[13] Perhaps this is a reason for the popularity of the large open wards; religious feelings already current would be even more intense among the ill or those about to die. To see the host lifted was para-

mount, or at very least to hear the words of the Mass.

The orientation of the chapel was a matter of concern. The altar usually faced east, but to allow for that on an awkward lot the chapel might project at right angles to the ward. We have chapels affixed to their wards every which way. The ward of the Byloke Hospital in Ghent (1234) is the second largest barrel-roofed ward remaining in Europe and belonged to an abbey. The chapel was a small parallel appendage to the ward—it is now used as a morgue (fig. 25). A large double arch in the long side of the chapel established at least an auditory connection with the ward, although only the few patients opposite could see the Mass. In the thirteenth or earliest fourteenth century, the arches were walled up and two small doors substituted. Van Puyvelde suggests that perhaps the sisters did not wish to be distracted at their night services by the noises of the ward![14]

The chapel of the Second Hospital of the Knights at Rhodes (1440–89) is in the long wall, which obviously faces east (fig. 26) This hospital on an island off the coast of Turkey was built by the military and nursing order, the Knights of St. John of Jerusalem, for members wounded while fighting the mainland Turks. We recognize immediately the simple, secular small windows of a rather dark ward and the flood of light through the ornate arch of the chapel (figs. 27 and 28). Rings for night lamps may still be seen embedded at the peak of the arcade arches. A very interesting feature has been added: a row of service rooms of varying sizes down both long walls of the hall (fig. 26), most of which have two doors. Some rooms are large enough to contain a bed; others consist of a brief curved passage from one door to the other and it is hard not to furnish them with a close-stool. No sight of sewers; furthermore, these are second-story rooms over solid stone walls. And no windows whatever in the little rooms. Some say they were for the sick knight's squire, who stood at attention behind his master's bed until he was called. On the ground floor beneath this ward were deep windowless chambers with one wide opening on the street (visible in fig. 28). It has been surmised that they were rented out as shops.[15] This would not be the first hospital or the last to make money that way.

Finally, we turn to St. John's Hospital of Bruges, founded by laymen at the end of the twelfth century. The plan (fig. 29) indicates how a large ward might accrue, section by section, from a small beginning. The first ward lay beside and was not much bigger than its chapel. Segments were added over the next two centuries until the chapel occupied only one

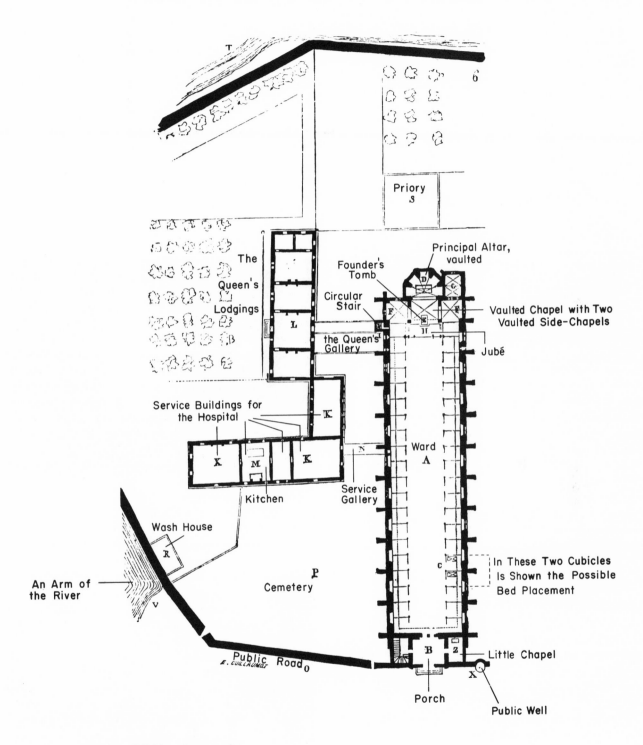

Fig. 24. Plan of the hospital in Tonnerre and its service areas, by Viollet-le-Duc.

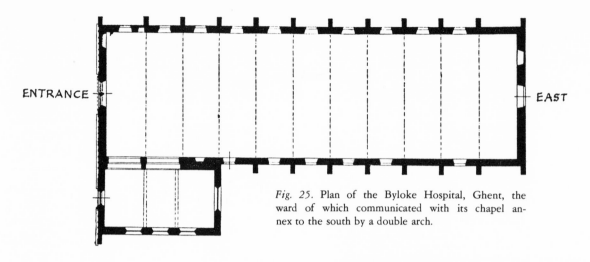

ENTRANCE

EAST

Fig. 25. Plan of the Byloke Hospital, Ghent, the ward of which communicated with its chapel annex to the south by a double arch.

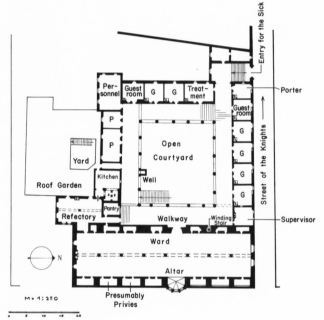

Fig. 26. Second-floor plan, Second Hospital of the Knights, Rhodes (1440–89).

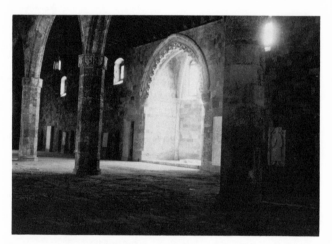

Fig. 27. Relative illumination of ward and chapel, Second Hospital of the Knights, Rhodes. Photo taken in 1968.

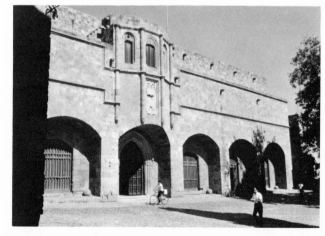

Fig. 28. Eastern facade of the Second Hospital of the Knights, Rhodes, in 1968, showing the exterior of the chapel windows in figure 27. The ground-floor openings are to deep, narrow rooms with only this entrance, which may have been used as shops.

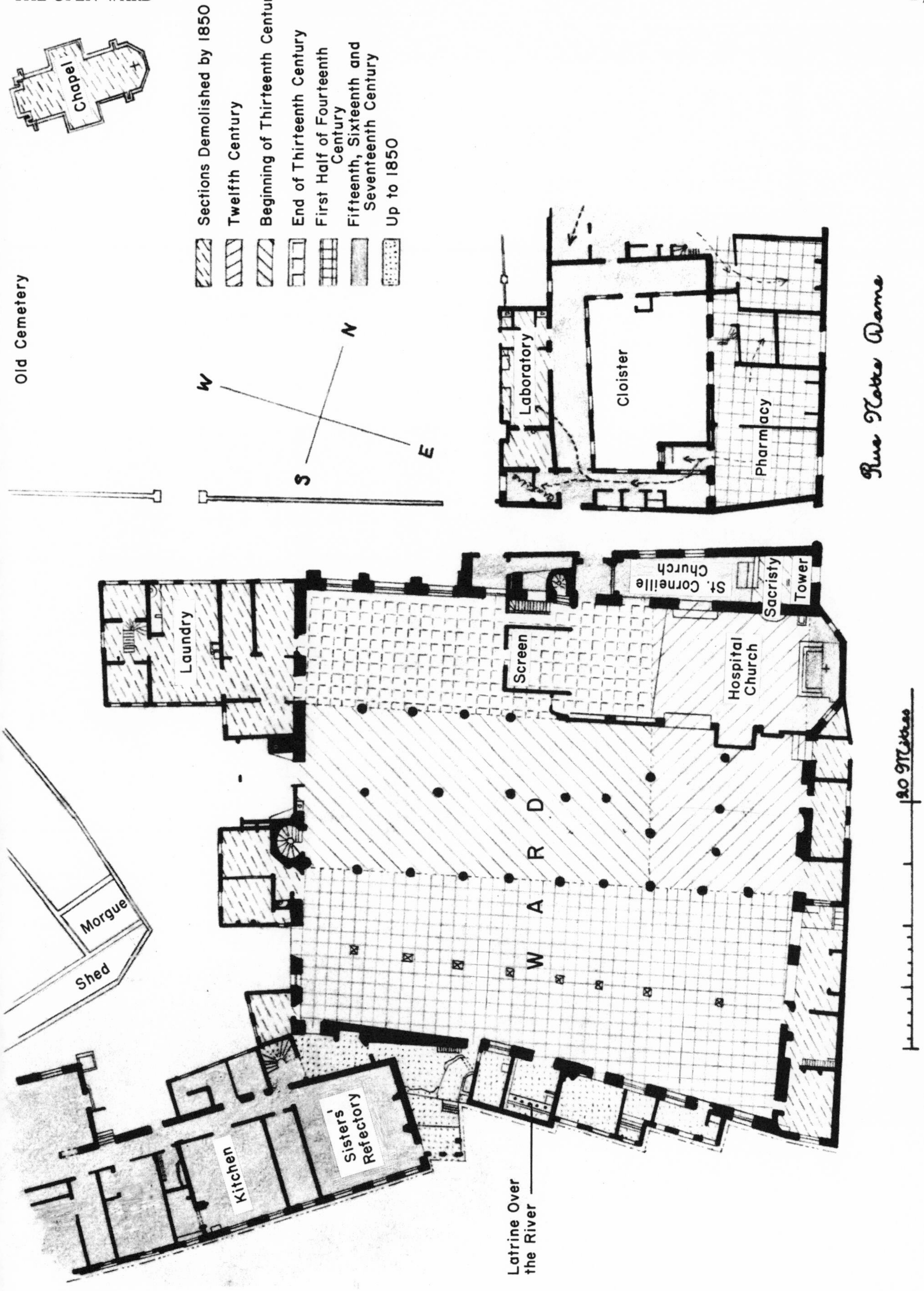

Old Cemetery

Chapel

Sections Demolished by 1850

Twelfth Century

Beginning of Thirteenth Century

End of Thirteenth Century

First Half of Fourteenth Century

Fifteenth, Sixteenth and Seventeenth Century

Up to 1850

N

W

E

S

Laboratory

Cloister

Pharmacy

Rue Notre Dame

St. Corneille Church

Screen

Sacristy

Tower

Hospital Church

Laundry

Morgue

Shed

Kitchen

Sisters' Refectory

W A R D

Latrine Over the River

20 Metres

Fig. 29. Plan of St. John's Hospital, Bruges, in 1850, showing successive stages in building from the end of the twelfth century. Redrawn by Bev Pope.

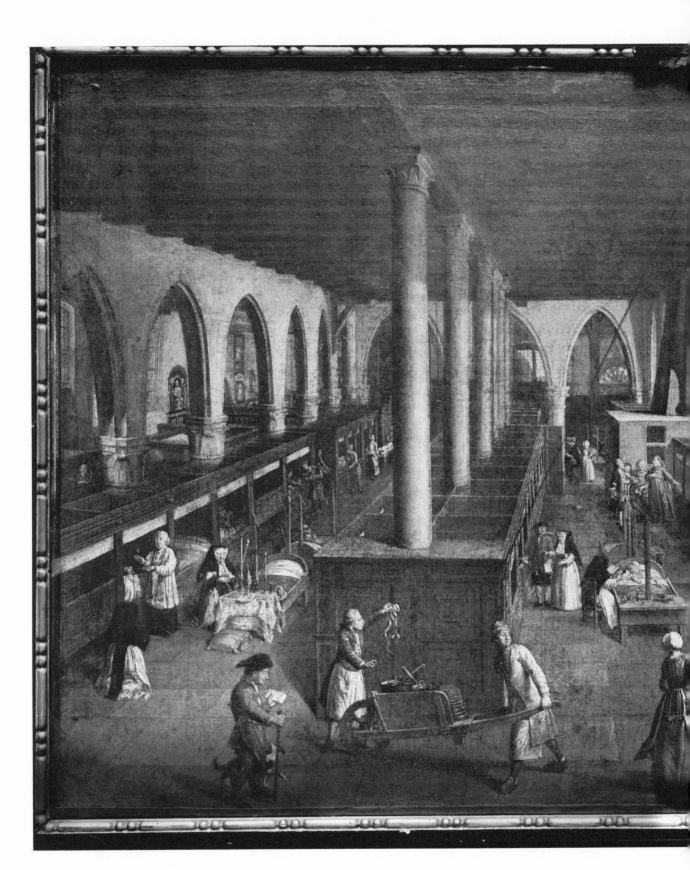

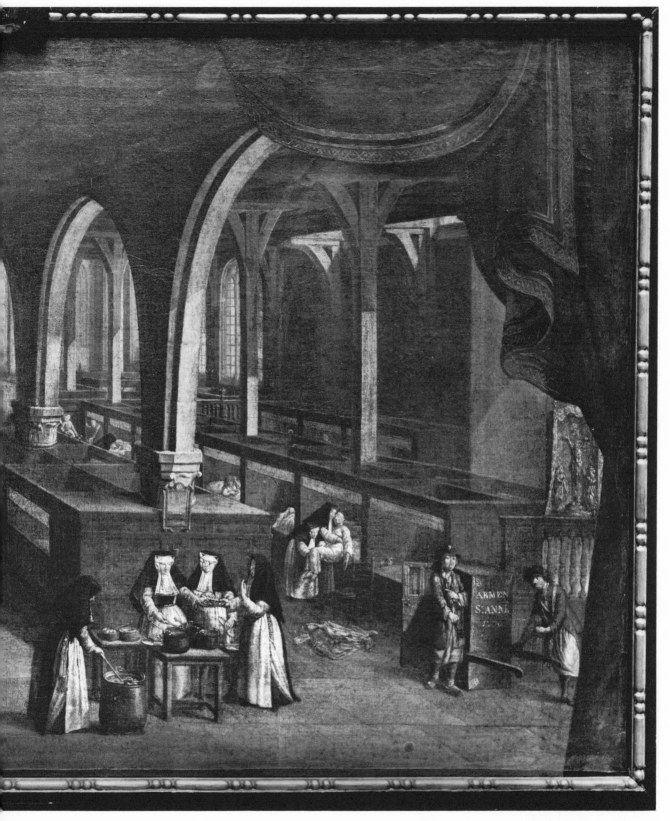

Fig. 30. Johannes Beerblock's painting *View of the Sick Ward of St. John's Hospital (Bruges)*, 1778.

corner of an open space about 5,000 square feet in extent and in its southeastern corner two stories tall. The chapel was open to the ward until very recent times. A remarkable painting, Johannes Beerblock's *View of the Sick Ward of St. John's Hospital, 1778* (fig. 30), shows everything cheerfully happening at once: from left to right, a patient receiving extreme unction, a bed being made ready for him to die in, medications being brought in, and at the far end of that aisle a corpse being carried out; plates and pails being taken away on a wheelbarrow, and a maid with a tray flirting with the young man at the wheelbarrow; a doctor feeling a patient's pulse, a convalescent being discharged, and a deathbed (right in the center of the picture); visiting clergy and a cleaning maid with her mop; dinner being served, and an emergency case being brought in by sedan chair ambulance. We see beds in cubicles, whose sides lift up and down as on a crib, while the square little house center rear is an inside necessarium flushed by water from a diverted stream.[16] The arcades look very much like those of the hospital at Rhodes. Beerblock's picture conveys the conservatism that preserved the forms of the great hall for 600 years and gives us some notion of the frenzied life therein—generic nursing and housekeeping patterns that never changed in any radical way until in the nineteenth and twentieth centuries medicine finally discovered what makes people ill and the chapel lost its power.

Cross Wards

Now picture the dilemma of a medieval administrator whose ward has grown too small for the crowds of those who call upon its charity. He has a beautiful chapel, properly oriented, and westward a large open ward in perfect visual and auditory communication with it. He will be tempted to double the length of the ward. But although the length of an open ward is in theory infinitely extensible (unlike its width, which must be limited by how vast a space can be spanned by current vaulting methods), he must soon reach the point of diminishing returns: patients at the far end will no longer be able either to see or hear the Mass. Therefore, when overcrowding occurred, builders began to think in terms of large multiple units. At the fifteenth century Hospital de Santa Cruz in Barcelona, three or possibly four large halls, opening into one another, were arranged around a court. Their architectural style is very much like that of the dormitory of Poblet Monastery a few miles away.

Sheer logic, however, led to a better solution. If the altar is placed in the middle of a cross, and each arm of the cross is the size of the original ward, four times as many patients will be able to hear and see the same Mass. The principle had been invoked in the

cross-shaped church (martyrium) of Qalat Siman at the end of the fifth century, which enclosed the venerated pillar on which St. Simeon Stylites lived and died (figs. 31a and b). Did its influence filter down

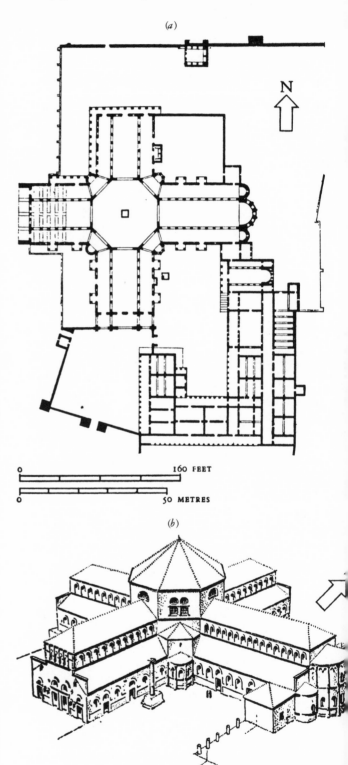

Fig. 31. (*a*) Floor plan and (*b*) isometric reconstruction of the cross-shaped church (martyrium) of Qalat-Siman, Syria (c. 470).

to the fifteenth century? One model was before every-body's eyes: the cross-shaped church. One hospital form in sixteenth-century Scotland was simply a church: "the nave formed the common room, the beds were placed in the transepts, and the whole was screened off from the eastern end of the building, where was the chapel."[17]

The Hospital of Santa Maria Nuova in Florence eventually assumed the form of two cross wards, one for women and one for men. But this came about through no dazzling stroke of logic. It was rather the result of a haphazard expansion: beginning with the hall and altar of the women's hospital (1315), which finally formed the lower arm of the cross, a right arm and perhaps part of the upper one was added in 1334, and finally in 1479 the left arm was built and the upper arm lengthened soon thereafter, with a church at the end of it and not at the crossing.[18] On the other hand, from the outset the Ospedale Maggiore of Milan was originally projected in 1456 in the form of two cross wards with chapel between and was minutely described in words, plan, and elevation by the architect Filarete in his *Tractate on Architecture*. Although the grandiose design took 350 years to execute in its entirety, the Ospedale Maggiore, almost from the time the first plans were published, took its place as one of the half dozen most influential hospital designs in the world. Contemporaries were vastly impressed, imitations sprang up within 50 years, and its influence can be felt in European hospitals right through the eighteenth century.

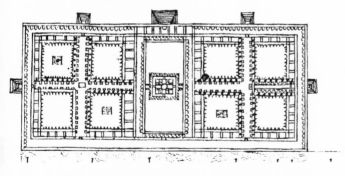

Fig. 32. Filarete's original design for the Ospedale Maggiore, Milan (1456).

Filarete's original design (fig. 32) shows the cross ward for men to the right, that for women to the left of an oblong court, in the center of which he placed the church. Eight smaller courtyards were formed by surrounding the two huge crosses with two stories of peripheral rooms for staff, for services, and "for gentlemen, who will be kept separate from the commoners through respect."[19] In execution, the central court was greatly enlarged and the church moved to the rear. The pinnacles and projections Filarete lib-

erally supplied were omitted, leaving an almost featureless front facade neither elevated, nor adorned with monumental staircases one and a half stories high. Filarete had planned to bring in supplies by boat at the rear, along the Naviglio (a canal probably the equivalent in texture and odor of the moat at Canterbury). He does not say how he will get carriages and patients up those stairs.

An eighteenth-century plan gives a better idea of what the Ospedale Maggiore looked like when fully built and functioning (fig. 33a). At the first press of overcrowding, Filarete's exterior arcades were filled in to form four more huge wards, thus closing off the peripheral rooms from the street. Basement rooms, under the rooms of the perimeter, only half buried, were used for services or rented out for shops and storerooms.[20] There was a full basement under the cross wards, half of it above ground, with light from four side doors and cross ventilation and walls thick enough for a fortress (fig. 33b). It was never used for patients, but wine and bread were made there, the laundresses worked there, and meat for the patients was brought in on the hoof and slaughtered at need in one of the basement rooms.[21] (Hens were raised in the women's ward.) Each court of the men's ward was given over to a separate function: pharmacy, icehouse (snow shoveled in during the winter packed down into ice), woodyard, kitchen.

The ceilings of the great wards were almost 33 feet high (John Howard's complaint in 1784 that the wards were "not lofty"[22] gives an idea of eighteenth-century expectations). The height of both stories of the peripheral rooms did not equal that of the open wards. The cross wards were to be ventilated by four fireplaces, one in the side wall of each cross ward close to the central chapel, and probably they were heated by a line of braziers down the median line. In the fifteenth century, beds were very wide, uncurtained, made of wood, with mattresses presumably of straw. Beside each bed was a cabinet with a drop leaf that served the patient as an end table. In a chest at the foot of the bed his or her clothes were stored, after being washed. All patients of the time went to bed nude. It has been calculated that Filarete intended 8 beds to a side, only 16 in one of the huge arms of the cross. The number of beds soon doubled; in later centuries another row of beds was even added down the center of the room, but a serious effort was made to let each patient lie alone. Only under very crowded conditions did they lie two by two, and then only temporarily.[23] When possible, contagious cases were sent to other institutions; the Ospedale Maggiore was chief hospital of a confederation of nine.[24] Men—even the priest—were strictly excluded from the women's ward.

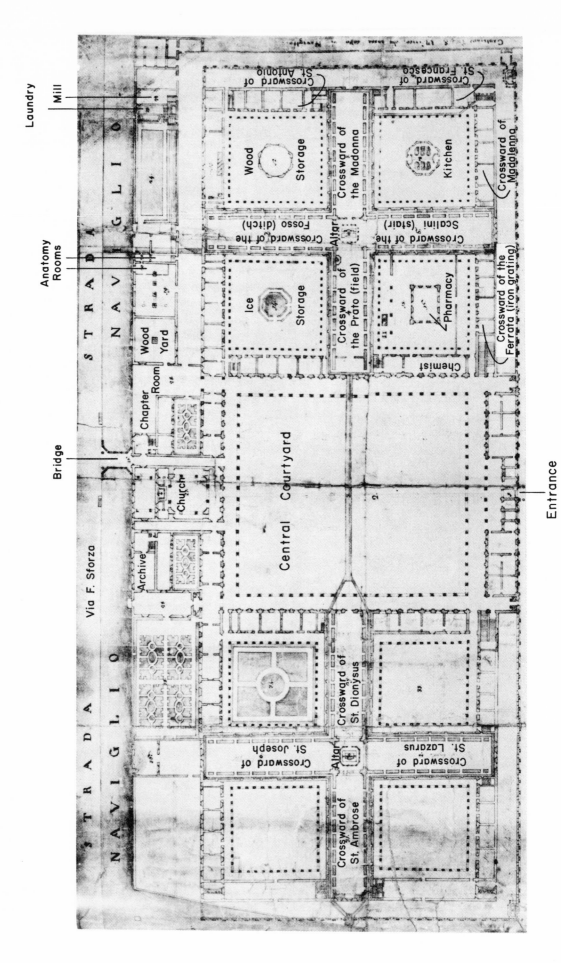

Fig. 33. (*a*) Eighteenth-century plan of the ground floor of both cross wards of the Ospedale Maggiore.

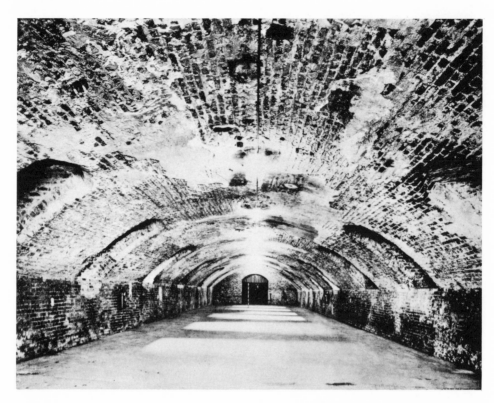

Fig. 33. (b) The cellar of one arm of Filarete's cross ward today.

Between every two beds was a door leading to a private privy. A floor plan by Hansgeorg Knoblauch conveys the arrangement (fig. 34a). A photograph of the privy corridor in the thickness of the cross-ward walls (fig. 34b), with sewer beneath, shows how much narrower these channels were than the ones at the monastery necessarium. On Filarete's drawing (fig. 32) a row of dots ran along the outside of wards to indicate the seats, for Filarete was very proud of his sanitary innovation. Water from the Naviglio, regulated by a series of sluices, was to sweep around the channel and "come out below the water level of the moat" (that is, the Naviglio; see fig. 34c). "It cleans the latrines and the road outside the city to the great advantage of anyone who owns fields in that direction."[25] Filarete proposed to do away with every last vestige of odor by spiracles every ten *braccia* (22½ inches), rising from the channel through the buttresses to the roof. The spiracles were supposed to work both ways: in dry weather bad air was to rise *up* them, in a rainfall they were to be rinsed by pure rainwater pouring *down* them. By 1695, only the intake of the privy system was in working order.

In a photograph of the men's ward taken in 1966 (fig. 35a), vestiges of the privy doors can be seen along the wall. The hospital was badly bombed in 1943. What one of these wards had looked like with patients in it can be seen in figure 35b. Today, completely refurbished, it serves as library of the University of

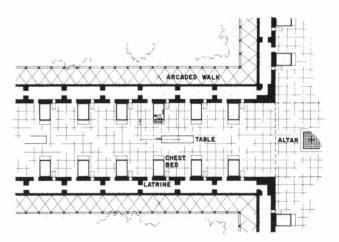

Fig. 34. (a) Floor plan of the privy system in a section of one arm of the Filarete cross ward; the dotted oblong beside each bed was a small end table that let down from a cupboard in the wall.

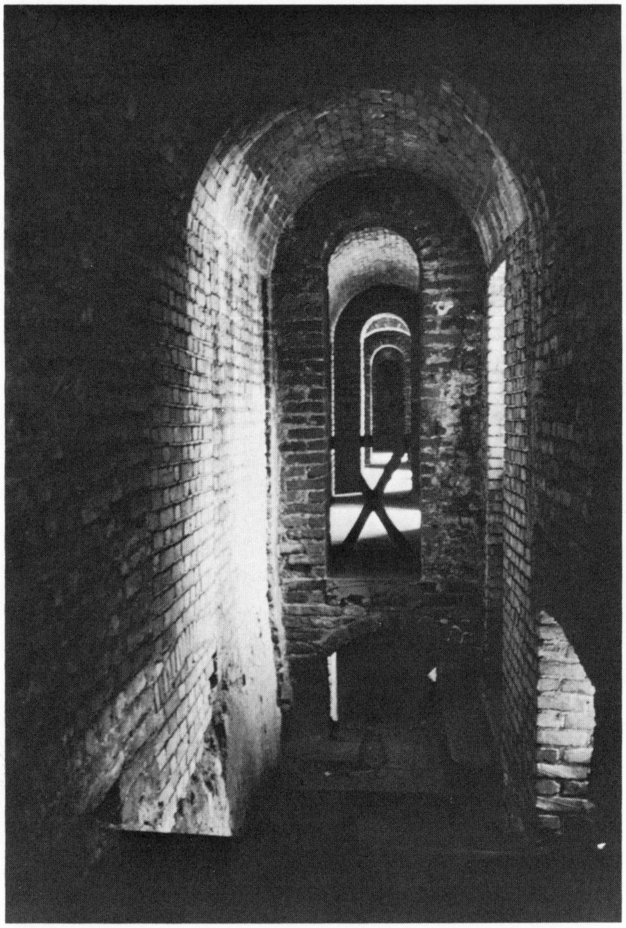

(b)

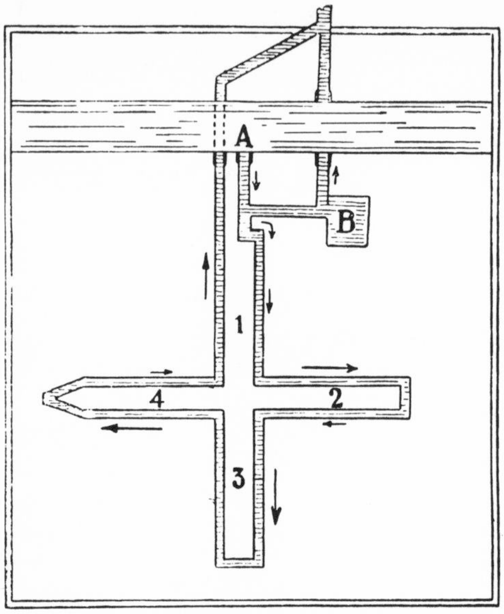

(c)

Fig. 34. (b) One privy corridor after bombing; photo taken in 1966;
(c) the course of the sanitary canal as indicated by arrows from
A, the entrance of the water from the Naviglio, on around the
four Filarete cross wards, named, respectively, (1) del Fosso
(of the ditch); (2) delle Donne, or Madonna; (3) degli Scalini
(of the stairs—the main stair from the street came up at the narrow end of this ward); (4) del Prato (of the field, referring to the
eventual destination of the valuable collected filth, on the other
side of the Naviglio). A branch of the canal from its source served
the laundry (B).

Milan, which occupies the entire reconstructed complex. Figure 35c, a transverse section by Liliana Grassi,
further clarifies the relationship of privy corridor to
ward and drain.

Imagination boggles at the burial arrangements of the
Ospedale Maggiore. Filarete spelled it out clearly:
he would have an upper altar in the church proper
and a lower altar in the church vault. "Above the
ground there are four columns where a Mass is said
every Monday for the souls of the dead. Below the
altar one can go down by this stair to the very bottom.
It has several openings above for putting in bodies."[26]
He describes "parallel iron bars, like a grating, where
the bodies are laid. This is almost at the level of the
water." We once asked the late Professor Robert
Herrlinger what services in such a church would be
like, as the smell wafted upward, and he replied, "I
fear that the problem how to do away with the corpses
was much more important than the problem how to
do away with the smell!"[27] But eventually the smell
daunted everybody. Spinelli is very tactful and avoids
mentioning gratings; however, he does describe overflowing vaults, an agglomeration of corpses 50 yards
from the infirmary that saturated the humus, common
trenches into which the naked dead were thrown in
times of pestilence, their remains eventually treated
with unslaked lime, and a desperate suggestion by the
tribunal of *health* to unstop the sepulchres toward
the Naviglio and let them drain into the city canal.[28]
In 1694 a new burial ground was opened well beyond
the city limits. Funerals left the Ospedale Maggiore
by two gates: the wealthy deceased in state by the principal portal; paupers by a back door over a little bridge
across the Naviglio that came to be known as the
"Bridge of the Poor."

Forty years after the laying of the cornerstone of the
Ospedale Maggiore, the Hospital General of Valencia,
Spain, was rebuilt in cross style (1492, 1512). Two
insane asylums, the Hospital Real de Dementes in
Granada (1504; note the differentiated ceiling of the
chapel in fig. 36) and the Hospital de Santa Cruz of
Toledo of the same year, were carried out as two-
storied cross wards for the separation of the sexes.
In such cases women were upstairs, probably to keep
the men from spying down on them. At Toledo the
crossing was two stories high because the hospital
possessed a splinter of the True Cross embedded in
a huge wooden cross laced with silver, and both men
and women would want to benefit from that. These
two hospitals were created on a regal scale, one of
them by a king, for "people from whom one could
expect no returns . . . people whom today's society
regards as a burden," as Dieter Jetter writes.[29] "The
incurably sick had the love of the people and the royal
favor, for heaven was open to them. So the hospital

becomes a Golgotha, and the sick became the precious possession of the community." This eloquent statement of the high purpose of these halls is qualified by a description of how they smelled when there were patients in them: night chaises, not properly closable and emptied at most once every twenty-four hours; perpetually damp mattresses of straw or seaweed crawling with bugs; unwashed patients and nearly unwashed floors, for water was fetched pail by single pail from the courtyard well; smoking blubber and oil lamps; kitchen odors—all combated in a rather hopeless fashion by fumigation and the sprinkling of perfumed waters.

Cross wards were built or projected all over Europe —in the eighteenth century John Howard termed them "the usual form of hospitals in many Roman-Catholic countries."[30] Of many we will mention the only cross ward in England, originally a palace which became in 1509 the Savoy Hospital of London—a Roman, not a Greek cross; the Hôpital des Incurables

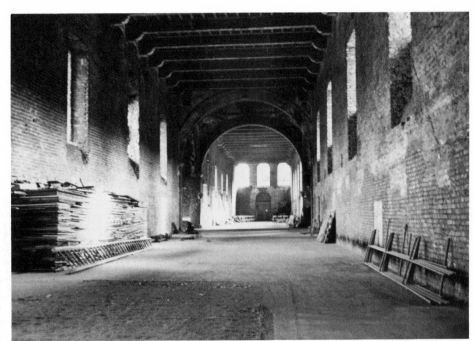

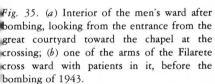

Fig. 35. (a) Interior of the men's ward after bombing, looking from the entrance from the great courtyard toward the chapel at the crossing; (b) one of the arms of the Filarete cross ward with patients in it, before the bombing of 1943.

Fig. 35. (c) cross section of one arm showing privy corridors and subterranean canals, with (right) the facade of another arm of the Filarete cross ward, Ospedale Maggiore (see diagram upper right for area represented); by Liliana Grassi.

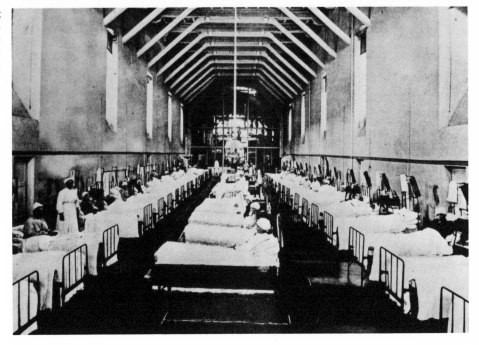

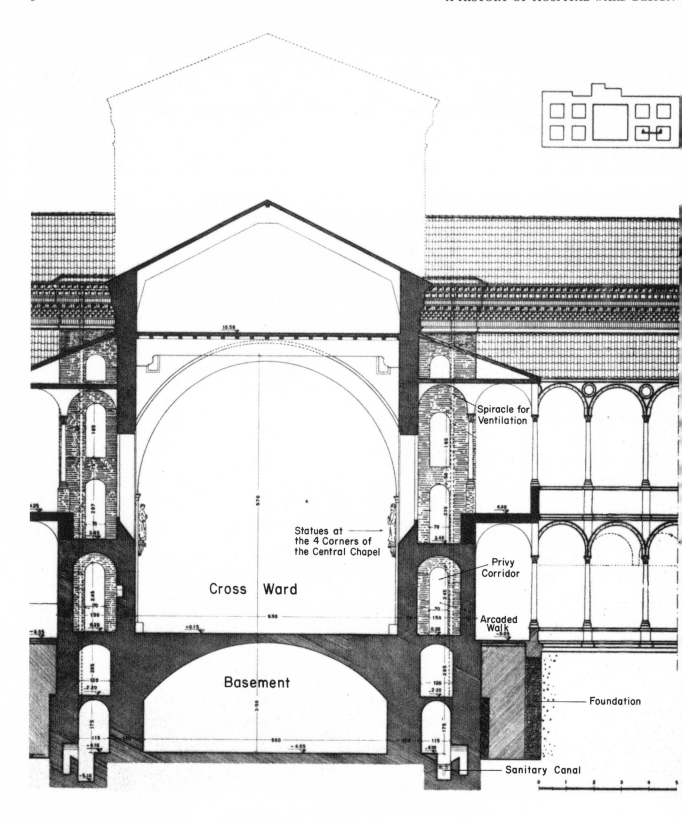

Spiracle for
Ventilation

Statues at
the 4 Corners of
the Central Chapel

Cross   Ward

Privy
Corridor

Arcaded
Walk

Basement

Foundation

Sanitary Canal

Femmes of Paris (1635–49), which like Filarete's plan for Milan shows two cross wards with a church between; and César Laure's cross ward for the Hôtel-Dieu of Lyons (1622–31), where the dome over the crossing was used for a nonreligious purpose: ventilation. It was hoped that poisonous air from the wards would collect there. The eighteenth-century architect Soufflot reported in a letter that he had been assured that birds would not approach the dome of the Hôtel-Dieu of Lyons, but if any did, they would fall down dead.[31] Ventilation was effected through the dome with such vigor that in 1842, in wards where big fireplaces burned all the time and there were one or two very large cast iron stoves, on winter mornings the temperature went down to 27½ degrees, and the dome area had to be partitioned off.[32]

An interesting French cross ward, planned by Philibert Delorme in 1561 but never built, groups the four large wards around an open, arcaded court, probably also for the sake of ventilation.[33] The sick rooms would have needed a powerful central whirlpool and stiff drafts from end to end since in this plan cross-ventilation is entirely cut off by side rooms.

We have no evidence that cross wards were actually built in Germany. One seventeenth-century architect, Joseph Furttenbach, was alive to their possibilities but lacked in Germany the stable centralized government necessary to support the execution of monumental plans, which therefore remained theoretical projects. Furttenbach spent ten years of his youth in Italy, including two years in Milan, and referred afterward to the Ospedale Maggiore as "the principal hospital of all Italy."[34] Even without that statement we know he was impressed. His plan for "A Hospital in the Italian Style" (1628) is explicit: there it all is, even a privy between every two beds. In Milan, before the building of the second cross, woman patients were kept strictly separate in the right arm of the men's cross. There was a chain across the entrance and the ward was off limits to all male personnel, even the administrator. Furttenbach likewise chained off the right arm of his "Italian" cross-shaped hospital.[35]

However, the climate of Germany is not the climate of Italy, and in his next plans Furttenbach turned to rectangular wards with 24 beds in four rows cowering in the middle of the room. A wooden partition lengthwise separated men from women.[36] Then Furttenbach combined his German interior with the Italian cross form to produce a "Grosses Lazarett" (1635; fig. 37). At the crossing he set a flight of stairs. Hospital historians who praise the designs of Furttenbach for their rationality fetch up against this staircase and are left speechless.

Not a single altar was included in the plans of 1635, but twenty years later Furttenbach more than recti-

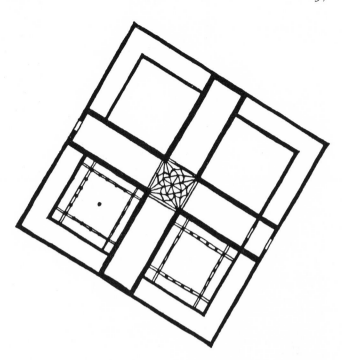

Fig. 36. Plan of cross ward of the Hospital Real de Dementes, Granada, Spain (1504), by Dieter Jetter. Note the ornate ceiling of the central chapel.

fied the omission in a plan shaped like a Roman cross (fig. 38). He said of it that the whole building should be thought of as a cross upon which Christ was crucified—he who "stretches out his merciful arms over the beds of the suffering, he who shares his merciful heart in the presentation of the Mass [the altar at the crossing being placed right at the heart] and in the place of the upper altar bends his holy head toward Christianity [the upper altar standing where his head would rest]. Thus we may see in this hospital building a lovable figure and be reminded constantly of the suffering and death of our own Savior and the one who made us holy . . ."[37]

Despite all this, there is considerable rationality in the plan. The arms of the cross may have held up the arms of Jesus but they also cut off the cold, wet winds from the west; the body of the cross was oriented to receive the morning sun, summer or winter, even though this meant facing the altar west. Windows were placed exactly opposite each other for cross ventilation. Christ's head on the altar was crowned, on the second story, by a kitchen!

So far we have examined hospitals where the cross form was exploited for religious purposes or—hopefully—to assist ventilation. A third virtue of the form was discovered: ease of supervision. In a cross, looking goes both ways. If in a cross ward four times as many patients can look *into* the crossing to receive religious consolation from an altar there, four times

38

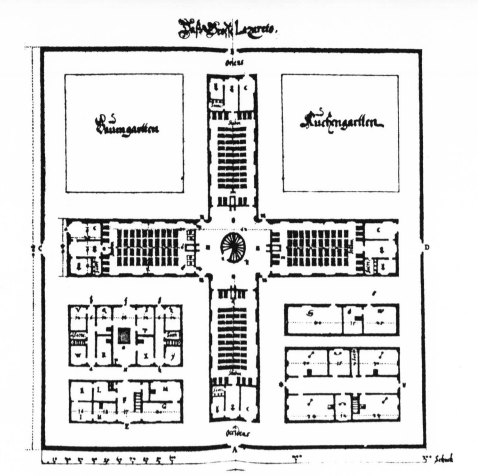

Fig. 37. Ground-floor plan of Furttenbach's "Grosses Lazarett," 1635, a cross plan with a stairway at the crossing.

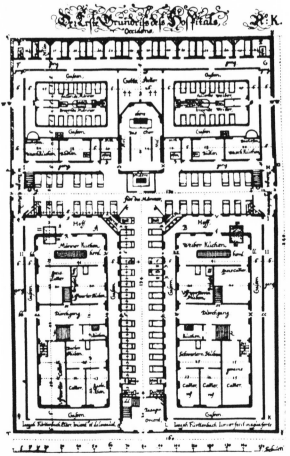

Fig. 38. Ground-floor plan of Furttenbach's hospital in the form of a Roman cross (1655).

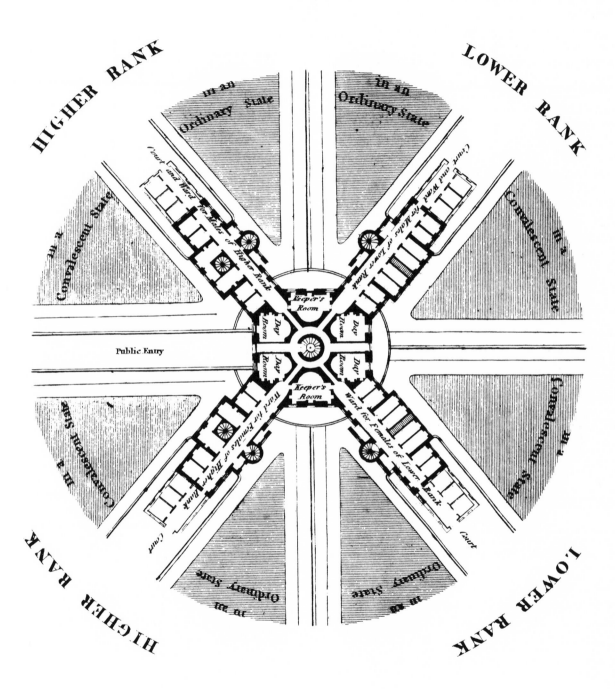

Fig. 39. Plan of the Glasgow, Scotland, Lunatic Asylum, 1810.

as many patients can be watched *from* the crossing
by the nursing staff. The cross form was a natural
for prisons and insane asylums and was enthusiastically
adopted in what were called "panoptical institutions."

"Panopticon" was a word invented in 1796 by Jeremy
Bentham, the English reformer and utilitarian philos-
opher, to describe an ingenious new prison plan he
had worked out: a perfectly round building within
which seven tiers of cells faced a central house for
the superintendent, who theoretically could see into
and thus supervise every single one. It had its practical defects (the superintendent's house as Bentham
conceived it would itself obstruct the supposed 360°
view) but enough merit to inspire a prison design in
Joliet, Illinois, 150 years later.[38] Bentham presented
this plan as suitable for adaptation to many purposes:
"punishing the incorrigible, guarding the insane,
reforming the vitious, confining the suspected, employing the idle, maintaining the helpless, curing
the sick, instructing the willing in any branch of industry, or training the rising race in the path of education."[39] Thereafter, designs based on the principle
of inspection from a central point were termed panoptical.

The panoptical cross ward of the Glasgow Lunatic
Asylum (1810; fig. 39) had a staircase at the crossing,
which made sense. The important thing was how easily
a supervisor could circle around the stairs to look
into the wards; note also that the staircase prevented
inmates of these wards from spying on one another.
In such a plan, useful triangular exercise courts are
formed that can very easily be supervised by an observer at the center of the pie.

The ultimate cross-shaped panoptical hospital plan
is the cross ward of the insane asylum in Erlangen,
West Germany (fig. 40). Built in 1834, it was already
too late for the high tide of panoptical building and
was regarded as somewhat archaic. Today it seems
pointless. The intriguing pinwheel effect produced
by an offset single-loaded corridor—that is, one with
rooms only on one side—is perceptible only in the
plan or from the air. The corridors are perfectly un-

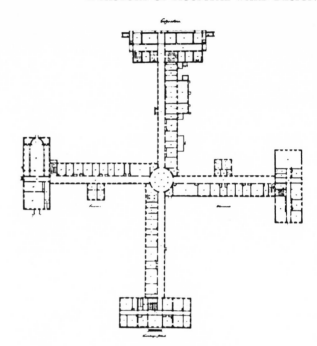

Fig. 40. Plan of the Insane Asylum, Erlangen, Germany
(1834–46).

remarkable, the crossing is completely ordinary, and
from the lawns the right angles formed by the walls
seem absolutely normal.

On Blackwell's Island, New York City, the Lunatic
Asylum for the Insane of Bellevue Hospital (1839)
was built as two arms of a panoptical cross (the central
section survives today.) But the completed building
was to be **C** shaped, not cross shaped, for the **L** was
to be repeated on the opposite side. As a final vestige
of the cross-shaped layout, Dr. Egill Snorrason refers
us to the site plan of the Gamles By (Old Folks' Home)
of Copenhagen (early twentieth century). The church
is at the head of the site, where Christ's head would
be. His arms would extend among the patients' pavilions; his feet are nailed to the administration offices at the entrance. His presence in the planning of
this hospital is about as tenuous as the smile of the
Cheshire cat; after this, he vanishes.

CHAPTER 3

Small Rooms and Private Rooms

Large Halls Subdivided

The progress observed in sick wards from smaller rooms in the ninth century to large infirmary halls in the eleventh and twelfth reflects a general tendency toward community living on the part of clerics and laymen. The great cathedrals were but one outgrowth of it. In the thirteenth, fourteenth, and fifteenth centuries a growing interest in privacy is testified to by the partitioning off of the lord's hall or the monk's dormitory. Enlart tells us that at a time when the "hall" constituted almost the whole of a private mansion, "compartments were created and delimited by partitions of woodwork or by simple curtains of cloth or out-stretched tapestry."[1] This was done only partly to combat drafts.

In monasteries there was a very slow drift toward privacy as such. It began in the dormitories. The monastic ideal was a dead level, no privileges, no possessions, but even St. Benedict considered separate beds a necessity, although all in one room if possible.[2] "But if their numbers do not allow of this, let them sleep by tens or twenties, with seniors to supervise them. There shall be a light burning in the dormitory throughout the night. Let them sleep clothed and girt with girdles or cords"—no doubt for moral reasons. "The younger brethren shall not have their beds by themselves, but shall be mixed with the seniors." A knife, a pen, a needle, were among the few conveniences doled out to each monk by the abbot —conveniences, not possessions, all personal property being forbidden. Since these are all sharp instruments, they were removed with the boots when retiring.[3] Very gradually from the twelfth century onward (as Dr. Charles H. Talbot described the process to us), a monk came to remove also the habit he had worked in all day and then his shirt, at which point he required a nightshirt and his own place to change in, for modesty's sake. Morality now implied privacy. So separate cubicles were installed in the monastic dormitory and the arrangements carried over to the infirmary, where people are also lying down: first a temporary wooden partition with a few curtains, later a permanent wooden cubicle.

The trend can be traced today in a monks' infirmary

and a bishop's hospital. The twelfth-century Infirmary Hall of Fountains Abbey, England, erected on the traditional site rearward and east of the abbey church, rested upon great piles that spanned a multiple drain leading from the River Skell (fig. 41). In the fourteenth century this hall, to judge from existing doorsills, was subdivided into fifteen rooms with stone walls and actual doors. Also English, a thirteenth-century cathedral hospital, St. Mary's in Chichester, enclosed a combined hall and chapel within the familiar vernacular form of a barn with very low side walls and a high-pitched roof whose eaves reach almost to the ground (fig. 42). The intervals of the upright posts facilitated its later subdivision into rooms by wooden partitions only as high as the side walls and open to the rafters on top (fig. 43). This structure (modernized in the seventeenth century by the introduction of fireplaces[4] and in the twentieth by the addition of individual kitchenettes and w.c.s) still survives as an old-age home for women.

The interior of the Holy Ghost Hospital at Nykøbing, Denmark (fig. 44) shows a third way of subdividing an open hall: by bunk beds, a feature northern hospitals used for the sake of warmth as well as privacy. Finally, we cite the cubicles added in 1820 to the great ward of the late thirteenth-century Holy Ghost Hospital of Lübeck, Germany (fig. 45). This too is an old-age home now—for pensioners of both sexes. There were always two corridors, one for men and one for women. In 1787 the open hall contained 61 beds for men and 66 for women, in four rows, plus 12 private rooms "in which they have one cupboard and one chest."[5]

Pensioners, Almshouses, Leprosaria, Plague Houses

Thus far we have considered subdivision as a device to grant greater privacy to all patients, but it must be recognized that certain categories of patients were thought of all along in terms of smaller rooms. There were few exclusions from the prevalent mélange of maladies within one ward, modest or immense, but the few may be traced back very far and these patients were often placed in small or actually private units:

42

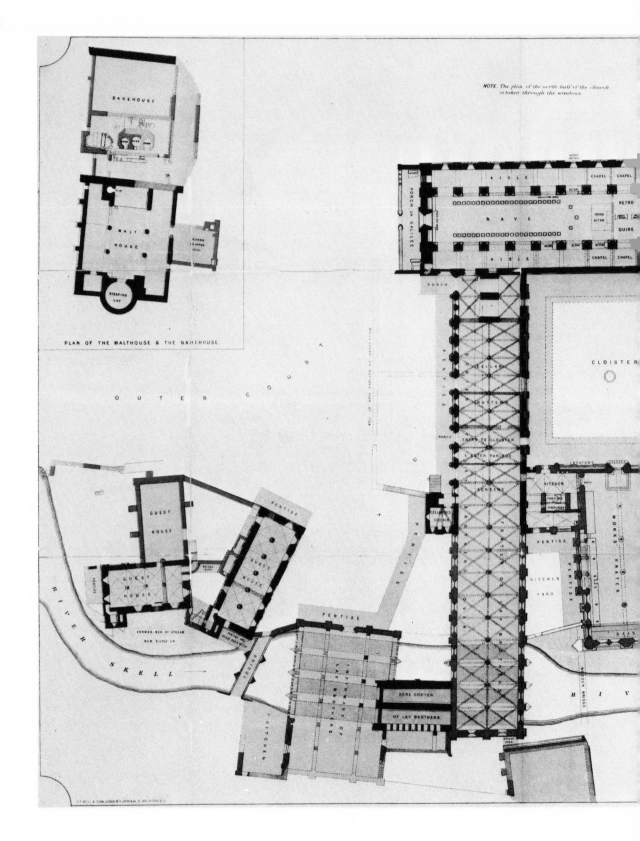

PLAN OF THE MALTHOUSE & THE BAKEHOUSE.

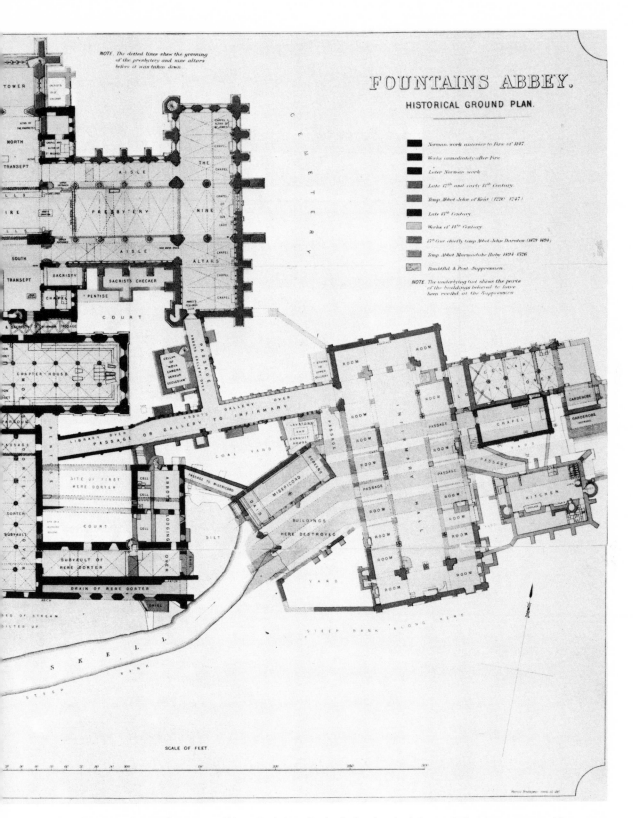

Fig. 41. Ground plan of Fountains Abbey, Yorkshire, England, showing the infirmary hall as later subdivided into rooms.

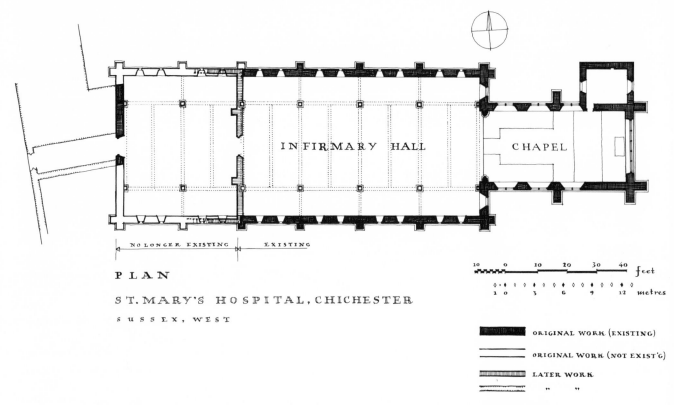

INFIRMARY HALL   CHAPEL

NO LONGER EXISTING   EXISTING

PLAN

ST. MARY'S HOSPITAL, CHICHESTER

SUSSEX, WEST

ORIGINAL WORK (EXISTING)

ORIGINAL WORK (NOT EXIST'G)

LATER WORK

"   "

Fig. 42. Plan of St. Mary's Hospital, Chichester, England (c. 1253), as drawn by Ernest Born.

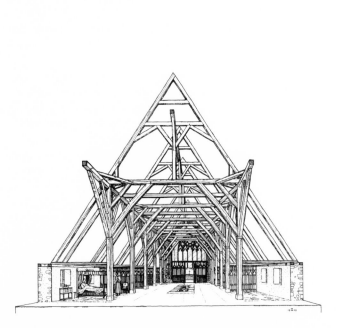

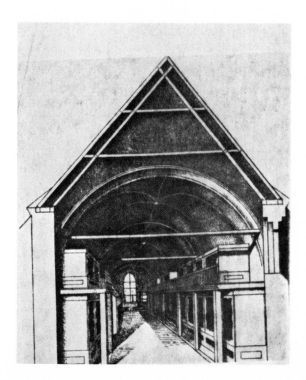

Fig. 43. Transverse section combined with perspective of St. Mary's Hospital, Chichester, as drawn by Ernest Born.

Fig. 44. Transverse section combined with perspective of the Holy Ghost Hospital, Nykøbing, Denmark.

the lepers, insane, and plague ridden; the superannuated; and the rich. The last two categories are not diseases, of course, but social conditions. Toward the end of the Middle Ages it was not uncommon for persons of moderate substance to arrange a kind of old-age insurance for themselves by signing over their property to a charitable foundation in return for board, lodging, and medical care for the remainder of their lives. The financial aspect proved so attractive to those responsible for nursing care that whole buildings were devoted to this type of patient, to the disadvantage of the truly ill and penniless cases for whom hospitals were originally founded. Even at Cluny, and as early as the twelfth century, Peter the Venerable lamented that many monks were professed who wanted only a retirement home in return for the dowry all monks must bring the monastery.[6] The practice continues in our own times: a problem today for the Danish Old Folks Home is the patient who gave his all in return for care and nursing until death—and then got better, thanks to modern medicine, and was able to move back into an apartment of his own for several years. What happens to the money then?

Superannuated pensioners were ambulatory so there was no need to put them into one room with the chapel; they could walk there. For this reason a large ward was unnecessary and also undesirable because rich people expect privacy. For at least half a millennium they have taken it for granted that they will be able to buy privacy. It is remarkable how far back one can trace the double standard: within one hospital, group wards for paupers coexist with private accommodations for those who could pay for them, and the single rooms might even have an anteroom for a private attendant. Specific instances can be pointed out in the context of individual hospitals (for instance, the 12 single rooms at Lübeck!) Here we may cite two early arrangements that reveal social discrimination. In one plan already discussed, Furttenbach's design of 1655 for a cross-shaped hospital (fig. 38), the two lower floors were to take the form of open wards of 52 beds to a floor, with 21 seats in the "secretos" of the ground floor for the men, 17 on the second floor for the women. The top story, intended for pensioners, was laid out as 30 private rooms that opened off both sides of the central corridors. There were to be 15 toilet seats, a slightly higher proportion per patient. At the St. Nikolaus Hospital in Cues, Germany (1447), actually built, class distinctions were nicely worked out, the north wing of the cloister forming an open hall for 21 commoners (it was cubicled at a later date), the southern and western wings composed of 8 single cells apiece for priests and noblemen.[7]

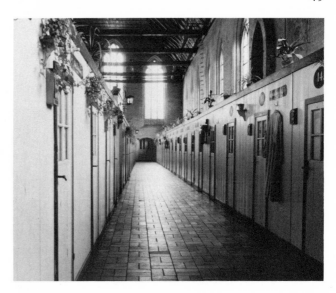

Fig. 45. Men's corridor, Holy Ghost Hospital, Lübeck, Germany, in 1967; a late thirteenth-century open hall subdivided by the eighteenth century into individual cubicles.

The tiny cloister of God's House in Ewelme, England (1436) for thirteen paupers (a number recalling, probably quite deliberately, Christ and the twelve apostles) is made up of two-story dwellings, living room below, bedroom under the eaves, and a stairway more like a ladder between them that is almost too steep for sick or aged persons to contemplate, let alone navigate. A schoolhouse downhill from the cloister and a church uphill(!) complete the beautiful complex, which is still intact today. Thus individual housing for the old was not always limited to those who could pay for it; benefactors too might think in terms of privacy. An earlier, larger, and more famous almshouse in the form of two-story dwellings is St. Cross, founded in 1132 by the Bishop of Winchester for the health of his own soul and the souls of the kings of England.[8] This cloister included its own church, a refectory hall, and lodgings for 13 "impotent poor men." If any recovered sufficiently to maintain himself, "he should be respectfully discharged, and another admitted in his place."[9] However, when the foundation was enlarged in 1444 by Cardinal Beaufort to include 2 priests, 35 brethren, and 3 sisters, it seems to have taken in a more exclusive clientele, for the cardinal was wont to call it "the almshouse of noble poverty," probably meaning decayed gentlemen. The more elaborate later units included sitting room, bedroom, scullery, and privy for each inmate. The latrines, flushed by a diverted stream, were and are "externally arranged as a series of gabled projections, thereby diversifying the otherwise unbroken line of the elevation toward the garden most felicitously"[10] (figs. 46 and 47).

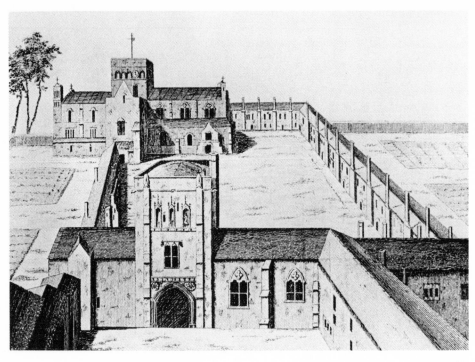

Fig. 46. View of the gateway, dwellings, and church of the Hospital (almshouse) of St. Cross, Winchester, England, as enlarged in 1444.

Figure 48 is a rather abstract model of the Amsterdam Beguinage in 1545. Today the enclosure is really quite charming; the blank squares before the individual houses are gardens. The Beguines were a female nursing order and a Beguinage more abbey than almshouse, but in the Low Countries, as in England, row houses in a straight line along the street, in two long lines facing a central courtyard, or in the form of a hollow square—usually with a church at the end of the row or somewhere in the middle of the square— were used as almshouses in the fourteenth to nineteenth centuries. *"Godshuizen,"* they were called in Flemish, an equivalent of "Hôtels-Dieu."

Look on that picture, now on this: the leprosarium of St. George in Stettin (Szczecin), Poland (fig. 49). The central, dominating church and the small connected houses around three sides of a square courtyard demonstrate that lepers too could band together in a kind of religious order. True, they knew their place and this detail of the Stettin city plan specifies it: "a stone's throw" beyond the city moat, walls, and gate for fear of contagion, yet directly on the main road into the city to receive alms from passersby. Somewhere in front of the requisite wall separating travelers from the infected community would be an almsbox, into which contributions were cast without bodily contact. Not all leprosaria were so highly schematized; many were a mere collection of scattered houses, any size and shape, with some kind of chapel.

This plan, that of the Amsterdam Beguinage, and that of the Almshouse of St. Cross suggest a common ancestor. One need not look far to find it. It was probably the Carthusian monastery, which in turn harked back to a collection of small huts grouped any which way around a common church, that is, to the very first monasteries. The earliest Christian ascetics rebelled against the license of pagan Rome by taking to the wilderness and living there as hermits. In the fourth and fifth centuries most of them had been organized as religious communities with a common Rule requiring, instead of private devotions and mortifications, public services in a central church around which were grouped the monks' dwellings. These dwellings might take various forms, as Krautheimer tells us:[11] a cluster of hovels or a loose arrangement of the component parts—cells, kitchen, refectory, church—around an open area, or a tight rectangular block with inner courtyard. From such prototypes the Carthusian Order (founded 1084) evolved a monastery plan to suit its special needs. The monks' living quarters were built as individual units because they were required to work, eat, and drink in solitude. At the mother house, La Grande Chartreuse near Grenoble, France, thirty-five monks' cells open upon the main cloister, each consisting of ambulatory, living–bed-

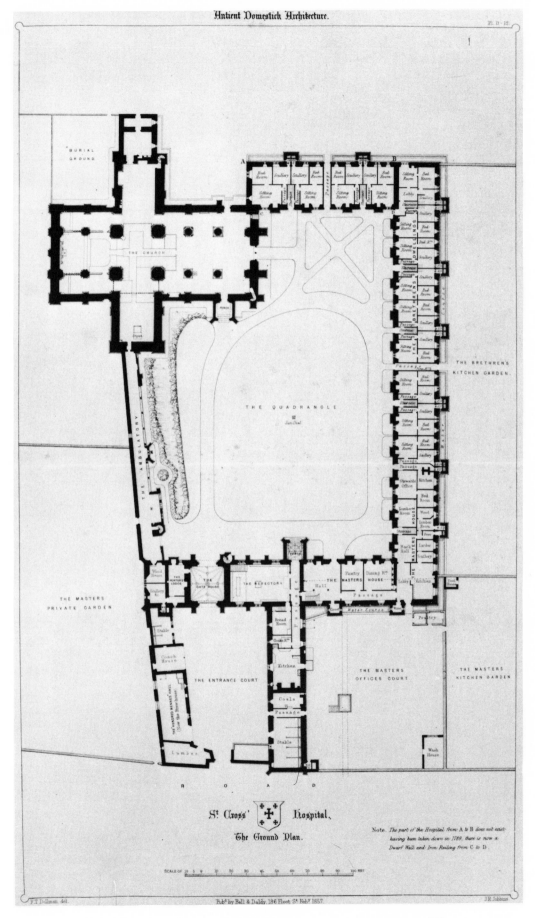

Fig. 47. Ground-floor plan of the Hospital of St. Cross, as enlarged in 1444.

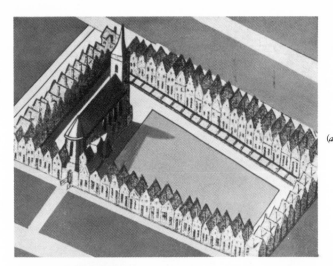

Fig. 48. (a) A stylized 1545 view and (b) a twentieth-century air view of the Amsterdam Beguinage: almshouses wrapped around a church.

(a)

(b)

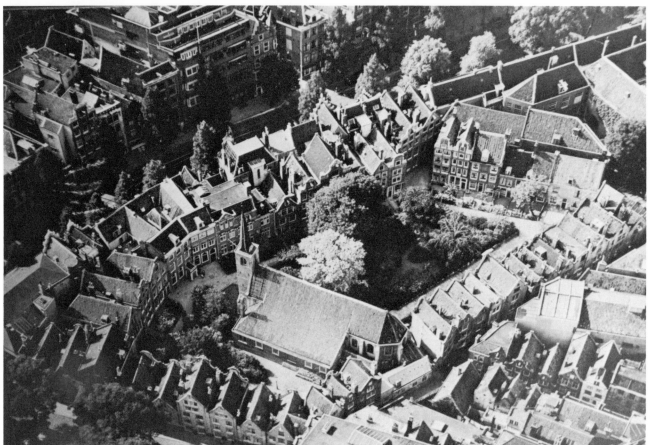

room, oratory, workshop, and private garden.[12] Figure 50, the *Encyclopaedia Britannica*'s basic plan for a Carthusian monastery (a reconstruction of a foundation of 1219), has much in common with our Beguinage, almshouse, and leprosarium.

It is possible to see what the units of such a leprosarium might look like. Camille Enlart gives us a glimpse of the exterior and interior of the two remaining units of one in Périgueux, France, which date from the twelfth century (figs. 51 and 52). They were

"situated along a river, in a remote but cheerful spot." Opening toward a courtyard, the little houses had at their rear, roadward, the merest slits by way of windows.[13]

Plague houses might be projected in similar form. Terror of contagion during plagues was even greater than it had been for leprosy (which, by the time of the great plagues, had considerably abated). True, leprosy was a loathsome, disfiguring, chronic disease; but plague struck suddenly, killed within the day or

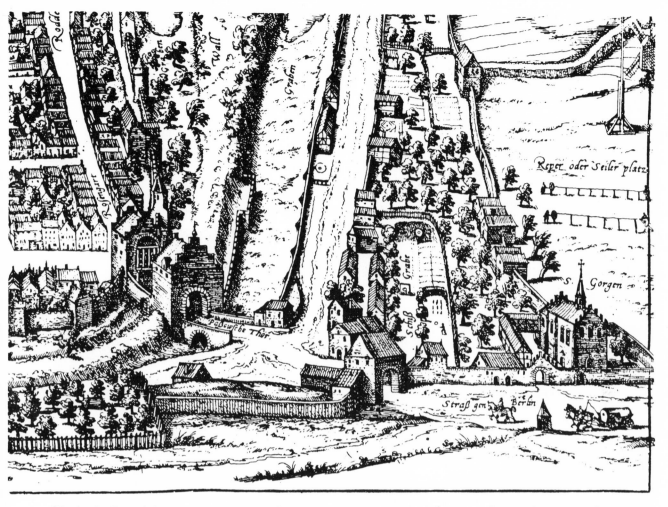

Fig. 49. St. George's leprosarium, Stettin, Poland, sixteenth century: on a main road into town but outside the city walls.

by week's end, and swept away whole neighborhoods. Malachias Geiger provides for the needful in a plan of 1634 for a plague hospital that was never built (fig. 53). A moat of running river water around the entire enclosure turns it into an island, isolates it from the healthy population, and serves a sanitary purpose. An octagonal chapel in the central court can be seen into from the windows of every room through the wide arcade arches and the arches of the chapel itself, for it is a mere gazebo open to the altar on all eight sides. Every room has a privy emptying into the moat. On each of the two long sides of the rectangle are 32 rooms with three beds each for the hoi polloi. Along the two shorter sides are rooms twice the size with one bed each. They, of course, were intended for plague patients with money. The private rooms stand back to back, and it is hard to see how servants were supposed to enter on the water side or how the privies worked in the rooms facing the court. The enclosure could only be entered by two bridges over the moat on either short side. Two roads were to run alongside the loggias from one bridge to the other (top and bottom of plan).

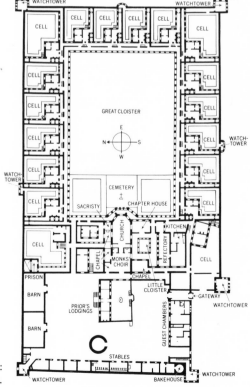

Fig. 50. Plan for reconstruction of a Carthusian monastery: Port Ste. Marie, near Clermont-Ferrand, France (founded 1219).

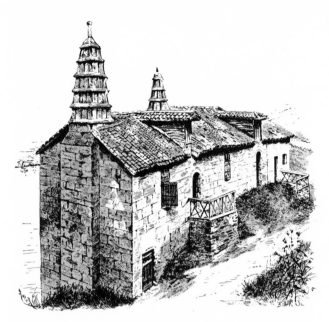

Fig. 51. Exterior view of two surviving units from the leprosarium of Périgueux, France (twelfth century).

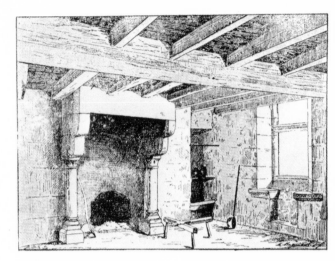

Fig. 52. Interior view of one unit of the leprosarium of Périgueux.

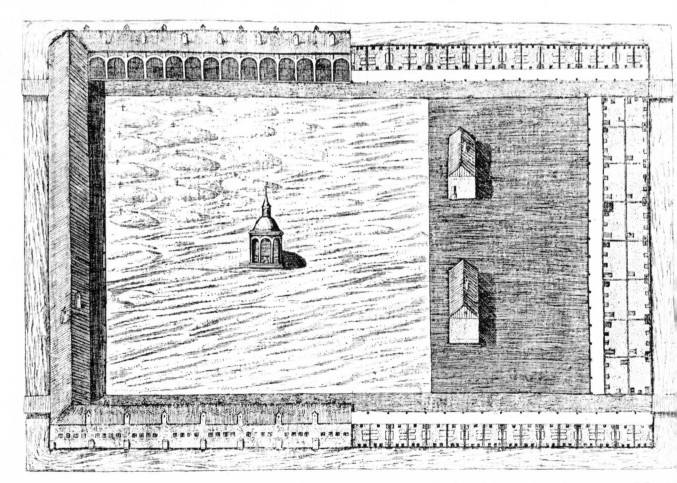

Fig. 53. Malachias Geiger's plan for a plague hospital (1634), showing an elevation for the left half of the patient rooms, and for the right half a plan.

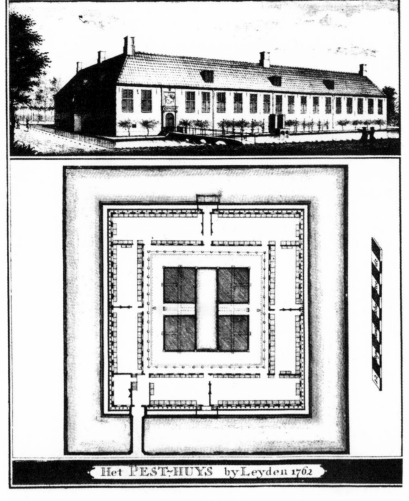

Het PEST-HUYS by Leyden 1762

Fig. 54. Elevation and plan of the Pest House of Leiden (begun 1635) in 1762; a hollow square of multiple-bedded halls surrounded by a moat and crossed by a sewer.

The Pest House of Leiden, the Netherlands (1635 or 1658–62;[14] fig. 54) again employs the concept of square open court and square moat but has eight large wards, two of them with as many as 31 beds laid end to end around the outer walls. Indeed, plague and pest hospitals are as likely to adopt large rooms as small. At Leiden a sewer crossed under the wards and courtyards from one side of the moat to the other —and there was no chapel.

The prototype for Geiger's plan was Milan's famous Lazaretto, the plague division of the Ospedale Maggiore. The first proposal for the Lazaretto of Milan called for 200 small buildings, one to a patient, scattered over a plot of 160,000 meters that had been willed to the hospital for this purpose.[15] What was actually built (1488) was an arrangement of 288 contiguous cells around an octagonal church (fig. 55). This is how Manzoni described the building, in *I Promessi Sposi* (*The Betrothed*):

> The *Lazaretto* of Milan . . . is a four-sided, almost square, enclosure, outside the city, to the left of the Porta Orientale, and separated from the

city wall by the moat, a surrounding road, and a stream encircling the building itself. The two biggest sides are about five hundred yards long; the other two perhaps fifteen less; all of them are divided on the outer part into little rooms of one storey; round three sides of the interior runs a continuous vaulted colonnade, supported on small, slender columns . . . there were only two entrances: one in the middle of the side looking toward the city wall, and another facing it opposite.[16]

He describes the chapel, "a building, as it were, in filigree,"[17] with no support but pillars and columns, so that "the altar erected in the center could be seen from the window of every room in the enclosure, and from almost any point in the camp." Into this enclosure, in time of plague, were piled 10,000 patients. Shacks were hastily erected in the vast courtyard; had they not been, 40 patients would have had to be stuffed into each of the 288 cells. "The dead are given more space underground," observes Spinelli. Man-

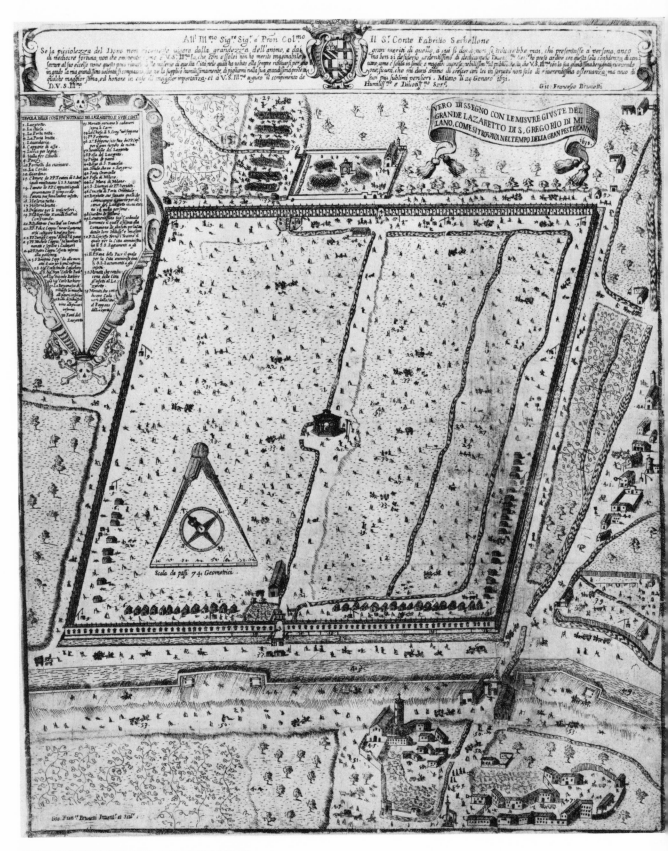

Fig. 55. The Lazaretto of Milan (1488) in 1630; an immense hollow square of 288 contiguous cells with an octagonal church in the middle

zoni pictures the Lazaretto with 16,000 plague victims in the early seventeenth century: "The whole area cluttered with cabins and sheds, with carts and human beings; those two unfinished ranges of arcades to right and left filled, crowded, with a confused mass of sick and dead, sprawling on mattresses or heaps of straw; all over this immense sty a perpetual movement like waves on the sea." A kind of alley was cleared from the entrance gate to the chapel in the middle and thence to the gate opposite. Women and infants were kept apart in a tract of cabins behind a kind of palisade fence, and among them weaved the she-goats, wet-nurses to the many weeping orphans.[18]

This description defines the fallacy inherent in the best-conceived plans for plague hospitals. In good times they stand empty, involving a community in huge expenses for maintenance. In time of plague even a vast prairie such as the court of the Lazaretto of Milan is inundated.

Insane Asylums

Insane asylums are a story in themselves. The crucial determinants in their design have been supervision and control. In response to the peculiar need, very different types of inpatient units were built with an emphasis on small or single rooms.

This patient population had something in common with prisoners because it must be restrained, and with lepers because it came to be looked upon with abhorrence as well as fear. The degree of fear and consequent restraint has always depended on whether a patient was dangerous or harmless. The degree of abhorrence in the eighteenth century rose to such a pitch that it cannot simply be explained by a long-prevalent conviction that to be insane was to be possessed by the devil. Perhaps Michel Foucault is right when he says that the madman fell heir to the superstitious horror inspired by the leper and that with the virtual disappearance of leprosy between the fourteenth and seventeenth centuries, this horror had been floating around in the back of peoples' minds looking for an appropriately detestable object.[19] Indeed one is forced to assume some strong irrational impulse to account for seventeenth- and eighteenth-century exclusion of the insane from the human species and their being treated worse than most animals.

This neglect continued right up to the twentieth century if one may call a purposeful campaign neglect. Principle was involved as well. While the sick were on principle received into the hospitals as suffering human beings, the insane were maltreated on principle. They were beaten during the Middle Ages in the name of love to drive out the devil within them and free them from his possession. They were imprisoned in the seventeenth century on a political principle: to re-

establish law and order after the anarchy of religious and economic disturbances that had so racked the sixteenth. And in the eighteenth century they were kept in unheated cells in the winter on a scientific principle: they were bereft of the light of reason that alone makes man human and therefore were supposed to be, like animals, insensitive to heat or cold. Lepers, however abhorred by society, could and sometimes did band together for mutual protection; the master of a leprosarium might himself be a leper. An insane patient was absolutely helpless in the hands of society; if no humanitarian spoke up for him he could not speak for himself. Thus, in the nineteenth century, did a violent patient receive his food at Aix-en-Provence:

> The floor of the cell was covered with broad stones, and a flagstone in the centre, somewhat thicker than the rest, was hollowed out into a round kind of basin about half the depth of the stone. Between the iron bars of the skylight, which shed an uncertain light upon this pestilent cell, the food-distributer introduced a tin vessel fastened to the end of a long handle, and upset its contents into the hole in the stone; this was the place which received the ration.[20]

Dieter Jetter writes:

> In America, there are continually reports of completely neglected insane until nearly the beginning of the twentieth century. Ever and again, the unsuspecting visitor looked through the small hole in the cell door and discovered a dirty straw bed "like the nest of a swine." And when he then met the gaze of the patient from eyes "like balls of fire," he was shocked to the core and asked the question that shakes a person to his very boots, "Is that a human being?"[21]

The philosophy of a large nineteenth-century English institution, Hanwell Asylum, is expressed in an inventory of instruments placed at the attendants' disposal: "Of restraint chairs, forty-nine; of restraint-sleeves of ticking or leather, seventy-eight; of leg-locks and handcuffs, three hundred and fifty-two; besides ten leather muffs . . . two extra-strong iron chain leg-locks; and two dreadful screw-gags."[22] A quarter of a century earlier, at the Asylum in York, ten female patients were

> each chained by one arm to the wall; the chain allowing them merely to stand up by the bench or form fixed to the wall, or to sit down on it. The nakedness of each patient was covered by a blanket-gown only. . . . In the men's wing, in the side room, six patients were chained close

to the wall by the right arm as well as by the right leg. . . . Their nakedness and their mode of confinement gave this room the complete appearance of a dog-kennel.[23]

Attempts to design functioning wards for the insane must be viewed against this nadir. Such was the status quo, which seventeenth-, eighteenth-, and nineteenth-century planners were trying to improve according to their lights. Generally speaking, in the seventeenth century, insanity was treated along with other social problems by incarceration in huge state institutions. At the end of the eighteenth century, humanitarian impulses began to play a role in the hospitalization of the insane, and in the nineteenth, architectural forms were modified by new scientific theories and treatments.

French Insane Asylums

Under the strongly centralized monarchy of Louis XIV the Hôpital Général was founded in Paris in 1656 to deal with society's less acceptable elements —old people, those with venereal diseases, epileptics, and the mentally ill, now no longer primarily objects of charity but victims of imprisonment by the state at the Hospice of the Salpêtrière (for women) or Bicêtre (for men). Able-bodied boys up to the age of twenty-five "who refused to work through laziness, or . . . girls who were debauched or in evident danger of being debauched"[24] were included by decree of 1690. It has been estimated that in a few years 6,000 Parisians had thus been removed from the city streets—about 1 percent of the general population.[25] What did society hope to gain? George Rosen defines the threefold purpose of the Hôpital Général: (economic) to increase manufactures, provide productive work for the able-bodied, and end unemployment; (social) to punish wilful idleness, restore public order, and rid Paris of beggars; and (religious and moral) to relieve the needy, ill, and suffering, to deal with immorality and antisocial behavior and to provide Christian instruction.[26] In time other Parisian charitable foundations were absorbed into the Hôpital Général, and the institution as a means of dealing with problems of poverty and disease was adopted by a number of large cities first in France and then in other European countries.

The Salpêtrière was adapted in 1656 for 4,000 "patients" and by the middle of the eighteenth century housed 7,800.[27] [Parenthetically, the planning implications of such numbers may be seen in a glance at a design for an eighteenth-century communal latrine at the Salpêtrière, of further interest to us as an elaborate, late development of the monastic necessarium over a diverted stream (fig. 56).] At the end of the

seventeenth century, "loges" for the insane were built. These asylums were not the first in Paris to be prepared for this category of patient; the hospice Petites Maisons drew its name from its loges or cells 9 or 12 feet square for the insane and a few old folk as well. At the end of the eighteenth century, 44 single loges were set apart for the furious insane whose relatives could pay 300 to 400 francs a year, while into the other cells (how many in all, the source does not specify) were crowded 400 crazy paupers.[28]

The first loges of the Salpêtrière were built at the end of the seventeenth century on marshy ground a little above the level of the Seine. Situated just at sewer level, they were prey to flooding and rats. La Rochefoucauld-Laincourt reported in 1790 that the loges were tiny, the courts between them narrow, and the air stank.[29] Madwomen in chains or in a howling rage mingled with the peaceable and quiet. Fairly tranquil patients and imbeciles slept two to a bed in unclean, stuffy quarters. "Finally, there exists no *douceur*," said La Rochefoucauld.

This repulsive but by no means unique state of affairs, created in part by seventeenth-century political expediencies, was ameliorated thanks to the humanitarian thinking of the late eighteenth century. In 1785 a book was published of "instructions on the manner of governing the insane." It called for pure air and water in insane asylums, "these precautions being all the more essential since most of the insane take very little solid nourishment, they only nourish themselves so to speak on air and water." There should be promenades with trees to give them some sense of freedom yet protect them from the sun. There ought to be several groups of buildings, all one story high and each group built around its own square court, to separate degrees and types of mental illness. Around all four sides of the square should run an arcade elevated three feet above the court. At the four corners of the court should be placed dayrooms, while the long low wings would be divided into loges eight feet square and lit by a grilled skylight in the vaulting. Each loge should contain a solid bed set into the wall with mattress and bolster filled with chaff, plus a covering; and to the bed should be attached several iron rings in case of need. Outside the door a bench of stone is to be set into the wall, inside the loge a smaller bench of the same type. And in the center of the court there would be a building for several stone bathtubs to which hot and cold water might be brought—for treatment, not cleanliness.[30] Cold douches were supposed to work wonders.

The following year (1786) Louis XVI ordered his court architect, François Viel, to build new loges at the Salpêtrière "so that the unfortunate insane shall no longer be exposed to injury from the air."[31]

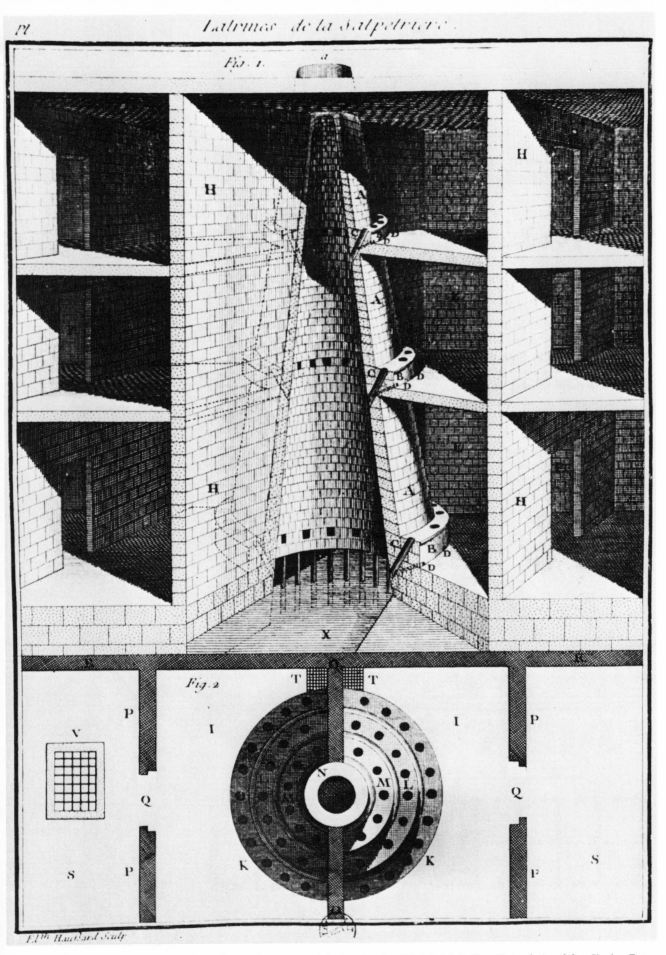

Fig. 56. Transverse section and view from above of a communal latrine for the Hôpital Salpêtrière, Paris, designed by Charles François Viel in 1786 when he was asked to reconstruct the madmen's quarters.

There were to be 600 loges and also two large buildings (one for 200 epileptics, the other for 150 de-
formed).[32] A start on the larger buildings was prevented by the revolution; the manner in which the
small cells were laid out may be seen on the plan
(fig. 57; hatched portions represent old loges not
torn down). The new small cells stood back to back,
and each court, barred at the narrow ends, took in
a different category of patient. The melancholy were
to console themselves among the trees of the central
garden, while the senile could walk around the periphery under the lindens. The cells themselves varied
in size. Some 14-foot ones undoubtedly served as
dayrooms, the average dimensions of the others being 7′6″ × 6′11″. Two of Viel's famous loges survive
to this day (fig. 58); Dieter Jetter's diagrams of the
elevation and section (fig. 59) reveal an extremely
effective ventilating system.[33] Viel carried out the
king's orders by taking care to avoid "injury from
the air" in more senses than one.

In a painting of the central court in 1824 (fig. 60),
the artist seems to have been particularly impressed
by the ventilating tower. This view of the *cour des
paisibles* shows also the stone benches set into the
wall, the high railing that separated one category
of patient from another, and the garden to cheer the
melancholy (who are represented as looking everywhere but at the trees).[34]

The original cells at Bicêtre were almost as bad
as the first ones at the Salpêtrière, lacking only the
river rats. In a cell 6 feet by 6 feet, with one door

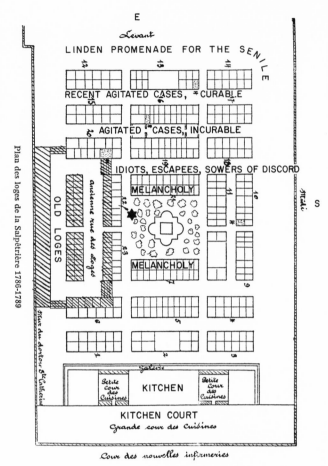

Fig. 57. Layout of Viel's loges at the Salpêtrière (1786–89).

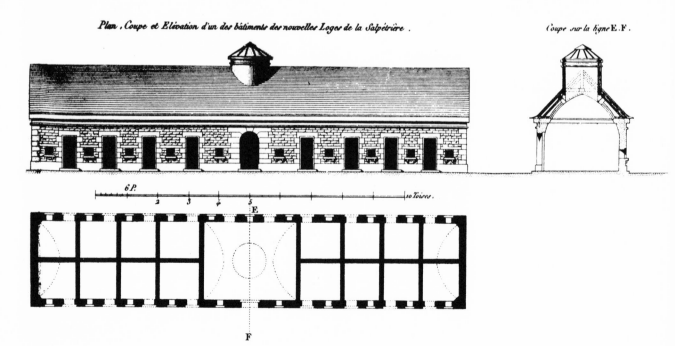

Fig. 58. Elevation, transverse section, and plan of the loges at the Salpêtrière by Charles François Viel.

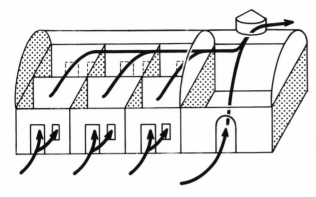

Fig. 59. Isometric view of the ventilation system of the Viel loges at the Salpêtrière, as diagrammed by Dieter Jetter and redrawn by Bev Pope, showing the air currents drawn through doors, windows, and ceiling apertures into the large vault of the attic and out through the ventilation dome of the roof. In some loges there was a large semicircular gable opening as well.

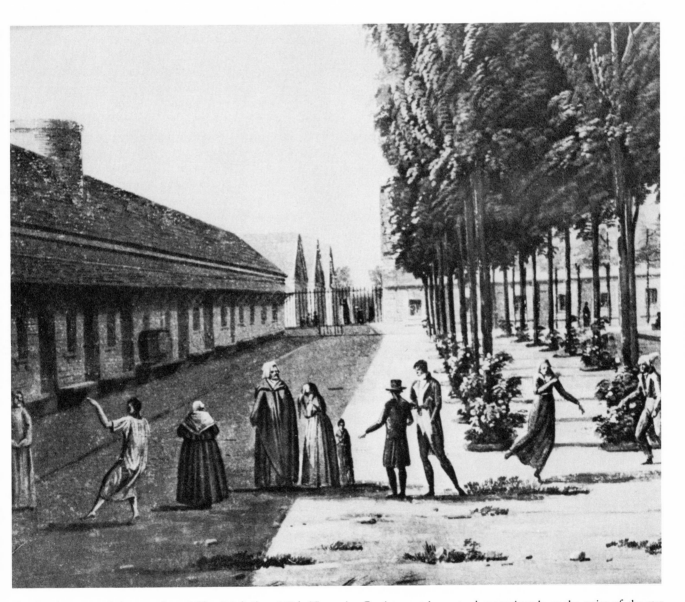

Fig. 60. A corner of the *cour des paisibles*, Salpêtrière, 1824. The artist, Bertin, must have stood approximately at the point of the star superimposed on figure 57. In the source this gouache is wrongly labelled as of Bicêtre. (Compare the ventilating tower with that shown in fig. 58.)

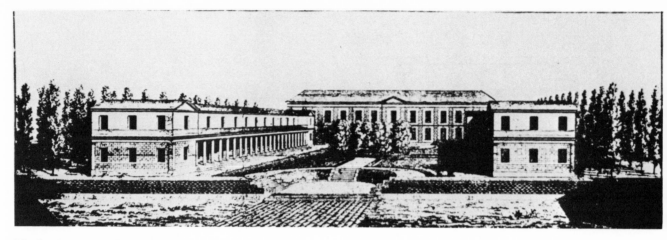

Fig. 61. New loges of 1822 at Bicêtre.

and a window only big enough to pass food through, the bed was affixed to the dank and freezing wall in such a manner that the sleeper had to press his body against wet stone. That bed, covered by straw, was the only furniture in the room. The agitated were bound to the bed with irons around their ankles, wrists, and even neck. The number of patients always exceeding the number of loges, they slept two to a bed—with the exception of paying patients, who had a bed to themselves and heat in the room and were allowed to walk in the inner courtyard.[35]

The new loges (fig. 61) looked quite different from those at the Salpêtrière and were a definite improvement. No longer were cells placed back to back, a layout that only aggravated dampness. Toward the court an open corridor offered a fair weather promenade overlooking quincunx and flower garden. A closed corridor along the rear was actually heated. A report of 1822 boasted:

> Never before was heating contemplated for the mad; in the coldest weather they were left without fire. No more do those belonging to this category suffer the rigors of winter; today they are warmed by two stoves placed in the closed galleries; this mechanism brings in ample drafts of warm air, which afterwards flows into the cells to preserve them from a humidity rarely avoided on the ground floor. They have floorboards instead of flagstones as is the common usage, and these floorboards have been elevated 18 inches above the ground, which is covered with paving stones.[36]

The double row of loges contained a hundred beds for convalescents and the more tranquil insane. The plan (fig. 62) shows ten single rooms on the ground floor with dayrooms in each corner pavilion. The planners lamented a congestion at the building site that left them no choice but to build in two stories

if they were to accommodate as many as they desired. Doubtless they regretted not being able to ventilate the cells through an opening in the roof.

The new plan caught on and was copied everywhere. By 1830 there were *carrés isolés* (as Jetter calls them, after a term used by the French psychiatrist Esquirol) in towns all over France.[37] The treatment of patients consigned to these squares took a turn for the better too. At the end of the eighteenth century, almost simultaneously in England, France, and Germany, a first attempt was made to substitute moral authority for whips and cloth binders for chains, while really unmanageable patients were temporarily confined in darkened padded cells in which they could not hurt themselves. Eventually attendants were forbidden to strike a patient even in self-defense—a far cry from the attendants ten or twenty years earlier who deliberately roused the insane to fury to make sure the paying spectators at the hospital got their money's worth. Philippe Pinel, attending psychiatrist

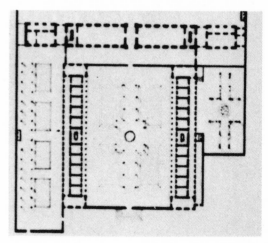

Fig. 62. Ground-floor plan of the new loges at Bicêtre, from an unfinished sketch dated 1836, showing a double row of 10 single rooms, dayrooms in the corner pavilions, and a heated corridor to their rear.

at Bicêtre, was profoundly convinced that all chains should be done away with, and Esquirol was able to put his master's theory into practice.

Patients were roughly classified. The convalescent were separated from the acutely ill, who might trigger a relapse. Broad categories of mental illness were grouped together "to enable," in the words of Pinel, "their officers to foresee and to calculate the wants of each class, and to make ample observations upon the symptoms and peculiarities of every case . . . to distinguish accurately between all the species and varieties of insanity; and finally, to establish such a system of treatment, as would be likely to meet the majority of cases." Epileptics were segregated; their seizures upset everybody. A work schedule was stressed: "I am convinced that no useful and durable establishments . . . can be founded except on the basis of interesting and laborious employment," Pinel wrote. "I am very sure that few lunatics, even in their most furious state, ought to be without some active occupation."[38] Melancholics were to be consoled by a change of scene and the ineffable solace of nature.

The carré isolé implements these principles admirably. In it the medical thinking of the time has been made flesh—or stone. It allows for relatively limited groupings of patients in interior corridors that must have been used as work rooms and in gardens and grilled courts within which there was freedom of motion but from which there was no escape. No wonder the unit was repeated so frequently, even within the same hospital. The great mental hospital of Charenton near Paris was built (1838–85) with no fewer than sixteen carrés isolés.

What that can mean in terms of sheer size is better imagined from a panoramic view (fig. 63) than from the plan (fig. 64). Completion of the original plans took nearly half a century, a reasonable span for a construction of this magnitude. The panoramic view, drawn in 1900, shows later additions. In the original design, the modules of the carré isolé and of the pavilion[39] were fitted into an overall plan characteristic of many hospitals of the eighteenth and nineteenth centuries, whether for mental or medical patients, whether built in the form of a single block or as an extended complex.

It is absolutely symmetrical, men on the left side and women on the right. At the center and head of the plot is the church, in this case an imposing neo-classical structure with pillars, the style in fashion at the time of building. At the foot of the plan, opposite the church, is the three-story administration building. The main entrance to the hospital is right in the center of it, and on the ground floor are rooms for porter, director, doctors, cashier, and staff meetings. In the wings are the patient wards and dayrooms.

The hospital is situated on a hill overlooking the Seine. The entry court—likewise a generic form, although in this case as big as a marketplace—is on the lower levels. The four courts on this level, reading from the entry court outward in both directions, were intended for (1) the melancholy, (2) idiots and the senile, (3) paralytics, and (4) epileptics; men on the left, women on the right. The open courts at the far ends are for the peaceable insane. On the upper level are the monomaniacs and *agités*, with four courts apiece. "Monomaniacs and maniacs must of necessity be isolated," said Esquirol.[40] The agités are in single cells, of course. They take the form of the unit of ten cells with square corner dayroom seen at Bicêtre, complete with a columned front and enclosed corridor to the rear, but there is no "dorter [dormitory] over." The cells are in one-story buildings for safety. A one-story uncolumned pavilion consisting of two assembly rooms divides the rectangular courtyard for the agitated (that is, uncontrollable) insane, forming two squares, or carrés isolés. Divide and conquer.

Convalescent men and women are tucked into the safest place, behind and to either side of the church. It was hoped they would benefit from the healing powers of the site and its miles of delicious walks down toward the river.

Central European Insane Asylums

The earliest cells for the insane, and for prisoners, in Germany were in the round towers of town walls, to which the violent were consigned by the town officials responsible for protecting citizens from insane or criminal attack. Even by the middle of the seventeenth century, hospital planning for mental illness was somewhat less than minimal. In Joseph Furttenbach's plan of 1655 for a hospital in the form of a Roman cross (fig. 38) it is interesting to observe the theoretical allotment of space in the four courtyards formed by the arms of the cross. In front, the two larger courtyards were to be filled to overflowing by the kitchen and rooms for staff; to either side of the apse in the rear were more staff buildings and behind them two 12-bed isolation wards for men or women with epilepsy, syphilis, and mange. A minute, wholly inadequate cemetery between them would have been a disaster if the plan had been carried out. Along the back wall of the lot there was to be a one-story building with 12 single cells for the insane constructed of thick oak planks and containing nothing but a sleeping bench and privy. Instead of a window, each would have a round porthole closed by iron bars.[41] At the far ends were ovens supposedly capable of heating the cells by means of warm-air ducts. A primitive concept, but ahead of its time.

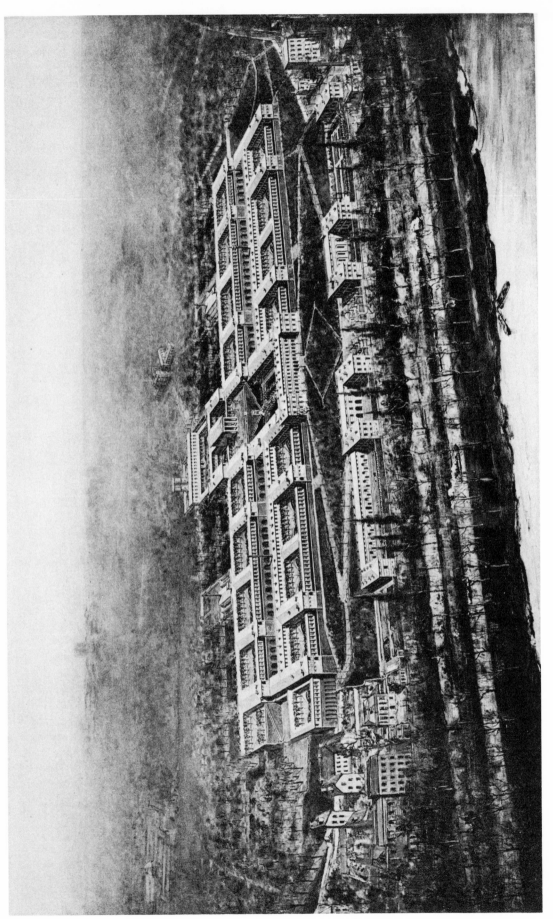

Fig. 63. Panoramic view of the Maison Nationale de Charenton, Paris (1838–85).

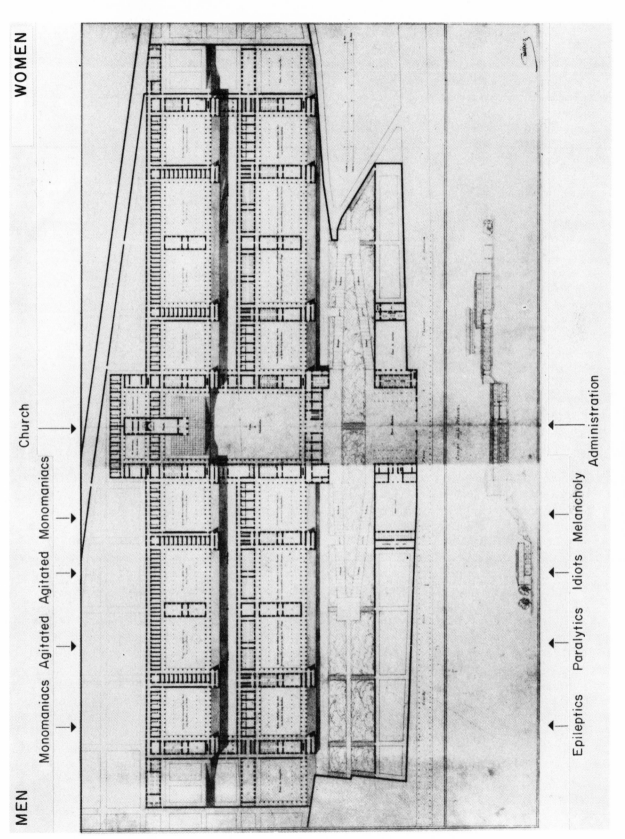

Fig. 64. Plan of the Maison Nationale de Charenton.

ARCHIVES NATIONALES, PARIS. SEINE 1181, NO. 3.

Its relative virtues shine by comparison with the plan of the "new" wing of the Simpelhuys of Brussels actually built nearly a century later (1741; fig. 65). This ill-begotten plan typifies the prison-mindedness of eighteenth-century insane-asylum designers. Cells on the basement floor were below street level. All cells were about 9 by 8 feet and opened on a corridor, the large barred windows showing on the elevation being corridor windows. The incredulous eye finds no windows in the rear walls of the cells and, since cell doors to the corridor were always locked, a patient received light from the corridor through an opening in his door 6 by 9 inches! Whatever door grille Furttenbach contemplated would at least have opened directly on the yard; he also took into account prevailing winds and orientation to the sun. At night the door orifice at the Simpelhuys was shuttered upon the patient and his corner privy (directly communicating with the city sewer). When it was opened next morning, "a cold, infected vapor poured out, visible to the eye." No attempt whatever was made to furnish heat.[42]

That progress in building insane asylums is not necessarily national or chronological is shown by comparing two other structures: the combined Prison and Madhouse of Celle, Germany (begun 1710) and the Narrenturm (Fool's Tower) of the General Hospital of Vienna, the Allgemeines Krankenhaus (1784). The later but more primitive form, the Narrenturm (fig. 66), seems to refer to those round towers in the city gates where the insane were originally incarcerated. It is all prison. The benevolent despot Joseph II took a personal interest in this hospital—he would mount to the attic of the Narrenturm to admire the view of Vienna. His benevolence was evidently directed not toward the patients but toward the citizens of Vienna, who were to be protected from their own insane. Situated behind the main body of the huge hospital, like Furttenbach's cells, the Narrenturm was a round fortress five floors high with twenty-eight cells to a floor. Each had one or two beds, a corner privy, and a corridor door made of thick oak planks reinforced with iron, with a tiny opening that could be locked by an iron grating. (fig. 67).[43] Patients could be chained to the wall and there were military guards besides. Though this building is circular, it is the opposite of panoptical. The court is bisected by a staff building, also of five stories. Neither staff nor guards could see more than a little way around that curving corridor.

One is relieved to find exterior windows in each cell. But John Howard reported (1791): "Though great attention was paid to cleanliness, the passages were very offensive; the form of the building causing the air to stagnate in its centre, as in a deep well."[44]

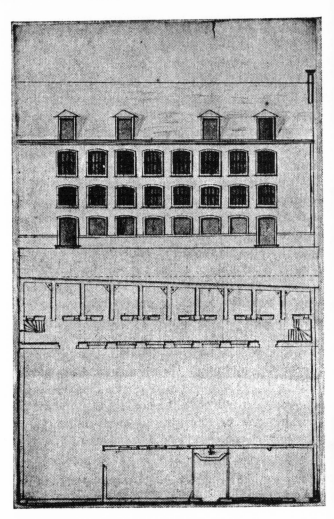

Fig. 65. Elevation and floor plan of the new wing of the Simpelhuys, Brussels, 1741.

During the first half of the eighteenth century the individual German states developed a type of madhouse that was combined with a penitentiary, a poorhouse, or an orphanage. At Celle (begun 1710; fig. 68) the functions of prison and madhouse were clearly differentiated by separate buildings—at a time when prisoners, patients, madmen, debtors, and prostitutes were not clearly sorted out in the Hôpital Général. The early date of this building is astounding. The arms of the madhouse at the rear embrace the prison in the foreground. Both are symmetrical—women left, men right—and once again the insane are in single rooms, not heatable but directly connected through corridors with heating rooms. To the cage-like grating of the doors galvanized copper bowls were attached with chains. Yet kosher food was available from a special kitchen for Jewish patients.[45] The entire area was probably patrolled by armed guards.[46] Privies in the corner of each cell connected to drainage canals flushed by a diverted river channel. An exercise court—spacious, airy,

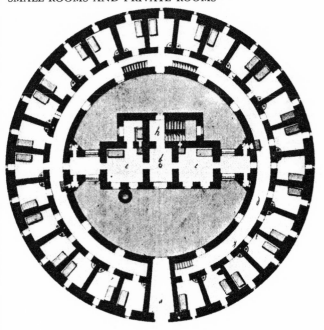

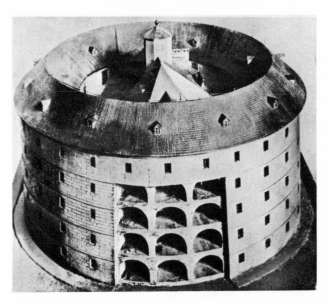

Fig. 66. (a) Plan of the Narrenturm, Vienna, 1784; (b) model of the Narrenturm with a section of the outer wall removed to show fortress-like construction of the individual cells.

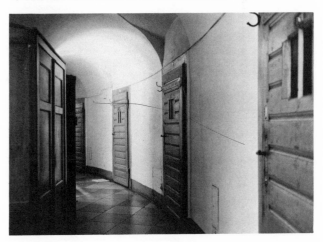

Fig. 67. Corridor of the Narrenturm in 1966, showing the prison-like oak doors.

and from which there was no escape—was formed by the three wings of the madhouse; the windows of the forty roomy cells looked out upon it. The doors opened onto an outside corridor.

The Insane Asylum of Schleswig, then in Denmark (1818; fig. 69), was a thoroughly worked-out solution in line with the thinking of the time. In describing the plan we paraphrase Dieter Jetter's conclusions.[47] The arrangement is again symmetrical, the men's and women's sides kept separate by entrance-ways along the center axis through the intervening wings. As usual, buildings to either side of the main gate are for the administration. (One instinctively glances across the court for the chapel; but no, only a throughway there.) The structure was conceived in terms of one and two stories that alternated. Corner buildings of the administration wing were two storied: to the left an apartment for the warden with the asylum kitchen on the ground floor; to the right an apartment for the resident doctor. This court resembles a carré isolé that predates any in France (it is known that Esquirol was asked to review the plans). But it has a fourth wing of one-story rooms for the concierge, gatekeepers, and turners and for the baths. The walkway on the court side of this wing was arcaded, like that at the Ospedale Maggiore of Milan.

The side wings were one story high and opened off corridors. Most of the rooms were double and meant for the higher class patient, who expects a private room, a fireplace, and a private attendant in the anteroom off the corridor. These rooms terminated in a large one on either side for a supervisor of the appropriate sex.

The wing across the back was again two stories,

arcaded toward the court. Cells for the poor opened off both sides of a dark central corridor. Since this hospital was intended for 150 insane and there are fewer than 50 single cells, the low-class insane must have been housed two and three to a room. Curable and incurable were mixed as long as both were harmless. The only segregation by medical diagnosis was of the violently mad, who were kept in single cells in a one-story rondel to the rear. After the towers in city walls and the famous Narrenturm of Vienna, round must have seemed an appropriate, safe shape for a ward of cells intended to control the uncontrollable.

In the cells of the rondel were corner privies emptied by hand from the inner corridor. The outer one may have been used as a sort of dayroom. Wedged in between two corridors, the cells must have been

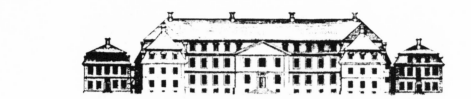

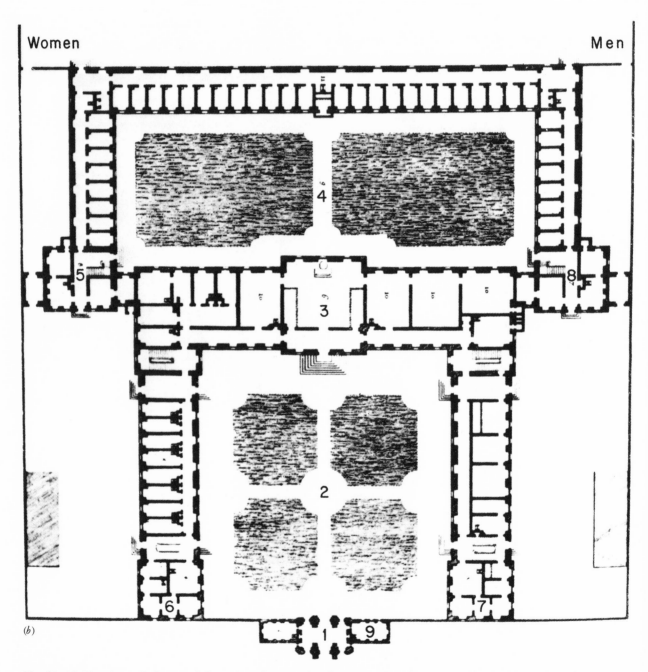

Fig. 68. (a) Elevation and (b) ground-floor plan of the combined prison and madhouse at Celle, Germany. The prison (1710, two stories) is in front, the madhouse (1731, one story and single cells) is in the rear. 1, Entrance; 2, court of the prison; 3, church; 4, court of the madhouse; 5, supervisor's quarters; 6, pastor's quarters; 7, warden's quarters; 8, food supervisor's quarters; 9, porter. On either side of the church were workrooms and reception rooms.

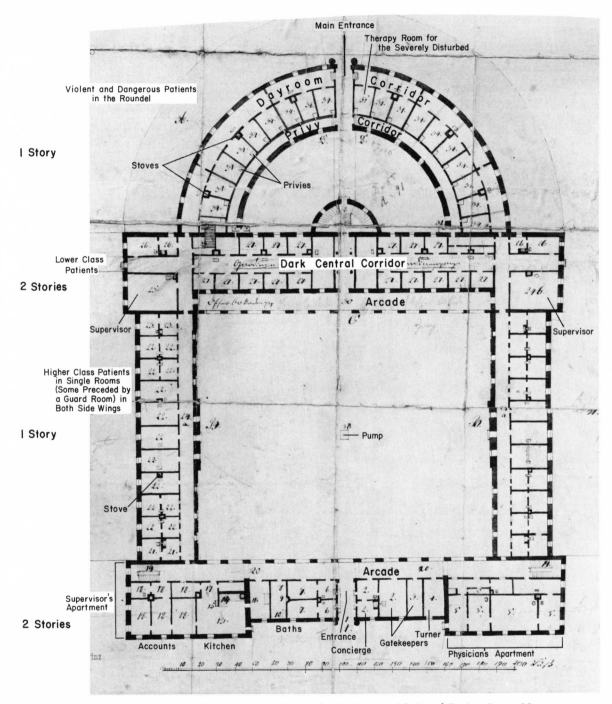

Fig. 69. Plan of the insane asylum at Schleswig, then Denmark (1818), with labeling following Jetter. Men were on one side, women on the other.

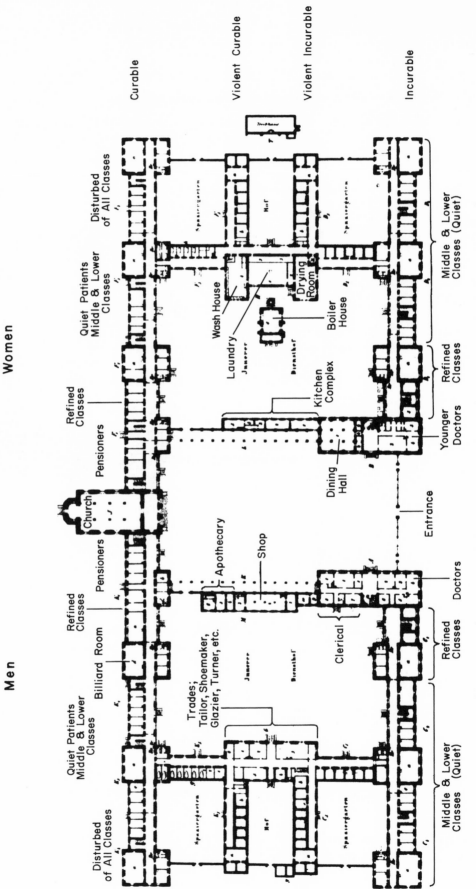

Curable

Violent Curable

Violent Incurable

Incurable

Disturbed of All Classes

Quiet Patients Middle & Lower Classes

Middle & Lower Classes (Quiet)

Refined Classes

Younger Doctors

Refined Classes

Pensioners

Women

Church

Pensioners

Refined Classes

Billiard Room

Apothecary

Shop

Dining Hall

Entrance

Doctors

Clerical

Men

Trades; Tailor, Shoemaker, Glazier, Turner, etc.

Refined Classes

Quiet Patients Middle & Lower Classes

Middle & Lower Classes (Quiet)

Disturbed of All Classes

Wash House

Laundry

Drying Room

Boiler House

Kitchen Complex

Fig. 70. Plan of the combined healing and nursing institution for the insane at Illenau, Germany (1837–42).

dark and stuffy; an attempt was made to heat them. On each side the outer corridor was divided by doors into three unequal segments, each with a stove stoked from the corridor that supposedly warmed all the cells and corridor space of that division.

Administrators and attendants who valued their lives early appreciated the necessity of differentiating the violent from all other mental patients and of treating them in another way. Not so self-evident was the desirability of separating curable from incurable insane to prevent a relapse, but Pinel and Esquirol, by precept and heartrending examples of recuperating patients that drooped and sank forever under the impact of an unfavorable encounter, established the principle in Germany as well as in France by the early nineteenth century. In France the architectural response was the design of the carré isolé. In Germany separate asylums were built for curable and incurable cases.[48] Eventually the two types affiliated and for each healing institution for curables there was a nursing institution for incurables, sometimes a hundred miles away. Since hard and fast diagnosis of curable or incurable mental illness is impossible even today, one can imagine the consequent trundling back and forth of difficult patients over the dismal nineteenth-century roads. Separate divisions were gradually established within the same town; finally it was decided to embody both divisions in a single institution. Such a combined Healing and Nursing Institution was built between 1837 and 1842 at Illenau (figs. 70 and 71).

Jetter calls Illenau a *relatively* separated healing and nursing institution. The violent have been siphoned off into single cells midway between the curable (at the top of the plan) and incurable (at the bottom). However, patients are otherwise not separated by diagnosis but by social class. Working outward in both directions from the church (in its traditional position, with men to the left of it and women to the right) we find: pensioners, who paid; the refined classes; the middle and lower classes; and the disturbed of all classes in single cells. Across from them were other single cells for the curable violent, which formed a three-sided court fenced in across the open end, a sort of imperfect carré isolé. To either side of the entrance were the incurable—no pensioners, but in the same order the refined and the middle and lower classes. At regular intervals dayrooms for the small wards occur, the one billiard room being strategically placed between the section for male pensioners and that for refined gentlemen. The trades wing on the male side balances the laundry complex on the female side. Left of the entrance is the administration wing and right of it the dining hall and kitchen.

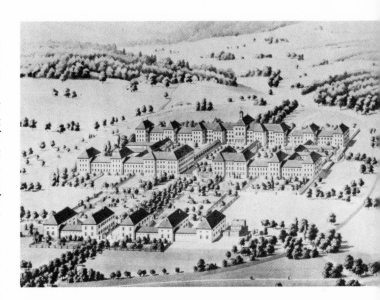

Fig. 71. View of the combined healing and nursing institution at Illenau.

For economic reasons, only the sections for the violent and the line of subsidiary rooms for the food and drug services were kept at one story. The imposing L-shaped entrance buildings and those for the communal halls were three stories high and sections for quieter patients two stories. If one did not know how tall the corner buildings are, one might assume from the plan that the corner courts were real carrés isolés.

A distinction between curable and incurable was faithfully carried out even in wards for the violent, who were treated as curable or incurable maniacs. No other diagnostic divisions were made. Yet Charenton, under the influence of Pinel and Esquirol, was built only a year later (1838) with separate sections for the melancholy, idiots, the senile, paralytics, epileptics, monomaniacs, and maniacs. The attempt to approximate a carré isolé for unmanageable patients at Illenau led to single-storied wings for the violent being placed exactly where their frantic howling might equally disturb curable and incurable patients. At an asylum built not much later in Halle, cells for the violent were as far removed as possible from the other buildings, and because of economic necessity they too were of more than one story. Jetter points out that this completely eliminated all Esquirol's influence as seen in Illenau and created a remarkably well organized and architecturally independent institutional style.[49]

English Insane Asylums: The Restraint System

Figure 72 is not a palace, though it looks like one. When it was built in London in 1676, the city laureate raised his voice in a paean of praise:

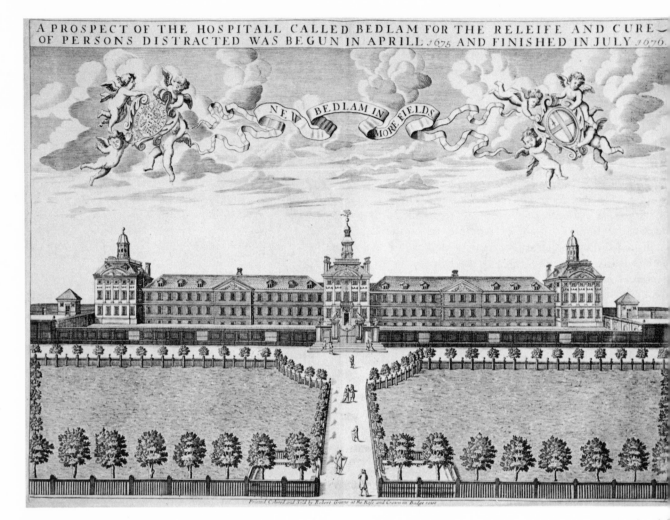

Fig. 72. Facade of Bethlehem Hospital ("Bedlam"), London (1676). A central administration building, ward wings to either side of and terminal pavilions.

This is a structure fair,
    Royally raised;
The pious founders are
    Much to be praised,
        That in such time of need
        When sickness doth exceed,
        Do build this house of bread,
        Noble new Bedlam.[50]

Yes, this is that famous, infamous Bethlehem Hospital, known as Bedlam, which gave its name to insanity itself. The building under discussion is its second incarnation, Bedlam in Moorfields. A hundred and twenty-five years later it was discovered that the foundation of this building was woefully inadequate, that the structure rested, without piles, partly on the soil of the city moat and partly on a Roman wall, that the side walls holding up the heavy roof had not been tied together, and that brick piers in the basement that carried most of the superstructure had been cut away to make room for storage. As a result, there

was not one floor that was level and not one wall that was upright (O'Donaghue, p. 287). And for a third time the hospital had to be relocated. But the nobility of the structure at Moorfields awed contemporaries, even foreigners. In 1788, when it was more than a hundred years old, a Frenchman saw there unbelievable freedom and cleanliness:

> The poor creatures there are not chained up in dark cellars, stretched on damp ground, nor reclining on cold paving stones . . . no bolts, no bars. The doors are open, their rooms wainscoted, and long airy corridors give them a chance of exercise. A cleanliness, hardly conceivable unless seen, reigns in this hospital. Five or six men maintain this cleanliness, assisted by the patients themselves, when they begin to come to themselves, who are rewarded by small presents (O'Donaghue, pp. 282–83).

A far cry from the odious reputation associated with

he name of Bedlam. Hospitals have a way of being
conceived in glory, executed with ingenuity and
humanity, then subjected in use to misuse and abuse,
finally to be overcrowded and understaffed and always and forever plagued by insufficient funds. A
hospital before death can become more decrepit
than a man. The man dies, but a moribund hospital
may live on for decades—and, what is so terrible,
filled to capacity.

A visitor entered this palace for the insane poor,
acute and dangerous cases preferred (p. 209), through
an iron gate in the high stone wall around the building. For a penny anyone could walk the wards with
unconcealed curiosity and amusement. Visiting Bedlam was something to do on an idle day, like going
to the zoo. A wide gallery ran across the north front
of the hospital and roomy cells opened off it, each
with a high barred window, unglazed. Some patients
were allowed "the liberty of the gallery" but most
were kept behind bars because the corridor was primarily for visitors, and the visitors were everybody
from gentlewomen going slumming to professional
thieves who stole from the patients. "I saw a hundred
spectators making sport of the miserable inhabitants,
provoking them into furies of rage," reported a news-
paper correspondent in 1753. O'Donaghue adds, in
his volume on the hospital from which these details
are taken, that the fair then turned into a pandemo-
nium, prisoners clanking their chains and drumming
on their doors in sympathy (p. 238). Bedlam during
visiting hours was a place of assignation for the lower
classes: "There was a Jack for every Jill: people came
in singly and went out in pairs." Only in 1766 was it
decided to call off the show. Three years later no
man except a governor was allowed access to the
women's side, a male visitor being permitted to see
a female patient only in the committee room, and
in the presence of a nurse (p. 240).

The galleries opened left and right from a grand
entrance hall in the central pavilion. On the second
story was a grand court room, reached by a grand
staircase. To the left of the hall was the room where
physicians and apothecaries saw patients on admission and discharge, to the right the office of the
steward (p. 206). Staff lived in attics, and kitchens and
other offices were in the basement, where extra space
was rented out to the East India Company for the
storage of pepper. The daily patient diet was supposed to be boiled beef broth and bread, with a pint
of very small beer. But in 1764, nurses were putting
aside the best part of it "for their ancient relations
and more intimate friends, who are to come and
visit them in the afternoon" (p. 263).

In 1766 it was ordered that men should occupy
the lower gallery and women the upper and "not be

suffered to lodge promiscuously" (p. 210). Later the
east wing was set apart for male patients. Strangely,
for a symmetrical plan, it was apparently not the plan
from the beginning. In 1729 an iron grille was erected
across the ward corridor to separate leaseholders
from freeholders (paying from charity patients) and
incurables from curables. In 1735 (a century earlier
than the plan of Illenau) new wings were added for
incurables, to the left for males and to the right for
females, on the site of airing courts where the patients
used to take exercise. There were 50 incurables of
each sex when John Howard visited in 1788, and a
waiting list. Their relatives paid for them "only *half
a crown* a week."[51]

Howard found no segregation by diagnosis: "The
patients communicate with one another from the
top to the bottom of the house, so that there is no
separation of the calm and quiet from the noisy and
turbulent, except those who are chained in their cells."
For 270 rooms on four floors he found only one vault
(privy), "very offensive." When Howard says a thing
is offensive, he means it stinks. And yet the rooms
were "quite clean and not offensive, though the house
is old and wants white-washing." He saw "sitting
rooms with fireplaces properly guarded with iron,"
but, he adds severely, "*no chapel.*"

O'Donaghue tells us that the foundation of St.
Luke's Hospital for the Insane in London in 1751
was prompted by evils at Bethlehem, particularly
the cardinal abuse alluded to in a St. Luke's regulation
that the patients shall not be exposed to public view
(p. 240). The present Governor of Bethlem Hospital,
L. H. W. Paine, believes that the bad days at Bethlem
can be dated from the building of St. Luke's. The stately
palace into which St. Luke's moved in 1786 (fig. 73)
is today completely altered on the inside, but its monumental shell survives as an appropriate casing for
the Bank of England's printing works. What it did
look like inside is preserved in a plate by Rowlandson
and Pugin for *The Microcosm of London* (fig. 74). George
Dance, the architect, also designed Newgate Prison.
"A grim theme," John Summerson suggests, "sometimes drew out the best in him. This gallery, with its
long thin windows, fantastically high cell doors and
iron grilles, might be a stage set for *The Duchess of
Malfi.*"[52] John Howard gives the cell dimensions as
10'4" × 8' × 13'3" high. The semicircular grille above
the door of the cell did however draw cross ventilation from its window. In the 15-foot corridor (same
width as at Bedlam) patients are helping out with
washing and rehabilitating beds, mattresses, and quilts.

The building was planned with one sex on either
side. In the center block were rooms for the administration. Each gallery had 32 opposite cells arched,
boarded, and wainscoted. Bed boxes with mattresses,

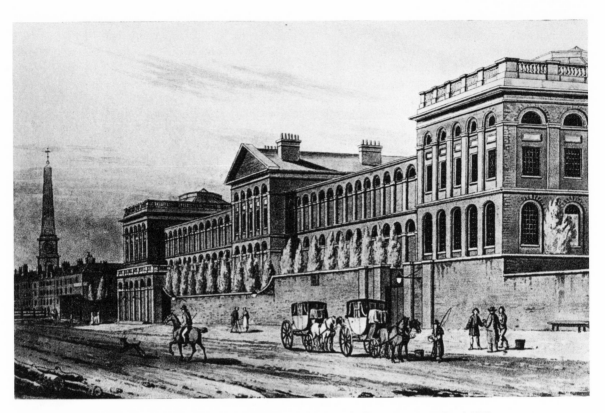

Fig. 73. Facade of St. Luke's Hospital, London (1786), from an aquatint dated 1815.

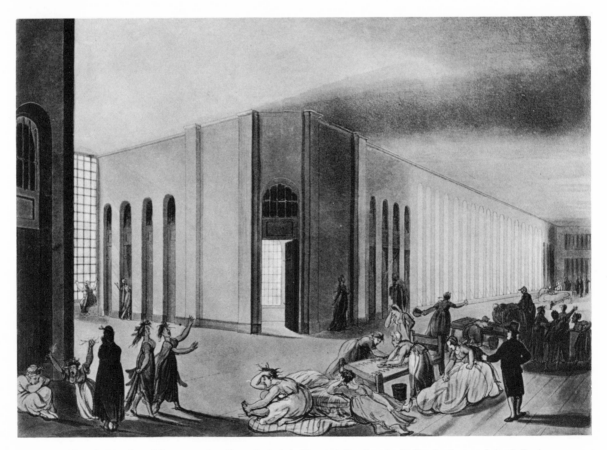

Fig. 74. Interior of the women's gallery, St. Luke's Hospital, London, by T. Rowlandson and A. C. Pugin.

or straw for the incontinent, lay at a slope and had false bottoms. Each gallery had two sitting rooms, one for quiet patients and one for the turbulent, who John Howard wished had been put in a place apart. Again, no chapel, not even for the recuperating. (Note that unlike general hospitals of the time, half our examples of asylum architecture lack the chapel.)

Amenities cost something; at St. Luke's a deposit of a hundred pounds guaranteed that the patient's friends would remove him when cured or at the end of a year's stay, whichever came first. Those remaining longer were classed as incurables and they paid, not half a shilling as at Bethlem, but *five shillings* a week.

This is how a forward-looking eighteenth-century asylum appeared to its contemporaries. In 1904 the medical superintendent of St. Luke's, looking back a hundred years, noted other aspects of the hospital as it must have been in 1803:

> The wards are shut off from the central portion by thick upright iron bars and heavy iron gates which accord a complete view of their whole length on each side. . . . The wards open directly into the wings, so that a classification of patients was not possible on any floor. There is no furniture beyond bare tables and wooden forms. The walls are not even white-washed. There are no fire-places nor any means whatever of heating the wards. . . . There are no infirmaries or places where sick patients can be treated apart from the others. . . . Each patient has a wooden trough-shaped bedstead fixed into the wall, and containing loose straw, which is covered with rough sacking in the cases of convalescing patients only. There are nearly three hundred patients in residence, two thirds being acute cases. The incurable patients are kept in the basement, many of them chained to the wall. . . . The noisy acute cases are in seclusion; those who are violent are chained to their bedsteads, covered only with a loose rug, or in the case of females with a loose blanket gown."[53]

And St. Luke's was among the best. No wonder William Tuke felt, after examining a local asylum infinitely worse, that fellow Quakers afflicted by "a malady, in many instances, the most deplorable that human nature is subject to" deserved better.[54] Public sympathy had been turned toward the plight of the insane by the long mental illness of King George III, and when Tuke finally succeeded in publicizing the deplorable conditions at York in 1814, the climate in England was ripe for reform.

English Insane Asylums: Moral Treatment

Moral treatment rather than chains was a solution arrived at in England, France (Pinel's *traitement morale et philosophique*), Germany (*psychische Curmethode*), and Italy (*cura morale*).[55] A precursor was the fear therapy of Francis Willis of Greatford. By inspiring sufficient terror of retribution in patients, Willis could allow them unusual liberties. He took mental patients into his home as early as 1750 and, when they overflowed, boarded them in cottages in the community, two to a cottage with a keeper for each.[56] The keeper was instructed to return blow for blow, and if the patient escaped he had to pay the cost of his recapture. Willis boasted of his ability to subdue a maniac by the mere power of his eye; when reproached with permitting his patient George III to use a razor, he retorted, "Place the candle between us, Mr. Burke. I should have looked at him—thus, sir—thus."[57]

The new method was at any rate an improvement on chains and lashes. Poor George III, when the straitjacket had to be used, called it his "best friend."[58] William Tuke dreamed of doing away with physical restraints in an asylum for Quaker patients but could never do so completely. However, Tuke's principles exerted infinite influence in Europe and America, while the institution embodying them, the Retreat at York, was much imitated and admired. Before describing the building we may summarize "moral treatment" as conceived of by the Tukes, William and Samuel, father and son.

Moral treatment has in it the element of fear, but fear of retribution should be inspired by the superintendent and attendants only to an extent that would enable the patient to control himself,[59] and punishment must never be expressed in the form of harmful force. If too much fear is excited, it debases the mind (Tuke, p. 143). There is in moral treatment also an element of bribery because good behavior was rewarded by added privileges, such as eating at the superintendent's own table, and respectful treatment as a result of which "the patient feeling himself of some consequence, is induced to support it by the exertion of his reason" (p. 159). If you take a patient at his word he will try his best to keep it (p. 160). He should be cajoled, argued, persuaded into a more rational state of mind, with utmost friendliness and above all with real kindness (p. 146). But coax patients only on points affecting their liberty or comfort. Don't try to reason with them on their particular hallucinations. That won't work and only irritates them (p. 151). Keep them busy; regular employment accompanied by considerable bodily activity is best (p. 156). The character of the attendant was the key to making the system work: a good attendant must be almost more than human. Samuel Tuke admits that "to applaud all [the patients] do right; and pity, without censuring, whatever they do wrong, requires such a habit of philo-

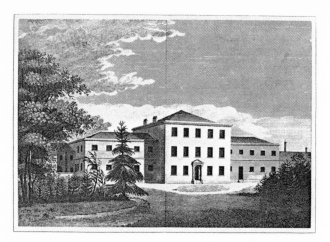

Fig. 75. Elevation of the Retreat at York, England (1813).

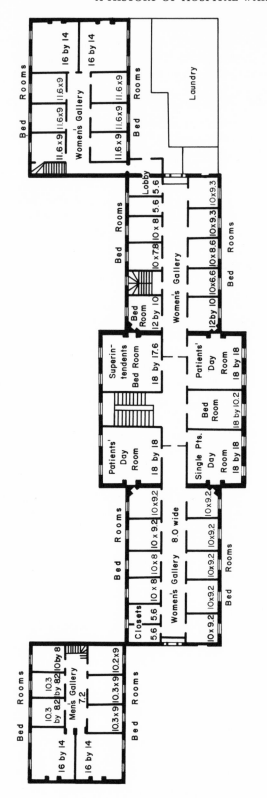

sophical reflection, and Christian charity, as is certainly difficult to attain" (p. 176).

Fortunately the Retreat at York was a small institution. At the time these words were written, 64 patients were organized as one big family. They came from all walks of life and were charged on a sliding scale (p. 49). The first building was planned for thirty patients simply because kitchens, parlors, exercise grounds, and personnel could not in any event be much reduced for half that number (p. 34). No particular claims were made for its value as architecture; in fact Samuel Tuke was dissatisfied with the final structure and would have preferred a panoptical design like that of the asylum later built in Glasgow (fig. 39) because it permitted better supervision (Introduction, p. 14). However, "an inferior plan well executed, may be more beneficial than a better system, under neglected management" (p. 47).

It was built of brick on a hill with a fine view in all directions (fig. 75). In front were only a fence and some gardens, both decorative and vegetable. The requisite 8-foot walls around the enclosed exercise grounds to the rear were made to seem somewhat less oppressive by being built at the bottom of a slope, and patients were taken for long free walks on the outside as soon as their condition warranted it. The front windows, 3½ by 6 feet, were ingeniously designed of iron frames and partitions; in each sash there were 24 glazed squares 6½ by 7½ inches (p. 98). They looked like ordinary house windows and nobody would have recognized the asylum for what it was, because it lacked window bars and a high stone wall. Windows of the patient rooms in the wings were smaller but framed the same way. Cross ventilation was made possible by a wooden slide across some of the window panes and a small wicket in the door, also used as a peephole. At night the doors of the patient rooms were locked.

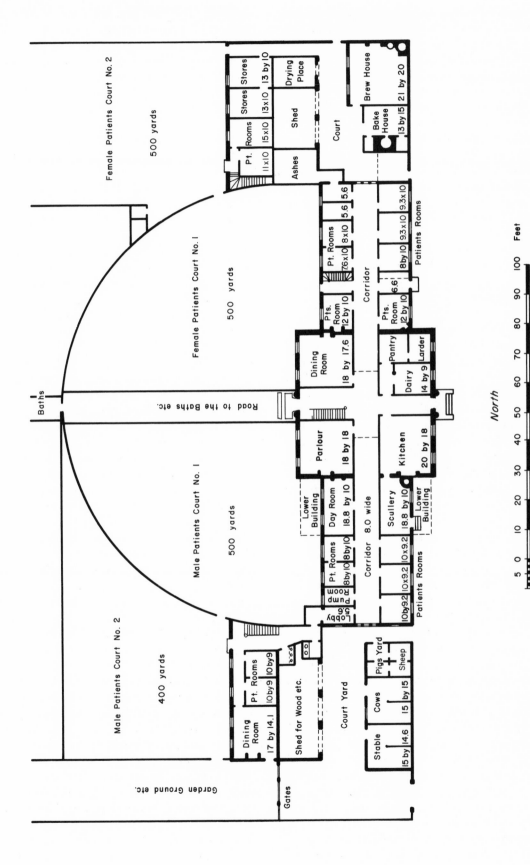

Fig. 76. Ground-floor plan of the Retreat at York.

The galleries to either side of the entrance block were composed of single rooms of a good size on both the ground and second floors (figs. 76 and 77). The central corridor was rather gloomy, lit only by windows at the far ends. Extensions set back on either side were for the violent—men to the left, women to the right. The bedrooms for male maniacs were upstairs and their dayroom downstairs, with two seclusion rooms next to it (the only ones in the house not directly lit by windows). Relative dark was thought soothing, and when the straitjacket was insufficient (padded cells had not yet been invented), the patient was confined to bed by a complicated linen restraining web that permitted him to change his position (p. 165). Tuke reports that of 64 patients in the previous year, on the average not two had to be secluded at any one time, not four to be restrained by any means (p. 167). The violent wing for women was similarly arranged. There were always more women here than men.

Division by social class was not neglected. Five or six quiet patients of the superior class were allowed to use the dining room of the central block as a dayroom. Their bedrooms were in its attic, and Tuke alludes to a fine view (pp. 100, 103) that, because the windows began 6 or 7 feet above the floor and went up to the ceiling, the patients must have enjoyed by standing on their beds. Socially superior patients were exempt from the institutional diet and lived in all respects as the superintendents (p. 124). And in the attic of the central block was a suite of two rooms for a male patient with a "distinct attendant." These rooms "would not be ineligible for the accommodation of a person in any rank of life" (p. 102).

To the rear of the ground plan are the baths. Tuke rather mistrusted the current medical treatment of insanity by drugs, emetics, purges, and bloodletting but said he got pretty good results from warm baths, particularly for the melancholy. On no account would he advise cold ones. Another innovation was the ample meal; in other institutions, patients were kept on spare diets almost to the point of starvation and were put to sleep at night with opium. Observing that in normal persons a full stomach induces indolence, reluctance to exert oneself, and sleep, he plied maniacal patients at bedtime with meat, or cheese and bread, and good porter, with excellent results (pp. 118, 124–26). He avoided the "mortification of the feet" prevalent in most asylums (where they had to wrap patients' feet in flannel and examine them morning and evening) by keeping the patients unchained and active and by warming the rooms (p. 119).

The question naturally arose whether such treatment would prove practicable in larger institutions. It was answered in the affirmative by John Conolly, who took over the administration of 800 to 900 patients in 27 wards at Hanwell Asylum in 1839 and in three years abolished every mechanical restraint in the house.[60] His courageous example transformed practice in other institutions; keepers of the insane could no longer make excuses based on fear. "He not only made the hitherto obscure movement a world-known success," observed Henry Maudsley, Conolly's son-in-law, "but he made reaction to it impossible."[61]

"Restraint," wrote Conolly in his *Construction and Government of Lunatic Asylums*, "was the grand substitute for inspection, superintendence, cleanliness, and every kind attention" (p. 28). In doing away with restraint, one could not leave a vacuum; one must restore the supervision for which it was the substitute and in the most minute detail. Building arrangements and the staffing pattern became of supreme importance, all the more because no real cure for insanity was known.[62]

Conolly preferred the projected plan for Derby Asylum (fig. 78) to that of Hanwell, which was an enormous, vaguely panoptical structure for 1,000 patients. Derby was laid out for 360, after which point "almost every desirable quality . . . becomes more difficult to be obtained or preserved. . . . The architect must sacrifice much to expediency, and the government of the establishment can scarcely preserve any uniformity of character" (p. 10).[63] At Derby two wings extend rearward, and two others are offset to either side, with single rooms on one side of the corridor that can be only "moderately perflated by every wind that blows" (p. 12). The wings are set back far enough to allow end windows to the corridor of the main block.

Conolly approves of the bay windows in those corridors, which are equidistant from both ends, well lighted, and opposite a fireplace. They make for a better-supervised dayroom than any separated space would be, yet are far cozier than the mere straight corridor used as a dayroom at Hanwell (p. 17). He likes a jutting administration building and a kitchen extending rearward to divide the court and to isolate the two sexes so they cannot look into each others' quarters. For essential communication he recommends a corridor running around the interior of the court and beneath the windows of the sleeping rooms, although of course this means placing bedroom windows on the ground floor so high that only from upper stories would there be a view (p. 19).

At Derby the insane are again divided by degree rather than type of illness: aged and infirm across the front, moderately tranquil in the side wings, and refractory in the wings extending to the rear, with airing grounds for each class. Workrooms and laundry close in the establishment at back, and Conolly approves their being detached from the wards a little

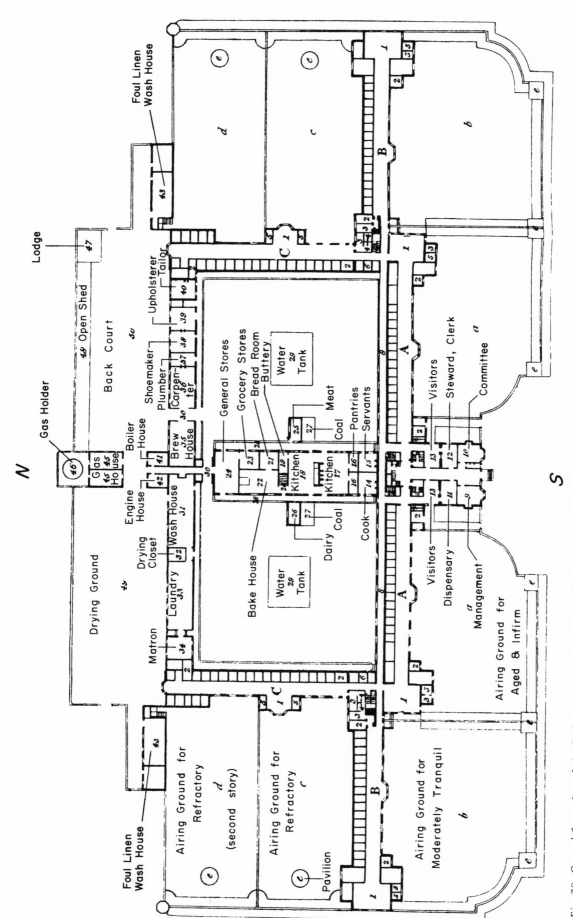

Fig. 78. Ground-floor plan of the Derby Insane Asylum (1851). Wings A, B, C have as airing grounds areas a, b, c, d (for second story of C). Ward features: 1, dining rooms; 2, attendants; 3, patients' washrooms; 4, patients' toilets; 5, attendants' sculleries and storerooms; 6, bathrooms; 8, communication corridors. Men on one side, women on the other.

to give patients a welcome change of scene during the work day.

Somewhat fewer than two-thirds of the rooms were singles. Conolly insists on at least two-thirds because he believes a private room is best for most mad patients. They will not disturb others, they cannot harm others, and the rooms may be more effectively cleaned and aired, especially those of the dirty patients. Furthermore, the orderly and convalescent desire nothing so much as a place where they can be quiet and alone. He is absolutely opposed to large dormitories because of their incredibly bad air and favors four- or five-bed rooms only for certain kinds of patients: the timid, the melancholy, and those disposed to suicide, who are safer not left alone (pp. 24–25).

Derby was a two-story building and Conolly will countenance no more than two stories. A third, besides being hard to ventilate, would be difficult of access and egress and thus becomes almost unavoidably neglected (p. 10). For the same reasons he wants no patient dormitories in attics or cellars. He insists on absolute cleanliness. "The provisions necessary for cleanliness are humble things to dwell upon," he said, "but they are the auxiliaries of health" (p. 38). Thus did he reason: Irritability is what we are combating in an asylum. Bad health makes people irritable. Therefore the bad smells, which produce "local malaria," must be done away with. No excuse should be admitted for a bad smell in any room or corner. If due to a defect in the building, it must be rectified at any cost. If due to neglect, as it usually was, one must speak to the attendants.

The attendants were what made Conolly's system work. They were to be an extension of his person and authority. If they were inferior, he could not use them; it would be like asking a doctor to use inferior drugs. They were his substitutes for the chain and straitjacket, yet even the best of them he never trusted with any detail that could be handled mechanically. Do not set the inspection wickets so high in the doors of the seclusion rooms that the attendants have to bring ladders to look in; the patients will never be inspected (p. 26). Do not put a spring lock on the fireguard; the attendant will leave the door ajar sooner than have to fetch the key to open it again an hour later (p. 43). And so on and on, but still most duties had to be carried out by attendants; if they did not, nobody would.

It follows that the attendants were well paid and well treated at Hanwell—according to the standards of the time. They worked a 14-hour day with a half-hour break for lunch and a good dinner at the end of it. After attending evening services, they had two nights off a week from six o'clock on. They sat up on the night watch, two by two, once every 12 or 14 nights

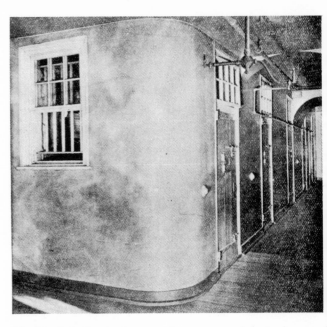

Fig. 79. Cells for the insane as first constructed in the basement of the original building, Pennsylvania Hospital, Philadelphia (1756). Below the outside wall of these cells ran a small moat like that in modern zoos, from the far side of which the public could watch the patients through their windows.

and next morning were permitted to start work at noon instead of six. An attendant could be summarily dismissed only for cruelty (p. 84). As the only sane person always with the insane, he must consider himself the friend and adviser of those who had no others (p. 110).

American Insane Asylums: The Kirkbride System

Conolly's principles and plans were officially approved in England. His approach was taken up in the United States, where treatment of the insane ran parallel to that in Europe: patients were housed in basement cells in 1756 at Pennsylvania Hospital, Philadelphia (fig. 79);[64] a Retreat was opened in 1824 in Hartford, Connecticut; finally, after a smashing campaign by Dorothea Lynde Dix against the prevailing hellholes, some thirty-two state asylums were built between 1841 and 1887.

Their pattern was set by Dr. Thomas S. Kirkbride, superintendent of the Pennsylvania Hospital for the Insane, Philadelphia, from 1840 to 1880. The Kirkbride system is a linear plan, fully executed as conceived at the State Hospital for the Insane of Alabama at Tuscaloosa (figs. 80 and 81). (The lot for Kirkbride's own hospital was not wide enough to receive it.) The three-story hospital of 250 beds could be used for both sexes, or, even better, one—assuming a similar building elsewhere for the other. An overcrowded hospital might expand by building a duplicate.[65]

The center building housed administration areas,

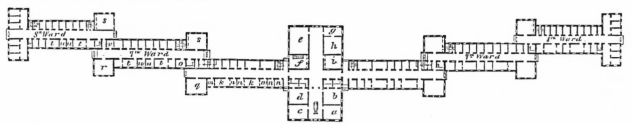

Fig. 80. Ground-floor of a Kirkbride "linear plan" hospital, the State Asylum for the Insane at Tuscaloosa, Alabama (1860).

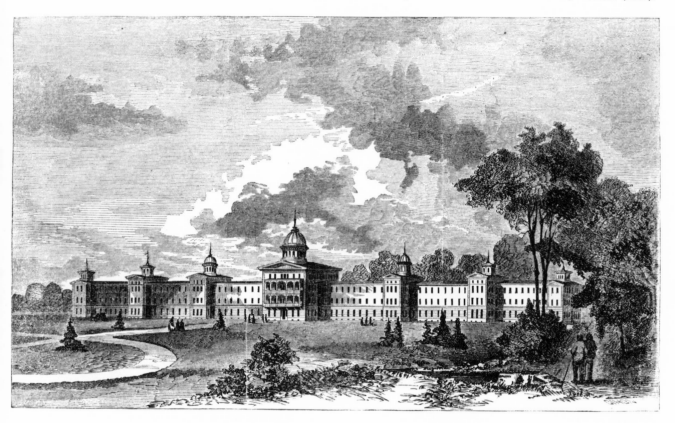

Fig. 81. Elevation of the State Asylum for the Insane at Tuscaloosa.

the superintendent's home was on the upper floor, and a water tank was hidden under the ornamental dome. The wings have been offset to the rear to allow a corridor open to sun and wind at both ends. A corridor of reasonable length, with bay windows in the middle, would permit the economic measure of locating rooms on both sides of it without detriment to light or ventilation (Kirkbride, pp. 138–39). Where the wings join the central structure a space ten feet wide is left free, with windows that can be opened running from floor to ceiling on both sides and on all stories. So sun and air are let into what is ordinarily the darkest corner of a hospital as freely as if the wards were separate buildings and with considerably greater convenience—one has here an all-weather passageway. Fireproof from cellar to roof and with fireproof doors, it makes an attached ward as safe as a separate annex. An ornamental grille guards

the windows on the inside and a very pleasant sitting area is created (pp. 59–60, 144).

The patients are to be medically classified with great care in wards of about fifteen beds (p. 58), the far wings being reserved for the excitable. Indeed, so important to the peace of the whole hospital is this section for the violent that Kirkbride would have an insufficiently endowed institution begin with the far wings and build toward the center because the first patients to be committed are sure to be the most unmanageable (p. 137). Six rooms at the end of the far wings are for temporary seclusion of patients who become violent (pp. 140–41).

Two-thirds of the patients should be in single rooms small enough (8' × 10') to make it impossible to add a single extra bed. It is really never either proper or safe to have two insane patients sleep in the same room without an attendant in it or in an adjoining one

(p. 65). Always assuming proper supervision, Kirkbride estimates that while one-fourth of all patients
may be lodged in groups of larger size without material
disadvantage, only about one-twelfth—the timid or
suicidal—really do better in associated dormitories.
"The great majority would strenuously object to such
an arrangement . . . just as much in a hospital as they
would in a hotel or boarding-house" (pp. 73–74).

He allows at least three large infirmaries on each
side for the physically ill or the dying, as well as one
or two large rooms in each ward for sick patients with
a private attendant or, simply, if friends of the individual desire a more spacious apartment than usual—
the price tag is assumed. Such amenities render a
state institution feasible for patients of all social classes.

They and their relatives will discover how much better
off they are than at home.

How practical, how respectable, how optimistic! Yet
as one thinks of surviving state asylums built on the
Kirkbride system, how pathetic, how naïve! George
Rosen points out the fallacy. The theory of curability
behind the optimism of doctors such as Kirkbride
simply did not work. Discharged patients broke down
again, returned, and became chronic. The so-called
back wards developed. There were not enough attendants—of any sort. Dorothea Dix lived to the age
of eighty-five, long enough to see the insane asylums
she crusaded to have built in the name of progress
and humanity become hellholes similar to those she
crusaded to destroy.

CHAPTER 4

Medium-Sized Wards from the Renaissance to the Nineteenth Century: Derived Plans

The Derived Plan

In chapter 2 we traced plans for large open hospital wards from prototypes in eleventh-century monasteries to eighteenth-century examples with an excursion into cross wards, which may be composed either of large open halls in the seventeenth century or small rooms at the beginning of the nineteenth. In chapter 3 we examined ward planning in the form of small or single rooms (a pattern originally found in monastery cells) as adapted over centuries to the needs of special patient populations: lepers, plague patients, pensioners, the superannuated, and especially the insane. With the Reformation a third type of accommodation was introduced. The church ceased to be the chief source of social assistance to the sick and destitute; the king, nobleman, or wealthy citizen of the new towns took over the responsibility and built mainly in medium-sized rooms for, say, twelve to twenty patients. Classification of hospitals by the size of ward employed is a useful descriptive device if while examining the evidence in this chapter it is remembered that large halls coexisted and persisted (as late as 1791, John Howard remarked that cross wards were the usual form of accommodation in many Roman Catholic countries)[1] and that building in private or single units for the rich or certain categories of patient continues to this day.

The first hospital discussed in chapter 1 was the Greek Asklepieion. We called it a derived form because it was simply a Greek stoa set aside for the sick. Derived forms are found among wards of all sizes when those responsible for housing the sick have commandeered any vacant structure or have built in contemporary style without functional adaptations. On the other hand, a designed plan is one in which some attempt is made to allow in advance for sanitary arrangements (orientation, ventilation, sewage), ease of nursing supervision, and economical administration. Derived and designed plans develop side by side. A given plan may be derived, designed, or a little of both. We have already mentioned completely derived plans (the open ward of the Hospital of Santa Cruz in Barcelona looks just like the dormitory of Poblet Monastery), plans taken from a recognizable model but adapted to a specific use (the cross wards of the Ospedale Maggiore derive from the monastic dormitory but are arranged around a central altar in order to accommodate the largest possible patient population, and rational sanitation has been provided for), and plans manifestly designed for a hospital purpose, as were the Celle and Schleswig insane asylums.

All the hospitals discussed in this chapter are derived plans. The function of caring for the sick has been fitted into an architectural form originally designed for some other purpose. Noble and bourgeois donors built for the sick poor in forms familiar to themselves that were so closely derived from palaces or country houses it is hard to distinguish a hospital from a gentleman's home. (Thus, Bethlem Hospital was conceived as a palace for the insane poor.) Extremely few modifications were introduced to facilitate group accommodation of a supine population. Like country houses, these derived structures had medium-sized rooms. Designed plans from the Renaissance to late nineteenth century (a parallel development during which the open ward was revived and took on sanitary significance) will be discussed in chapter 5.

As much pride, intelligence, and care might go into building a derived as a designed plan. Honest attempts were made to install adequate heating, lighting, ventilation, and toilet arrangements in wards indifferently or stupidly laid out. Nor were designed plans necessarily futuristic; they conformed to current fashion and the facade was always à la mode. The difference between the two types of plan is that in the first the architectural pattern dominated, and in the second, concern for a sanitary environment.

We have already met in several plans with one characteristic of Renaissance, baroque, and eighteenth-century plans for hospitals: like the palaces and mansions they imitated, they are strongly symmetrical. A practical planning aid, resulting from new theories of art and admiration for Greek and Roman models, was

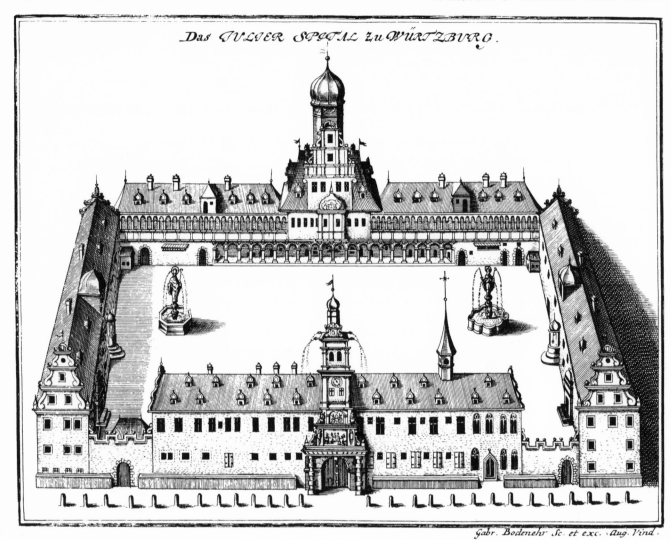

Fig. 82. The first buildings of the Julius Hospital, Würzburg, Germany (1576–85).

thus placed at the disposal of insane asylums and of general hospitals as well. Having half the building a mirror image of the other came in very handy for separating the sexes. Unfortunately, other characteristics of the classical building tradition were not appropriate. Insistence on the grandeur inherent in a sweeping view down the full length of a block or wing led, in mansions, to an alignment of doors.[2] This meant complete disregard of privacy because one could arrive at an end bedroom, for instance, only by trooping through all the others; in hospitals it meant that goods, food, medications, or personnel directed toward wards in the wings had to pass down the center aisle between the beds of every intervening ward.

One can watch the strong urge toward centrality materialize in the first Julius Hospital of Würzburg, Germany (1576–85; fig. 82). The building of the front (south) wing is basically a medieval ward–chapel combination. The chapel points east and has large church windows; the traditional little steeple marks a division between sacred and secular areas. The wards were built in two stories, both opening into the chapel, with a balustraded walk on the second story between the two rows of chapel windows for weakened patients of the upper floor to save their climbing stairs. At the western end, where the barred window is, was the pharmacy.[3] Upon this familiar layout has been superimposed a central gatehouse so ornate and compelling one has to look twice to recognize the essential asymmetry of the building. A parallel structure in the rear for aged pensioners fully achieved the transition to symmetry.

The Holy Ghost Hospital of Ravensburg, Germany (1448; fig. 83) compromised in another way between old forms and the new symmetry. The floor plan is irregular. The ground floor includes the traditional elements: large open sick ward, chapel, kitchen. On the upper floors off a wide central corridor was a series of rooms for paying oldsters.[4] No indication of what is going on inside can be gleaned from without. In the Middle Ages a special structure was planned for each function (for instance in monasteries), or at the least there were individually designed outbuildings or wings. The kitchen was kept longest in a separate building because of danger from fire. But at Ravensburg all functions however dissimilar have been packed under one roof, windows of the large ward and the chapel are identical and from the outside one half the building mirrors the other, with the exception of an inconspicuous but necessary door direct to the chapel (a similar door is found at Würzburg). Ravensburg might be called a forerunner of what was later known as the "block hospital."

We have seen plans for insane asylums that were fully symmetrical inside and out. A good model of a general hospital in this form is the Hospice of St. Jacques du-Haut-Pas, founded in 1780 to serve the poor of that Parisian parish by the Abbé Cochin, and later called the Hôpital Cochin. Extremely detailed plans exist (figs. 84–86) together with a longitudinal section of the second story (fig. 87) and an elevation (fig. 88). The architect is Charles-François Viel, who was responsible for the *petites loges* of the Salpêtrière. Characteristically, the ground floor is used for services and offices: admissions, clothing storage, discharges, kitchen, morgue. The second is the main floor, the *piano nobile* as it was called in Italy, where this convention originated. In Italian cities narrow streets were necessary for protection against the summer sun and the winter cold, but cramped streets and a jostling crowd led to riots, brawls, and nocturnal depredations. Therefore the nobility took to living on the upper floors of palaces, the principal floor being the second. The ground floor was devoted to services in Italian palaces, English country houses,[5] French chateaux, and in this palace the Abbé Cochin built for the poor of the parish of St. Jacques.

The two-story central chapel is situated directly above the morgue (as it was at the Ospedale Maggiore of Milan; also at the cross ward of the Hôtel-Dieu of Lyons, 1631). Sixteen canopied single beds in open wards on either side of the chapel were for the poor. In the left-hand ward for men, six beds were reserved for the sick, ten for the infirm.[6] Ventilation was effected in the open wards by windows high above the beds, other windows onto a corridor, and four narrow chimneys, two marked "ventilator," opening above the roof. The placing of two latrines on the second and third floors probably made the front courts stink and rendered the corridor windows unfit for ventilation. On the top floor, entirely reserved for women, was a five-bed dormitory for the nurses (*religieuses*). Single rooms (a sure indicator of private incomes) were reserved for women with extraordinary

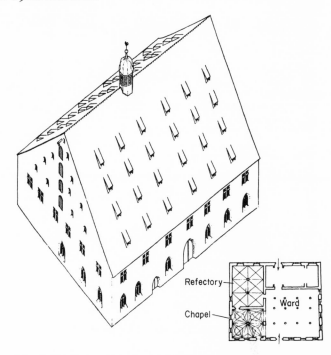

Refectory

Chapel

Ward

Fig. 83. Isometric reconstruction and plan, Holy Ghost Hospital, Ravensburg, Germany (1448), drawn by Ulrich Craemer.

infirmities or maladies who could pay an annual pension of 450–500 *livres*, whether or not they belonged to the parish. That there seem to have been no fireplaces for the parish poor may be one reason for the ventilating shafts since fireplaces were used to draw out foul air as well as to radiate heat. In each private room is a fireplace to perform both functions, and there are fireplaces in the two-bed wards in the wings of the principal floor. (It is interesting to observe that in 1780 the proportion of patients in semiprivate or separation rooms to patients in the open ward was two to sixteen.) Rich patients upstairs must have received private attention from the chaplain, since they were given no direct connection with the chapel.

The Hospice of St. Jacques du-Haut-Pas conforms in every respect to specifications for a mansion or palace of the Italian Renaissance: (1) three stories of considerable height; (2) a symmetrical axial plan, (3) windows placed above each other and equally spaced horizontally, so that their regular rhythms control the entire facade;[7] (4) concatenation of the parts and their integration into the whole; (5) one ruling part and a differentiation of the parts by distinguishing between dominant and subordinate.[8] Should one ask how the practice of medicine fitted into so highly formalized an architectural pattern, the answer can only be: the best way it could; and the same applies to patients.

The plan of the Hospice of St. Jacques du-Haut-Pas, although not outstanding, is as typical of eighteenth-century block hospitals as the skyscraper is of hospitals

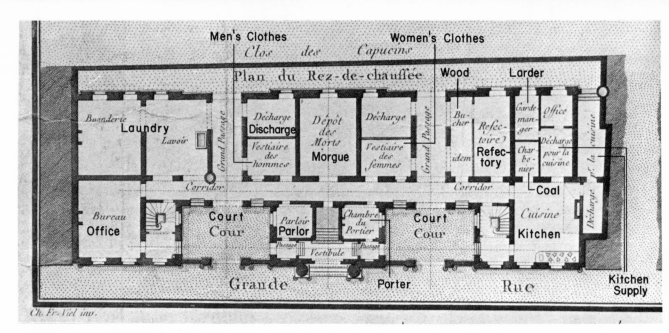

Fig. 84. Hospice of St. Jacques du-Haut-Pas, 1780, design by Charles François Viel; ground-floor plan.

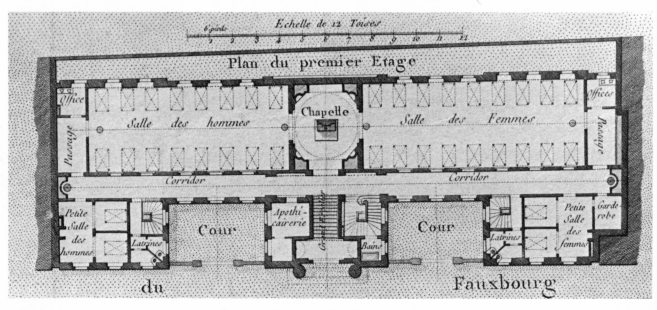

Fig. 85. St. Jacques du-Haut-Pas, second-floor plan.

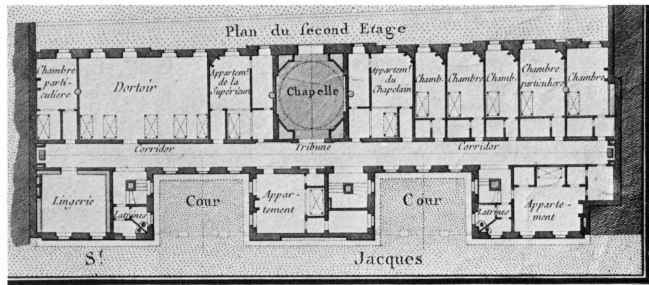

Fig. 86. St. Jacques du-Haut-Pas, third-floor plan.

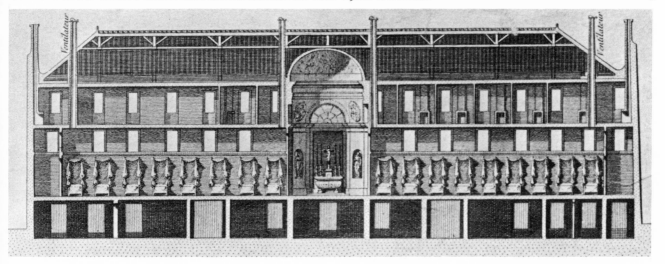

Fig. 87. St. Jacques du-Haut-Pas, longitudinal section.

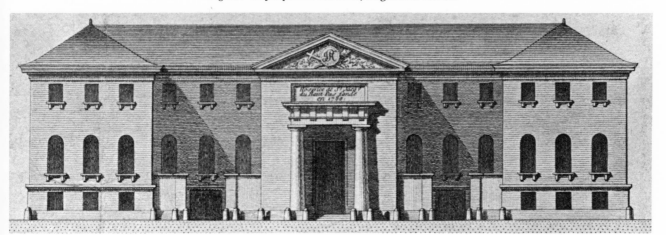

Fig. 88. St. Jacques du-Haut-Pas, elevation.

today. A classic front, projecting wings—which can be recognized in eighteenth-century England, Spain, Denmark, Germany, France, and colonial America— set a norm. But it is not the norm of the Middle Ages. In the second half of the eighteenth century, after a transitional period of about 300 years, during which the open ward and chapel combination continued to be built and the cross ward maintained its popularity, a new architecture for hospitals finally took firm hold.

British Voluntary Hospitals: Courtyard Plans

The ancient and notable monastic hospitals of Britain met an untimely death during the Reformation. By order of Henry VIII, church lands were usurped, stained glass windows smashed, lead stripped from the roofs of the great halls, and the buildings abandoned to be quarried by neighbors or gutted by rain. A not inconsiderable number of Catholic hospitals had fallen into corruption and had misused endowments intended for the sick poor, but now the sick poor were worse off than ever: though promises of re-

lief were made, for nine years no alternative arrangements were actually undertaken. From 1536 to 1544, London lacked all forms of social assistance. Beggars, lazars, cripples, soldiers and sailors returning maimed from the wars, and paupers pitifully ill crawled through the streets. A committee of the substantial citizens of London, under the lord mayor, put an end to the intolerable situation by petitioning the king for the return of the city hospitals, whose operating expenses they promised to pay out of their own pockets. St. Bartholomew's, St. Thomas's, Bethlem, and two other London foundations were restored, partially endowed, as "Royal Hospitals," the king taking credit where credit was not due.

St. Bartholomew's, or Bart's, founded 1123, and St. Thomas's, founded sometime before 1173, were ancient institutions. With the Reformation they became in effect a new kind of hospital: the crown and not the church was the sponsor, the bourgeoisie and not the church paid the bills. The citizens of London were moved by pious impulses—all the inscriptions say so. But their chief motives were to make the city a healthier place to live in and to institute a manageable system of social aid.

> An order was issued by the City of London in 1569 for the Preventing of all Idle and Begging People, whether Men, Women, or Children, or other masterless Vagrants . . . to take them all up, and to dispose of them in some of the four Hospitals in London, by the sixteen Beadles belonging to the same, who had their several Standings and Walks in every Ward. Those that were Vagabonds and sturdy Beggars, they were to carry to *Bridewell*. Those that were aged, impotent, sick, sore, lame, or blind, to *St. Bartholomew's* or *St. Thomas's* Hospital. And all Children under the Age of sixteen to *Christ's* Hospital. And this order was made at a Meeting of the Governours of all the Hospitals.[9]

Gone was the assumption that any "poor object" might be the Lord Jesus Christ in disguise. Payment, as a tax, of what had been a charitable offering for the good of one's soul became compulsory. The helpless and sick were to be sent back to their own parish, there to be supported by contributions from parishioners that were extorted either by persuasion on the part of the church authorities or, if that failed, actual imprisonment until a reasonable sum was offered (1562).[10]

Bart's and St. Thomas's were rebuilt in the eighteenth century on the original sites. The new buildings of Bart's will be discussed under the heading of designed hospitals. The buildings of St. Thomas's, which were repaired by the Corporation of the City of London when they were purchased in 1551–52, were not substantially altered for 140 years; wards and church were literally crumbling away when they were replaced (1693–1709) by a succession of courts remarkably similar to those of an Oxford college or the Inner Temple of London (fig. 89).

Below the bottom border of our picture would be found the western gates to the hospital; two large ones of iron for carriages, two small ones for pedestrians. The ornamental frontispiece that originally adorned this entrance, with statues in niches of Edward VI and four cripples, was moved to the entrance to the second court. The foremost court was entirely for women, who were given six wards in the block on the north and south sides, three wards one above the other on each side. Ground-floor wards were narrowed and darkened and their capacity considerably diminished by a paved arcade that ran around the interior of the court with stone benches for patients against the walls at intervals.[11] Every other window of this court was bricked in to avoid paying a tax

on windows (1696) that applied even to hospitals!

The second court was given over to services, religious or useful. It was entered under the frontispiece through a sixteen-foot gap in the first cross building, in which the kitchen, kitchen personnel, and butler's apartment were located. The steward's apartment was in the northern wing of the second court, then came the chapel and chaplain's residence. Every convalescent was required to repair to the chapel before discharge to "return thanks to the Almighty for the benefits he has vouchsafed to grant them, and to join in prayers for the pious founder, the subsequent benefactors, and the present supporters of the charity" (pp. 216–17). The southern wing of the second court incorporated the parish church of St. Thomas's and the treasurer's house. An accident entrance between them was open from 9:00 A.M. to 9:00 P.M., or 10:00 P.M. at the latest, "except on a very great occasion" (p. 201). (The main gate was open from 10:00 to 4:00.) In the second cross building, half the ground floor was taken up by the counting house, conveniently adjacent to the treasurer's apartment, and half was left open as a wide colonnaded passage to the third court. The entire upper story was given over to the Great Hall. In each of the three wings of the far court were two wards for men, and two of the six were the largest wards in the hospital. In 1819 there were said to be half as many women's beds as men's—114 to 226—because "the habits and ways of life of the latter expose them to a greater number of casualties and diseases than women" (p. 132). Admissions and surgery were on the ground floor of the men's quadrangle. Throughout, staircases were set at the angles of the buildings.

Off the men's wards, in a side court irregularly shaped, were the four "foul wards," one for women with 30 beds, three for men with 30, 30, and 23, respectively, for "the victims of a disease so degrading to humanity." Syphilitics were not admitted to most other hospitals, and St. Thomas's seems to have been the first hospital in London where wards were assigned specifically to them, though such patients were sometimes slipped into the clean wards as if suffering from some other complaint (p. 133). (Special lock hospitals were planned for this type of patient.) Around the court for syphilitics and under their wards were rooms for the brewhouse, bakehouse, warm and cold baths, carpenter shop, and morgue.

In every ward of St. Thomas's Hospital the following charge to the patients was prominently displayed

THE INTEREST OF THE POOR AND THEIR DUTY
ARE THE SAME
FOR
CLEANLINESS GIVES COMFORT;
SOBRIETY BRINGS HEALTH;

E.

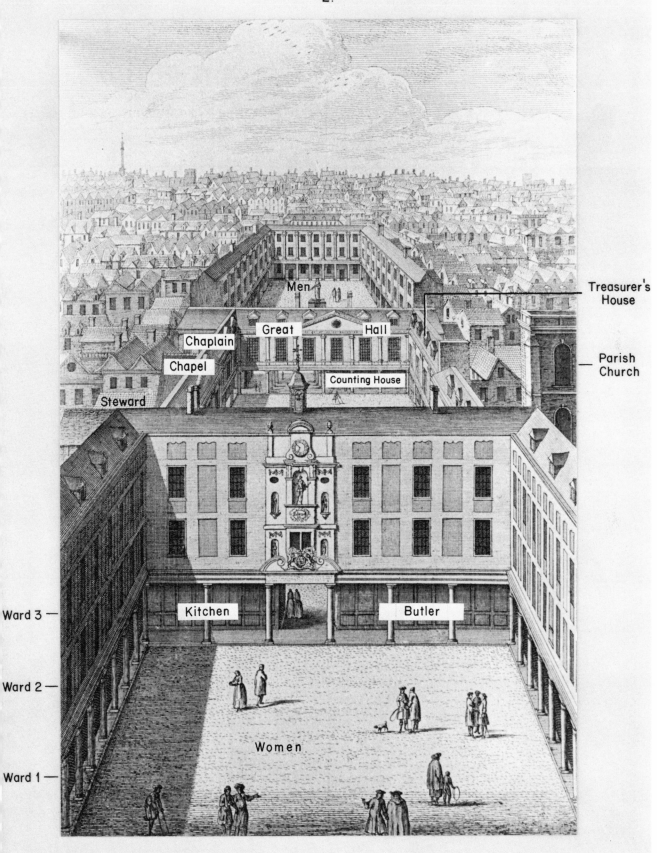

Treasurer's House

Parish Church

Men

Great Hall

Chaplain

Chapel

Counting House

Steward

Ward 3

Kitchen

Butler

Ward 2

Women

Ward 1

Fig. 89. The courtyards of St. Thomas's Hospital, London, in the first half of the eighteenth century.

INDUSTRY YIELDS PLENTY;
HONESTY MAKES FRIENDS:
RELIGION PROCURES PEACE OF MIND,
CONSOLATION UNDER AFFLICTION,
THE PROSPECT OF GOD'S BLESSING, THROUGH CHRIST,
IN THIS LIFE, AND THE ASSURANCE OF
ENDLESS HAPPINESS AND GLORY
IN THE LIFE TO COME.

(p. 138)

This may be paraphrased as follows: It is not enough
for the poor to be miserable; they must be virtuous
as well.

More than a century after they were built, the quad-
rangles of St. Thomas's struck at least one physician
as eminently satisfactory. By 1819, people were beginning to condemn the plan as fatal for the free circulation of pure air, but Dr. Benjamin Golding, in his
Historical Account of St. Thomas's Hospital, quotes
no less an authority than Francis Bacon as praising the
facility of communication that can be maintained with
all its connections. Sir Francis, it seems, proposed a
similar plan for a royal palace. Golding affirmed that
no establishment could possibly be better calculated
for a hospital than St. Thomas's—and for what reasons?

> The whole design of the building gives it a bold
> and commanding appearance. It is constructed
> upon a magnificent scale. . . . The white stone
> pilasters in every square afford a pleasing con-
> trast to the red brick body of the building, and
> relieve, with a peculiar lightness, what would
> otherwise appear not so agreeable. Instead of
> that heavy sombre appearance, which is so fre-
> quently complained of as making an hospital
> resemble a prison or place of punishment, and
> striking a repulsive awe in the sufferers who apply
> for relief, it bears a striking similitude to an agree-
> able private mansion (pp. 120–21).

Golding may have been a physician but he was think-

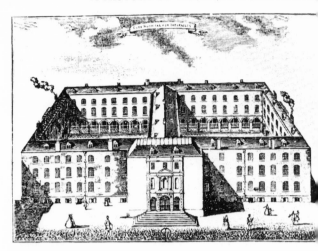

Fig. 90. Guy's Hospital for Incurables, London. Figures 90, 91
and 92 are from an engraving by Thomas Bowles, 1725.

ing of the patients in terms of architecture. "The
beautiful colonnades surrounding the different courts,"
he continues, "give them an air not merely of elegance
but grandeur; and the harmony and magnitude of the
whole building entitle it to the character of a chaste
and stately edifice." Thomas Guy was still under the
spell of St. Thomas's colonnaded courts when he
endowed the hospital called by his name. In fact
the two courts of Guy's Hospital are colonnaded on
three sides and separated by a cross wing with two
stories of wards, as at St. Thomas. The ground floor
of the cross wing is colonnaded throughout (fig. 90).

A vivid "prospect of one of the wards" at Guy's
has come down to us from the year of its opening
(fig. 91). The ward has two fireplaces and in the outer
wall a few long windows irregularly placed with no
relationship to the row of wooden bunks. Beside
each bed is a bench—movable, one trusts; three
quarters of a century had elapsed since a complaint
was lodged with the governors of St. Thomas's that
six great wards there were rendered "much offensive
by unwholesome smells occasioned as is conceived by

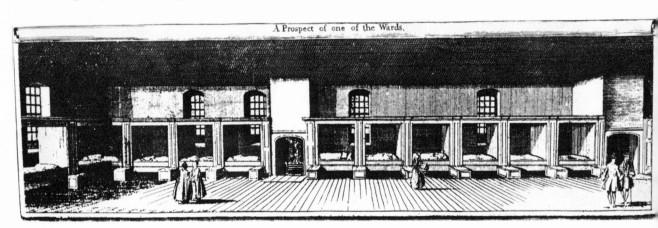

Fig. 91. "A prospect of one of the wards," Guy's Hospital.

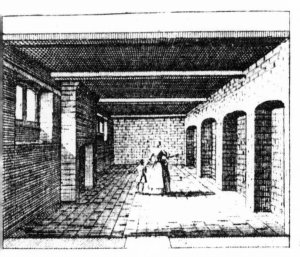

Fig. 92. "One of the rooms for necessarys below stairs," Guy's Hospital.

the settles fixed to the bed-steads therein, wherein under the beds cannot be washed nor swept."[12] As at St. Thomas's, all the patients at Guy's who were fit joined the nurses in "scouring and making clean . . . the beds and floors of the whole ward, passages, stairs, and garrets, and cleaning all foul bedding and washing all foul rowlers and rags, none of which were to be wasted or destroyed through neglect."[13] Despite the efforts of one cleaning squad forty years after the hospital was built, bugs were said to be "a greater evil to the patient than the malady for which he seeks an hospital"[14] and remained so until iron bedsteads were substituted for the ample wooden bunks, which accommodated more than one patient. The print of 1725 gives an invaluable glimpse into "one of the Rooms for Necessarys below Stairs" (fig. 92), and to bring the subject to its ultimate conclusion we reproduce the letterhead of a bill presented to Bart's Hospital (fig. 93) by one of that profession whose task it was regularly to remove the hospital's accumulated "night soil" and sell it for fertilizing the fields.[15]

Guy's Hospital was built opposite St. Thomas's for patients "thought capable of relief by physick or surgery" but excluded from St. Thomas's as incurable "by reason of the small hopes there may be of their cure, or the length of time . . . thought necessary."[16] It was therefore intended as a supplementary hospital to St. Thomas's for chronic cases and the mentally ill, a designation that did not long persist. As early as 1732 the governors seized upon ambiguous phrases in Mr. Guy's will to justify discharging the very patients for whom the hospital was founded in favor of acute cases (such as were accepted by every hospital) whom *they* thought capable of relief by physick or surgery. A century later a small panoptical ward for twenty lunatics was discontinued. When the governor of Guy's was recently asked, as he must often be, "What about the

incurables for whom the hospital was really founded?" he smiled and retorted, "*All* the diseases we now know how to cure were thought incurable in Thomas Guy's day."

In the chapel of Guy's Hospital was inscribed the following tribute to its founder: "After administering with extensive Bounty to the claims of Consanguinity, He established this Asylum for that stage of Languor and Disease to which the Charities of Others had not reached. He provided a Retreat for hopeless Insanity, and rivalled the endowments of Kings."[17] In building this kingly mansion for the pauper sick, Guy followed the precedent of Greenwich Palace, which had been converted in 1694 to a hospital for the use of disabled seamen, and the Chelsea Royal Hospital, constructed 1632–90 on a regal scale for disabled soldiers. Foreigners visiting England were said to remark that "her charitable foundations were more fitted, by their grandeur and extent, for the residences of kings; while her palaces, by their external appearance, seemed better calculated for the reception of the needy and unfortunate."[18] One cannot doubt that a considerable residue of Christian piety was still operative, though the donors themselves no longer washed the feet of a symbolic number of paupers on state occasions.

But straitened means and an emphasis on the rational modified its expression. During the first half of the eighteenth century a number of voluntary hospitals were founded in Britain without support from a very wealthy donor, without royal endowment, and subject to the new and sobering theory that, as Marc Antoine Laugier put it, "Houses destined for the poor should have in them something of poverty." The scale became much less grand, ornamentation less flamboyant. In 1755 Laugier wrote:

> Hospitals should be solidly but simply built. There should be no building where sumptuousness runs contrary to propriety. . . . Magnificence announces either superfluous funds in the foundation or very little economy in its administration; it is therefore a very much misplaced magnificence. . . . Too much beauty in a house . . . will no longer attract the interest of the charitable. . . . The poor must be lodged like the poor. A great deal of propriety and usefulness, but no ostentation.[19]

The age of the palatial hospital thus ended.

British Voluntary Hospitals: Block Plans

Most plans for eighteenth-century voluntary hospitals are block plans bearing a striking similarity to an agreeable private mansion—*how* striking one may judge by comparing the plan of the Rotunda Maternity Hospital of Dublin (1757; fig. 94) with that of Houghton Hall, Norfolk, England (begun 1722; fig. 95). The

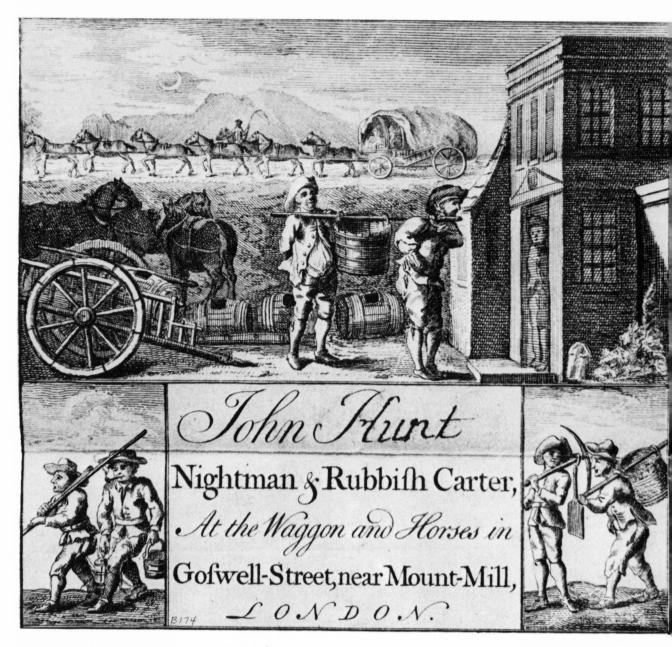

Fig. 93. Night soil men at work, heading of a bill submitted for work done for one of the houses owned by the Hospital of St. Bartholomew, London, January 26, 1757 (2 tons) and September 13, 1757 (8 tons): cost £2.

elevations are likewise similar up to the line where the domes or steeple begins (figs. 96 and 97; Summerson informs us that the plan of Houghton by Campbell and Gibbs became a standard plan in the 1740s and 1750s and that the corner domes, added by Gibbs after Campbell's death, seem never to have been imitated).[20] In its turn, Houghton Hall roughly derives from certain plans in Palladio's *Four Books of Architecture* (first published in 1570) for "country houses belonging to some noble Venetians," which also were symmetrical, pillared, porticoed, with two wings connected by porticos to the main blocks so that one can go everywhere under cover.[21]

The Rotunda Hospital drew part of its income from social affairs in the round hall that gave it its name (adjoining the right pavilion but not included in fig. 96). They say the hall produced "a grand effect on public nights, when illumined and filled with the native beauty and fashion of the country: the orchestra projects into the room, and is generally filled with the best musical abilities the city can afford."[22] Funds for the building were raised by public entertainments in the garden, laid out along the lines of the Vauxhall Gardens in London, which was busily devoted to musical soirees, banquets, and breakfasts before ever the designs had been completed for a hospital on the

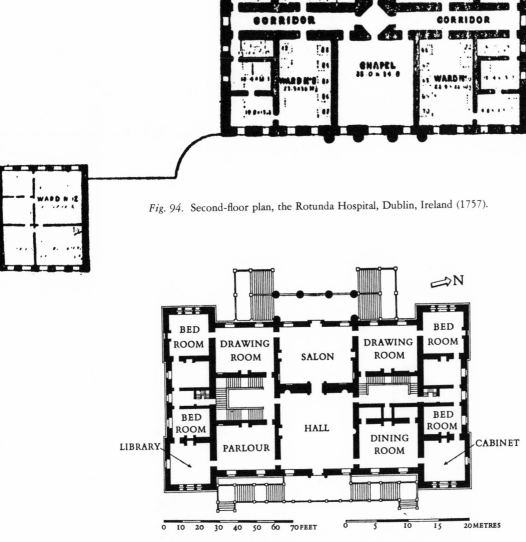

Fig. 94. Second-floor plan, the Rotunda Hospital, Dublin, Ireland (1757).

Fig. 95. Plan of the principal floor, Houghton Hall, Norfolk, England (1722).

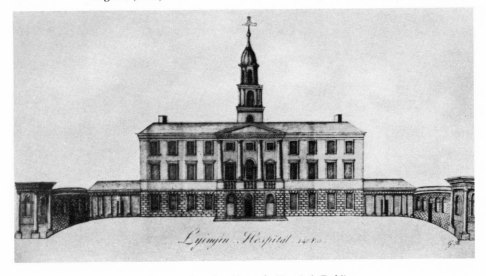

Fig. 96. Elevation, Rotunda Hospital, Dublin.

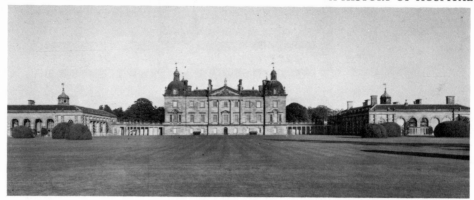

Fig. 97. The garden front of Houghton Hall, Norfolk, begun 1722 (domes from 1729).

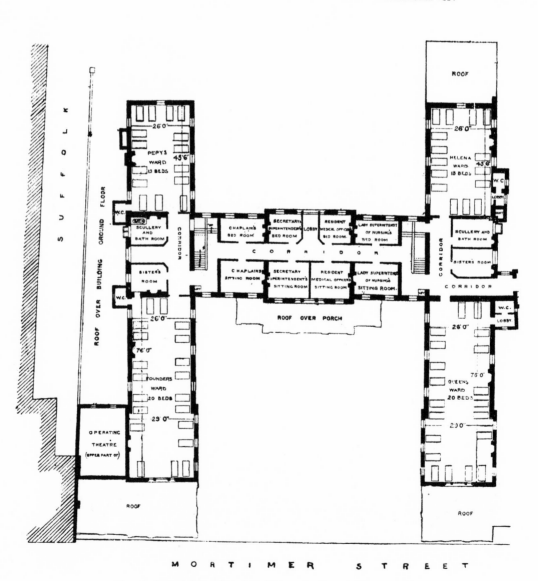

Fig. 98. Second-floor plan of Middlesex Hospital, London (1755).

site (Browne, *The Rotunda Hospital,* p. 10) When the hospital chapel was completed, the governors sold pews to the highest bidder (p. 18) and by such commercial ventures managed to keep beds operating, though every now and then Parliament had to lend a hand.

In 1818 the hospital contained 87 beds. In one ward 31 by 23 feet there were 8 beds, plus 4 others in adjoining apartments "appropriate for women of a better description" (p. 31). The interior was said to possess "that kind of merit which is suitable to such an edifice, solidity, convenience, and neatness, without that display of ornament which, however graceful, is at the expense of charity" (p. 29). However, ventilation of these neat but not gaudy wards posed a problem because late eighteenth-century practice demanded that doors and windows be kept tightly shut. It was thought that wounds become infected from a miasma in the air; sealed windows and heavy curtains around the beds were relied upon to protect the patient. One administrator of the Rotunda in the 1780s insisted on having 1-inch holes drilled in ward doors and window frames, though he was warned about the pernicious character of drafts. He also introduced the ventilators invented by Stephen Hales and discontinued the practice of assigning two women and their babies to one bed. As a result, infant mortality fell from 1 in 6 to 1 in 19.3 (pp. 33–34).

Puerperal fever was an ever-present menace in lying-in hospitals, and the only way one could combat it was by sanitary measures. By 1858 there was a better understanding of and strong emphasis upon sanitary techniques at the Rotunda and elsewhere. The Rotunda Hospital then had 103 beds in 11 wards, 9 of them for the reception of labor patients, 1 a convalescent room, and 1 for women with diseases of the sexual system. Each labor ward consisted of 1 large room for deliveries and nursing and 2 small ones for infectious cases and isolation. A system of rotating the labor wards was introduced. Admissions were directed to a single ward until it filled up, which took between 24 and 48 hours; then admissions were sent on to the next one, whereas in the first all patients were kept a standard 8 days and discharged. If for some reason any must remain, those women were removed to the convalescent room. The empty ward was thoroughly scrubbed and scoured and aired, and not filled with admissions until its turn came again after two or three days (pp. 47–48).

But we have been lured ahead of our story by this interesting nineteenth-century instance of the rotation of wards. To return to the eighteenth century: the country residence of a British nobleman, almost invariably symmetrical, might assume the shape of an H, U, E, or C; so too the voluntary British hospital. In the following examples one can assume a central block between two wings, a central entrance with columns somewhere about it, and a triangular pediment. An H-shaped floor plan adapted to hospital purposes would suggest service areas in the crossbar and wards in the wings, as at Middlesex Hospital, London (1755). Burdett's plan of the interior indicating wards and beds (fig. 98) dates from nearly 140 years after the hospital was opened and more than 80 years after the famous Rowlandson print of the interior (1808; fig. 99). Yet by comparing the two one can guess that the room Rowlandson portrayed must be Queen's Ward.

Note in the etching the surprising amount of space in the center of one of these informally arranged medium-sized rooms. Note also that each bed has a half-curtain attached to a canopy, from which also hangs the kind of stirrup we see in hospitals today. The patient in the right rear corner is using one to hold herself in a sitting position while a doctor examines her or adjusts her pillows. We assume that the person in pants is not her husband, since other visitors to this women's ward are women and the only males are two doctors arguing a case in the foreground and one of their helpers [wearing an apron like auxiliary personnel in Bruges a century earlier (cf. fig. 30)]. The head matron, with the keys, is listening in. Individual medications are kept on a shelf above the patient's head, and from the number of bottles it is clear that dosing was as copious as one would expect in an age of heroic remedies. The chamber pot was kept under the bed and presumably used behind curtains. Though Rowlandson included only a token number of these appurtenances, they were probably standard equipment for all. On this sunny day, two windows are open and linens are being aired on a windowsill, yet a coal fire is roaring up the chimney. The fire would be needed all year round for ventilation and to heat wash water, tea, or soup. The garment the nurse is holding up before the fire to dry seems to have holes for sleeves and to resemble an overgarment the patients are wearing. The occupant of the extreme right-hand bed is enjoying a cup of tea (or, if that was too expensive, cocoa) from the teapot on the grate. Those well enough to get out of bed may have taken their meals at the tables. The inscription over the fireplace might be ward rules, a diet chart, or a pious reminder to the poor of their interests and their duty such as the one at St. Thomas's.

A U-shaped hospital was the London (1752; fig. 100), where two wings ran back from the main block. A detail from a plan of 1893 (fig. 101) describes the double wards prevalent in eighteenth century hospitals. By dividing lengthwise a ward as wide as that at the Middlesex with a wall pierced in two places by doors to

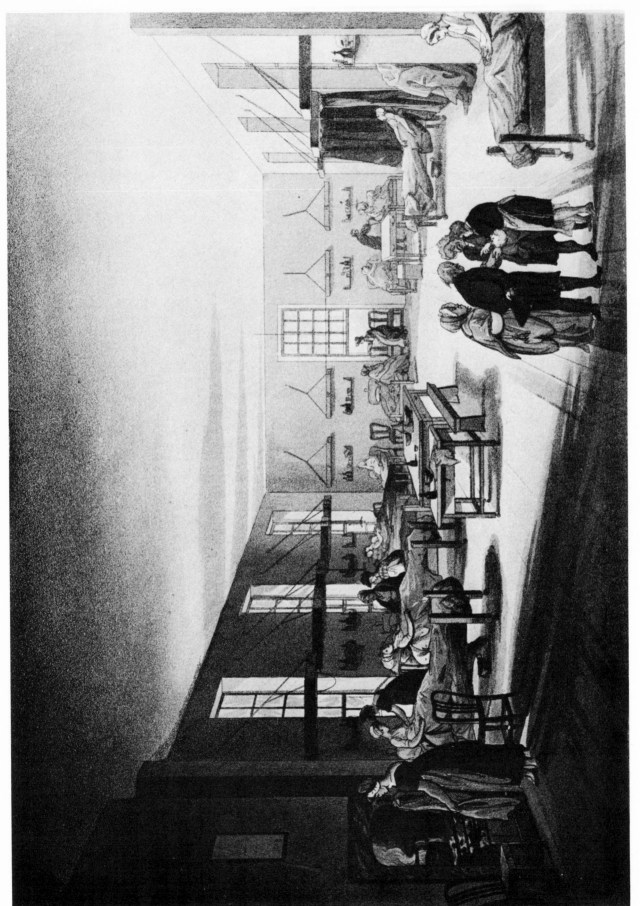

Fig. 99. Ward interior, Middlesex Hospital, London, an etching by T. Rowlandson and A. C. Pugin, 1808.

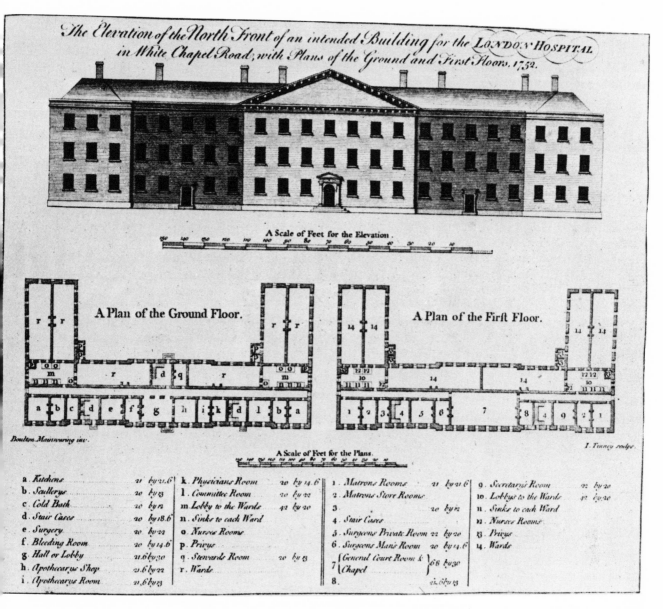

The Elevation of the North Front of an intended Building for the LONDON HOSPITAL in White Chapel Road, with Plans of the Ground and First Floors. 1752.

A Scale of Feet for the Elevation.

A Plan of the Ground Floor.

A Plan of the First Floor.

Boulton Mainwaring inv.

I. Tinney sculp.

A Scale of Feet for the Plans.

a. Kitchens	21 by 21.6	k. Physicians Room	20 by 14.6
b. Scullerys	20 by 13	l. Committee Room	20 by 22
c. Cold Bath	20 by 12	m. Lobby to the Wards	42 by 20
d. Stair Cases	20 by 18.6	n. Sinks to each Ward	
e. Surgery	20 by 22	o. Nurses Rooms	
f. Bleeding Room	20 by 14.6	p. Privys	
g. Hall or Lobby	21.6 by 30	q. Stewards Room	20 by 13
h. Apothecarys Shop	21.6 by 22	r. Wards	
i. Apothecarys Room	21.6 by 23		

1. Matrons Rooms	21 by 21.6	9. Secretarys Room	22 by 20
2. Matrons Store Rooms		10. Lobbys to the Wards	42 by 20
3.	20 by 12	11. Sinks to each Ward	
4. Stair Cases		12. Nurses Rooms	
5. Surgeons Private Room	22 by 20	13. Privys	
6. Surgeons Mans Room	20 by 14.6	14. Wards	
7. General Court Room & Chapel	68 by 30		
8.	21.6 by 23		

Fig. 100. Elevation and floor plans, the London Hospital, 1752.

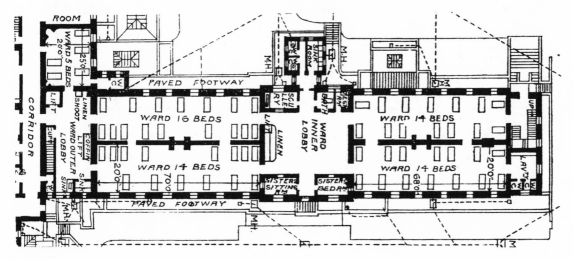

Fig. 101. Plan of one ward of the London Hospital.

serve as passageways, one could find room for twice as many beds in the same space. One could also drastically reduce cross ventilation, and if the two halves were given over to different diseases one could more than double the risk of infection.

A late E-shaped plan for Westminster Hospital (1834; fig. 102) assigns the middle stroke of the E to the chapel and finally replaces walk-through wards with a corridor. A C-shaped design was chosen for the Royal Infirmary of Edinburgh (1738; fig. 103). Above the entrance pillars and under the dome was the motto, "I was sick and ye visited me" accompanying a bas relief not of a prostrate figure in bed being cheered by friends but of a figure seated in a chair and having his leg dressed under the directives of his physician.[23]

Medicine was slowly coming into its own. Accumulation of a large number of pauper sick in hospitals proved a godsend for the doctors. They need not waste their strength traveling all over town to treat patients, and they could begin to specialize. At last they could find under one roof numerous instances of the same condition and compare cases. Though private patients still expected treatment at home of any disease they contracted, if the physician had any strength left after making a living off his private patients there was literally no end to the variants on

the diseases of one particular organ that could be studied in the hospital.[24] They could watch the progress of a disease from its inception and after death check the body for lesions. As doctors began to learn directly from living material, they taught at the bedside, at first instructing only their apprentices who "walked the wards" and were told to keep out of everybody's way but later whole classes of eager students who gathered even from across the ocean. In the mid-eighteenth century, when medical training at Edinburgh was the best in the world, American students flocked to the Royal Infirmary and brought its clinical approach back to the colonies. Now medicine was no longer a matter of memorizing authoritative texts. One might try this treatment or that on actual patients and compare results.

Even surgery was becoming respectable, centuries after having been abandoned by the learned doctors to barber surgeons who were the only ones actually to operate upon patients. In the eighteenth century, barber surgeons were accepted to train in medicine, while physicians were trying to learn surgery in order to earn the good money that had gone to barber surgeons up to that time.

At Edinburgh a flourishing medical school came first and the hospital was deliberately planned to accom-

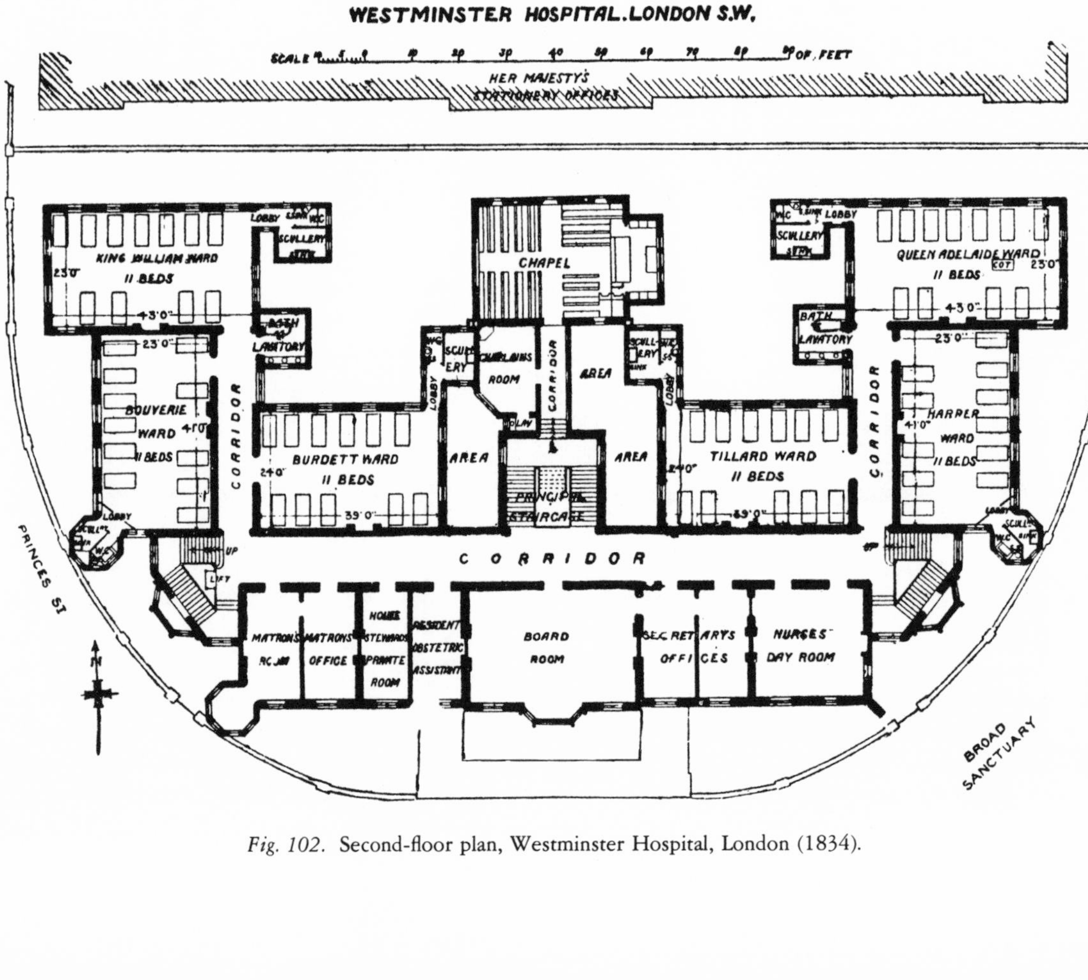

Fig. 102. Second-floor plan, Westminster Hospital, London (1834).

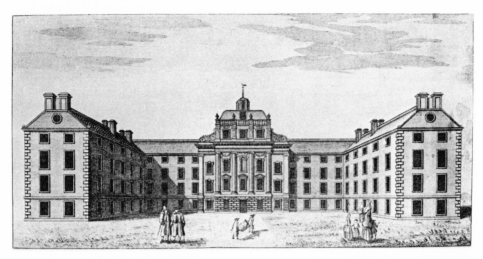

Fig. 103. Royal Infirmary, Edinburgh, Scotland (1738).

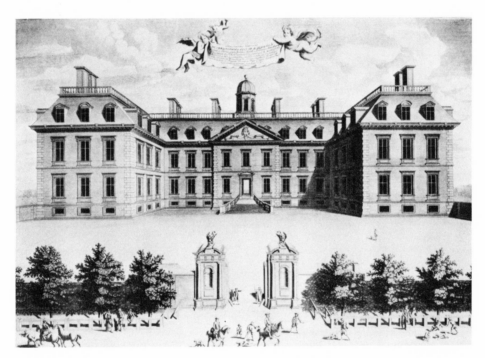

Fig. 104. Clarendon House, London (1664–67).

modate it. The hospital directors, "foreseeing that its interest would soon be interwoven with that of the university . . . resolved to adopt every measure that could tend to facilitate medical education, and to render it compleat. They, therefore, permitted all students of medicine, upon paying a small gratuity, to attend the hospital, that they might have all the benefit that could be derived from the practice of the physicians and surgeons." The managers further-more "gave liberty to the professors of medicine to lecture on such cases of the patients as they should find most conducive to the instruction of the students."[25]

The layout of the Edinburgh Royal Infirmary, storage bin for so much valuable case material, was most un-

remarkable. The Infirmary seems to have been a late descendant of Clarendon House in Piccadilly (fig. 104), built for the Lord Chancellor in 1664–67 and de-molished only sixteen years later, but influential as a design.[26] Plans for the upper three stories of the Edinburgh Infirmary (the fourth, or attic, floor is given in fig. 105, the others being nearly identical) show open walk-through wards with the beds arranged in pairs: 24-bed wards to either side of the central hall, 12-bed wards in each wing; men to the left, women to the right. Auxiliary services were kept on the ground floor as usual (which here was above ground at least) and so, as noted earlier, were single cells for the howling insane (fig. 106).[27] In private courts, on the

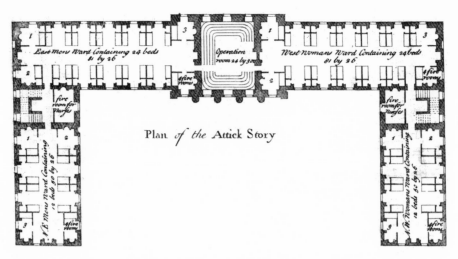

Fig. 105. Fourth or attic floor plan, Royal Infirmary, Edinburgh.

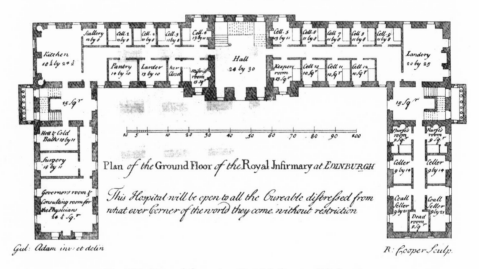

Fig. 106. Ground-floor plan, Royal Infirmary, Edinburgh.

ground floor only, were the necessary houses. This 200-bed hospital magnificently professed itself "open to all the Cureable distressed from what ever Corner of the world they come without restriction."

The managers were not unaware of the hazards of a large open ward and girded themselves to counteract them. If there was a single case of an infection, smallpox for example, that was nowhere else in the house, the patient should be at once removed to one of the small rooms in which there were two beds and was to be shifted from one bed to the other. The empty mattress was to be frequently turned or if necessary removed, and fresh bedclothes supplied. The room must be freely ventilated and "the air ought likewise to be corrected with the vapours of warm vinegar." If, however, the infection was general, it was hard to decide what to do: "It will depend upon the judgment of a physician to make the best arrangements he can; for separate rooms cannot be found

when many patients are in the disease." The rather hopeless suggestion was made that perhaps it will help to move infected patients to the end of the ward, where the fire is and where a draft up the chimney may divert the infectious vapors from the other patients.[28]

Three Early American Voluntary Hospitals

As we have seen, in seventeenth-century London the first secularized poor relief took the form of returning the unhappy recipient to his own parish and there compelling contributions from the parishioners. George Rosen reminds us that, by the eighteenth century, cities had grown too big and migrations of individuals too complicated to send the poor back home again.[29] The early voluntary hospitals of London and elsewhere that we have been examining were of the new mold in accepting "strangers," that is, sick or needy nonresidents, "from what ever Corner of the world they come without restriction." Hospitals of Britain's colonies in America followed suit.

Of the three earliest hospitals in the American colonies, Pennsylvania Hospital, New York Hospital, and Massachusetts General, only the first had a floor plan at all resembling that of the Edinburgh Royal Infirmary. Pennsylvania Hospital (founded 1751) assumed a modified H plan facing south. The terminal wings, instead of reaching wholly forward like those of Edinburgh, were centrally placed so that the north and south fronts looked nearly alike (fig. 107a). As usual, the central block was for administration and the apothecary. But one cannot jump to conclusions about the wings; *both* lateral wards of the first floor were assigned to men and both those of the second floor to women. Each large ward (fig. 107b) had four fireplaces plus ventilators. Cells for the insane were again in the basement (fig. 79), together with baths and the latrines. The attic was broken up into servants' rooms and isolation rooms for patients of both sexes. The attic terminal wings were used for overflow: storerooms, extra kitchens (the main one was in the basement of the center block), and "private apartments for such patients as may be improper to receive into the great wards."[30] Cupolas on the roof served as excellent ventilators. Though the first half of the structure, the East Wing, was completed by 1755, building work lagged for lack of funds and was interrupted by the Revolutionary War, so that the whole structure (still standing) was not completed before 1805 (fig. 107c). First the wards went up, afterward the less necessary administration area.

The provincial Philadelphians looked askance upon the concept of a central, community-supported hospital for strangers and the sick poor. Dr. Thomas Bond, who had studied in Edinburgh, could not arouse the interest of his countrymen in such a foundation until he persuaded Benjamin Franklin to act as his public relations man. In that colonial outpost, it was scarcely a question of amassing teaching and research cases for doctors to work among, but the town had grown to a size where there was real need to find adequate quarters and nursing care for stricken strangers (citizens would naturally be nursed at home), single persons without families, paupers, and the unmanageable insane. Franklin recognized the need and found the means. Seeing that subscriptions were going to be insufficient and that the assembly would have to pitch in, he invented the device of matching funds: when contributors had raised a capital of £ 2,000, the assembly must agree to sign an order for 2,000 more. Franklin wrote:

> This condition carried the Bill through, for the Members who had oppos'd the Grant, and now

conceiv'd they might have the Credit of being charitable without the Expence, agreed to its Passage; And then in soliciting Subscriptions among the People we urg'd the conditional Promise of the Law as an additional Motive to give, since every Man's Donation would be doubled. Thus the Clause work'd both ways . . . And [he adds, chuckling] I do not remember any of my political Manoeuvres, the Success of which gave me at the time more Pleasure. Or that in after thinking of it, I more easily excus'd my-self for having made some Use of Cunning.[31]

That some early hospitals in the American colonies and the early Republic took in pay patients from the first may be derived from the following rule: "Those who are taken into the Hospital at a private Expence, may employ any Physicians or Surgeons they desire."[32] But the chief beneficiaries were the poor, excluding only the incurable, the infectious (with smallpox or itch), and young children. The chief benefactors were the people at large rather than a few rich men. As Franklin put it,

> Incapacity of contributing can by none be pleaded; the Rich only indeed can bestow large Sums, but most can spare something yearly, which collected from many, might make a handsome Revenue, by which great Numbers of distress'd Objects can be taken Care of, and relieved, many of whom may possibly one Day make a part of the blessed Company above, when a Cup of cold water given to them will not be unrewarded.[33]

Franklin's formulation reads like a medieval otherwordly bribe in a refurbished Protestant version. The poor are once again presented as an instrument to save men's souls. In his noble and dignified cornerstone inscription, Franklin flattered all concerned:

IN THE YEAR OF CHRIST

MDCCLV

GEORGE THE SECOND HAPPILY REIGNING

(FOR HE SOUGHT THE HAPPINESS OF HIS PEOPLE)

PHILADELPHIA FLOURISHING

(FOR ITS INHABITANTS WERE PUBLICK SPIRITED)

THIS BUILDING

BY THE BOUNTY OF THE GOVERNMENT,

AND OF MANY PRIVATE PERSONS,

WAS PIOUSLY FOUNDED

FOR THE RELIEF OF THE SICK AND MISERABLE

MAY THE GOD OF MERCIES

BLESS THE UNDERTAKING.

This cornerstone was deposited in the southeastern corner of the Pennsylvania Hospital "with due formality and with Masonic rites."[34]

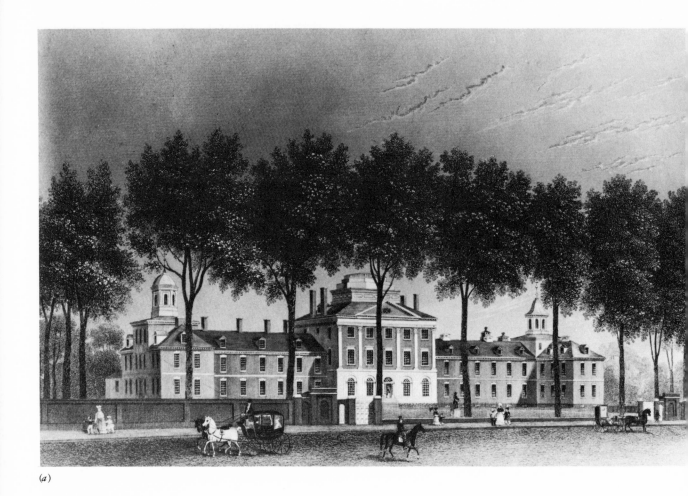

(a)

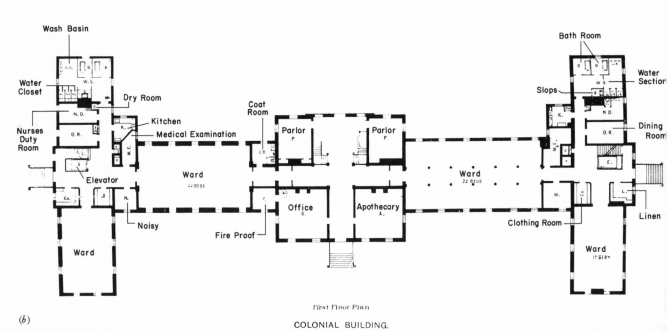

(b)   First Floor Plan

                                       COLONIAL BUILDING.

Fig. 107. Pennsylvania Hospital, Philadelphia (1755). (*a*) Elevation; (*b*) ground-floor plan; (*c*) stages in building the Pennsylvania Hospital: A, the first colonial building; B, after the Revolutionary War another L-shaped building was added; C, the two wings were joined by an administration building at the beginning of the nineteenth century.

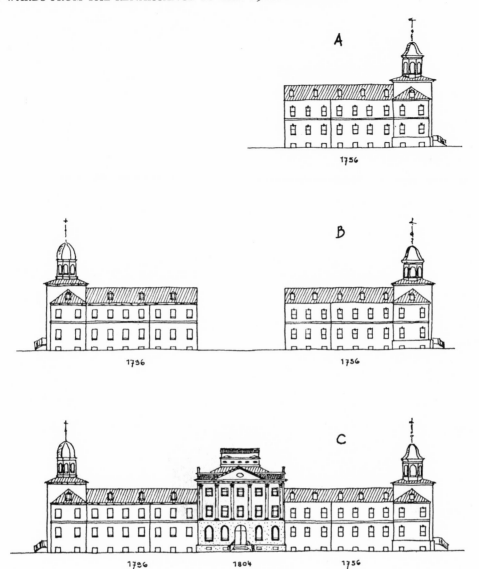

Fig. 107 (c).

The New York Hospital (figs. 108 and 109) was built in 1773–75 in a regular H form with wards in the wings. When barely finished it caught fire and was almost completely gutted. It was repaired just in time to be captured by the British and used as a barracks. Not until 1791 were the first civilian patients admitted. The plan and elevation are taken from a hospital report of 1811; a third story had been added in 1803.

Cells had been made ready for the insane in the basement of the destroyed building, but before any patients could be admitted, the whole wooden part was reduced to ashes in a single hour.[35] In the rebuilding of 1791 the insane finally emerged from the basement and from the building to occupy their own smaller H-shaped building off to one side. This lunatic asylum offered rooms of all sizes and of a degree of elegance to fit any income, for it was entirely a pay hospital. All rooms were heated in winter by seven large stoves spaced at intervals along the basement, whose pipes ascended at a corner between every two rooms conveying heat to both of them. Rooms (ceilings and walls) were built entirely of brick so that the patients could in no way set the place on fire. Sixty cells served 80 patients—which very nearly adds up to private rooms.[36]

The hospital itself catered mainly to paupers. Those able to pay, wholly or in part, were expected to do so. Convalescents unable to pay anything must donate their services, nursing others, washing and ironing the linen, washing and cleaning up the rooms, or doing whatever else the superintendent or matron required. Every Sunday at 10:00 A.M. and 3:00 P.M., one patient in each ward was put to work reading the Bible to the others, "who are to attend thereto with decency and sobriety" (*Account of the New-York Hospital*, pp. 47–48). Excluded from the wards were

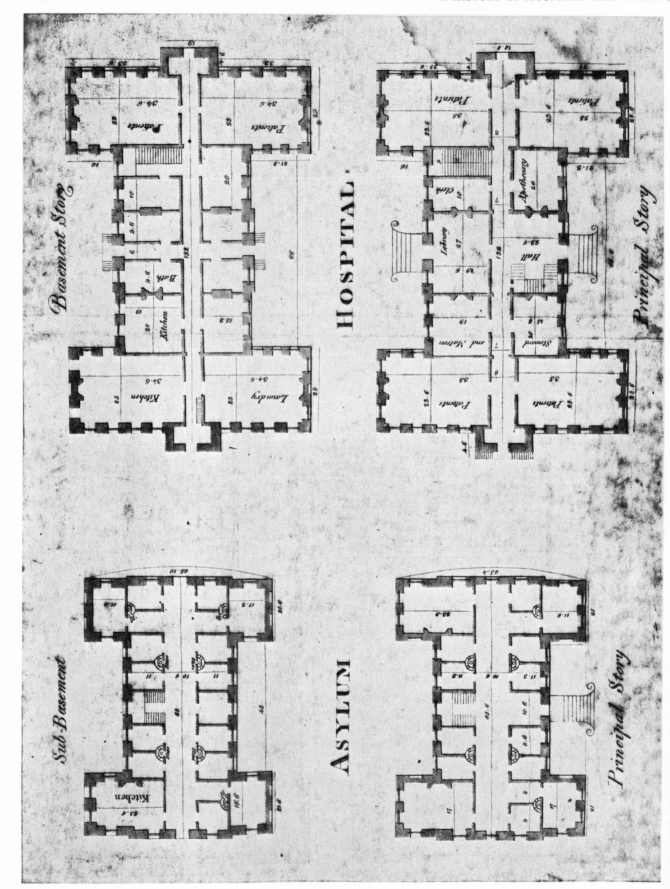

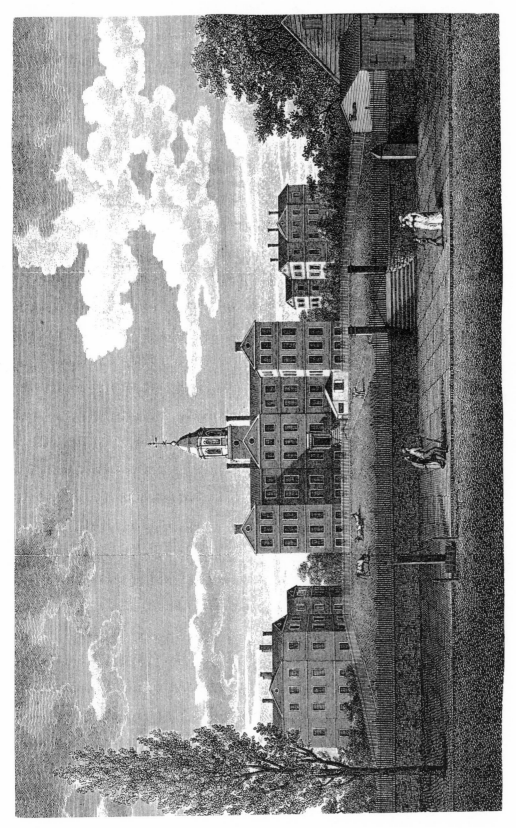

Fig. 109. Elevation of the New York Hospital and Asylum.

smallpox or measles victims, and incurables. Young children were not permitted to accompany their mothers unless they were sick too. "Patients whose particular disease renders it necessary to remove them from intercourse with others" were temporarily put up in two wards in the basement (*Account*, p.11). Every patient—pay, partial pay, pauper, and lunatic—may be described as a reluctant one, for the general account of the patient population for the years 1792–1810 excuses a mortality ranging from 7 to 19 per 100 as follows:

> It may be proper to observe, that few patients apply for admission into the Hospital, until every other resource has been exhausted, and their diseases advanced to their worst stages; and many, who meet with sudden accidents, are often brought to the Hospital, in an incurable state, and die of their wounds or fractures, a short time after their admission.   (*Account*, p. 58)

The site of the hospital, between Broadway and Church Street, was lofty and airy. The 14 wards, their dimensions a little less than the 36 by 24 feet of those of the gutted building, with 10- to 14-foot ceilings instead of the original 18 feet, took in twice as many patients as had been contemplated by the founders. A famous colonial physician, John Jones, suggested 8 patients as a maximum for the original wards,[37] but in 1811 the 14 wards contained 300 patients. Allowing for 75 patients on the added third floor, this works out to 16 patients per ward. The plan that came down to us—that of the earlier building was probably consumed in the fire—allows ventilation of the wards from three sides. A door in the fourth side opened into a corridor swept from north to south by breezes from the Hudson River 600 feet away.

The circular window in the pediment gave upon an operating room on the top floor because the surgeons requested oculus lighting rather than a skylight (*Account*, p. 11). No chapel in sight, but the statement of purpose is genuinely religious and democratic. Said the governors of New York Hospital to the governor of the Province in 1771:

> Our professed object is to find means for the recovery of the poor diseased, who are so indigent as to be helpless without the public aid, and our care is to extend relief with the most indiscriminating impartiality to the sick and distressed poor amongst us of every character, without the most distant regard to National, Civil or Religious distinction. This is the Godlike design of our patent, and it shall be executed upon principles of the most liberal and extensive charity.[38]

The promise was kept. Between 1792 and 1811, this hospital of the port of New York received patients from Asia, Africa, America, Algiers, Denmark, England, the East Indies, France, Germany, Holland, Ireland, Italy, Norway, Prussia, Poland, Portugal, Russia, Scotland, Spain, Sweden, and the West Indies, and ten patients whose origin was never known (*Account*, p. 56). The New York Hospital was so situated as to be able to carry out in practice the high-flown ambition of the Edinburgh Royal Infirmary: it really did treat the "Cureable distressed from what ever Corner of the world they come without restriction."

The third voluntary hospital in the United States,[39] Massachusetts General Hospital of Boston, admitted its first patients in 1821. The two doctors who proposed it be founded in 1810 still felt they must justify the usefulness of the hospital as an institution. They undertook to answer two questions: (1) whether the relief afforded by hospitals is better than can be given in any other way, and (2) whether there are in fact so many poor among us as to require a hospital of this sort.[40] In answer to the first question they point out that some lying-in women have no other recourse, that for most mental patients there is no alternative, and that the almshouse, having had to take in the community's least desirable members, the debauched and profligate, was a place that would cause respectable poor folk to want to die rather than enter.

In answering the second question they explain that hospitals are not meant merely for lazy and dissolute beggars. (Laziness was a cardinal sin in Yankee America.) An honest working man on a borderline income who lives in an attic or garret must lie in the cold when he is sick without proper food or conveniences and worry about how he is going to pay next month's rent, his sufferings aggravated by the cries of hungry children. Decent women abandoned by intemperate husbands have nowhere to turn when ill. The young apprentice has not had time in a short work life to lay by money for an emergency; he is caught unprepared by accident or illness, and it is no real remedy to collect the sick of this class in one room, sheltered from the weather and merely being fed. Such persons would do well to enter a hospital even if they must pay the expense of their maintenance. This class of workers includes domestic servants, who can scarcely be adequately attended if they are sick in their rooms at the end of the house while the mistress has all their work to do herself and must nurse them besides. "Persons of these descriptions would not be disposed to resort to a hospital on every trivial occasion. But, when afflicted with serious indisposition, they would find in such an institution an alleviation of their sufferings, which it must gladden the heart of the most frigid to contemplate."

The Commonwealth of Massachusetts offered to

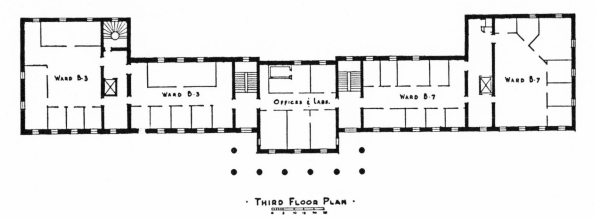

· THIRD FLOOR PLAN ·

Fig. 110. Third-floor plan of the Massachusetts General Hospital, Boston (1848), adapted from an augmented plan of 1941. The original open wards survived until 1975.

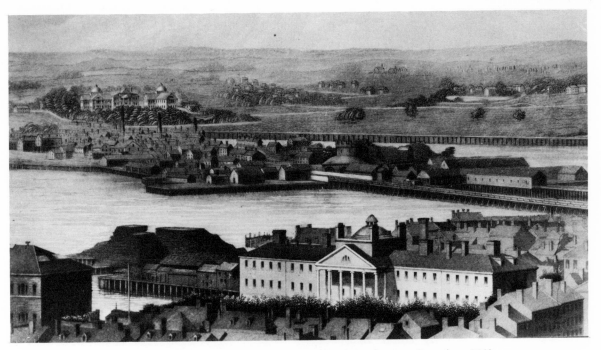

Fig. 111. View of the Massachusetts General Hospital and surroundings about 1853.

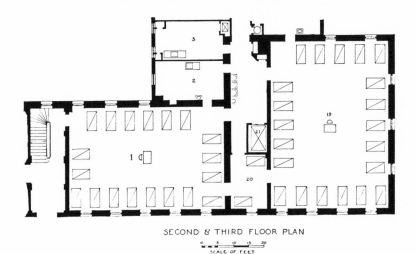

SECOND & THIRD FLOOR PLAN

SCALE OF FEET

Fig. 112. Bed pattern in 1924, Massachusetts General Hospital.

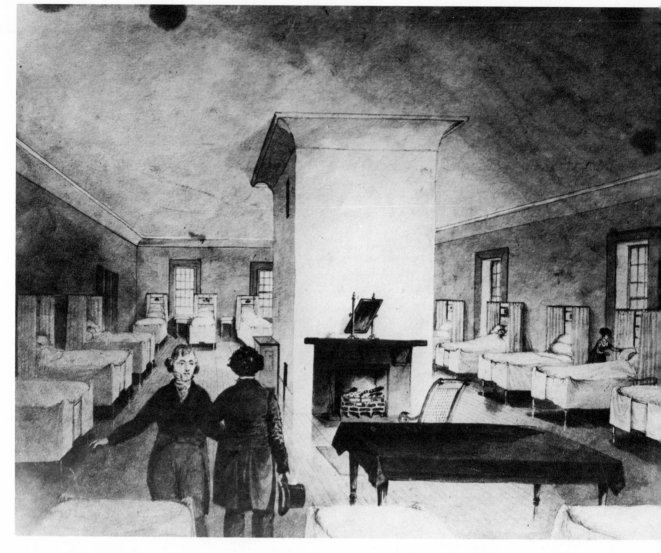

Fig. 113. Interior of a ward of Massachusetts General Hospital, 1845.

donate a valuable mansion to the hospital if $100,000 were raised by subscription. A door-to-door canvass in 1816 that obviously knocked at the right doors netted almost $95,000 in one week, and the same year the Grand Lodge of Free Masons of Massachusetts laid the cornerstone. From the first, this building did not include the insane; a separate structure was planned for them in another town. Our plan and elevation (figs. 110 and 111) show the hospital after it was enlarged in 1848 by the addition of two well-ventilated end wards but before a distinct brick building was added behind the administration core for the laundry, storerooms, cellars, and a kitchen that was connected with the wards by a covered passageway and dumb-waiters.[41]

Figure 112 shows the bed pattern in 1924 in the wards of the Bulfinch Building, as the original building of the Massachusetts General Hospital is called. One can prove that tradition persists a long time in America too, or else that there is only one logical way to lay out beds in a square ward, by looking at an interior scene of 1845 from the hospital archives

(fig. 113) of what can only be the right-hand ward of the plan in fig. 112, looking up from the bottom of the page.[42] The beds are "blacksmith beds," copied from England. Their framework was wholly composed of iron, even the hoops that stretched from one side of the bed to the other and held the mattress up were iron ("more elastic than wood, and cleaner than the common sacking"). These beds were in use at the Massachusetts General Hospital for more than a hundred years.[43]

About 1864 there were "seven private rooms of different sizes and grades situated in different parts of the institution. . . . Some of these rooms were fitted up quite luxuriously, and very little about them suggested a 'sick room.' The heavy damask lambrequins, surrounded by gilt cornices, and the lace draperies and soft carpet dispelled all thoughts of a patient's room in a hospital."[44] Ventilation was by large open fireplace, here and in the twenty-bed wards.

Many elaborate ventilation systems were in use by then. A doctor from the Massachusetts General Hospital, writing home from London in 1857, described the large tubes communicating with the external air by which most hospitals were ventilated, "from which branches are carried to the different apartments and introduced into these apartments at convenient places by a multitude of *very small* apertures, so that the air is received without any inconvenient blast. The air of the room is conveyed away by apertures larger than the first, all of which terminate in the chimney by metal tubes."[45] In addition to which "in most of the London hospitals fire is kept in one fireplace thro' the summer." All elaborate ventilation schemes seemed in the end to rely on the useful fact that a roaring fire sucks air out of the room and up the chimney. It was admitted in 1838 that "probably the best ventilator is an old-fashioned open fire-place, but everyone knows that it is not the most economical way of warming a room."[46] Furthermore, as soon as it was warm enough to do without a fire but too cool at night to keep the windows open, or on winter nights when the fire was allowed to die down, not only did ward air grow foul but erysipelas raged.

At the Massachusetts General Hospital the authorities improved the ventilation by improving the contact with the outer air. Ventilators were arranged so they could not be closed by patients or nurses, and the upper panels of the doors to each ward were removed so that the unheated air of the entries could pour in all winter long. If a ward did become infected, it was cleansed in the following manner:

> They moved the patients out. They fumigated the furniture and articles to be washed with sulphur in a closed room for three days, for one day exposed to the strongest fumes of chlorine or oxy-muriatic gas. Then they exposed the room to a free current of air, day and night, for at least a week, the articles, particularly the beds, to be turned occasionally and their position changed in order to subject them more fully to the cold air. The walls were whitewashed, the floors and woodwork scoured, then fumigated and exposed to a current of air, day and night, for as long a time as possible. The cellar was cleaned and put in perfect order.[47]

This was in 1827.

Eighteenth-Century Hospitals of an Enlightened Absolutism in Central Europe

By the eighteenth century the number and well-being of a nation's subjects had come to be a matter of concern to its rulers. Mercantilism placed a high value upon a large, industrious population as the basis for state power and unity.

Men were needed to labor in the fields and the mines, to work in the manufactures and on the ships, to provide soldiers and sailors and to people the colonies. The birth rate should be raised by maintaining a prosperous peasantry, by providing employment in industries and elsewhere, and even by the proper arrangement of taxes and bounties.[48]

One manifestation of this increased concern was large-scale hospitals. Of the three to be considered in this section, the first was built in Copenhagen in 1758 by King Frederik V of Denmark, the second in Vienna in 1784 by the Holy Roman Emperor Joseph II of Austria, the third in Bamberg in 1789 by the German Prince-Bishop Franz Ludwig van Erthal. The three rulers shared a conviction that state power is fittingly expressed in the erection of a magnificent palace. Its ultimate expression had been Versailles in the seventeenth century, and if later monarchs built on a smaller scale it was because of less absolute power or a limited access to funds, not because of more temperate ambition. And they provided on a princely scale for the poor by building the new hospices and hospitals as palaces.

This was baroque architecture, a form that English philanthropists had been forced to renounce in the eighteenth century and that the American republic that took shape in the eighteenth century never knew. But an absolute monarch no less than an American hospital board had to keep in mind certain economic and medical realities. Financial problems at Frederiks Hospital of Copenhagen being much the same as those of the Pennsylvania Hospital of the same date and medical developments no respecters of national boundaries, the solutions evolved were remarkably similar.

The plan of Frederiks Hospital (1758; fig. 114) is essentially a hollow square to which has been added four 2-story separate pavilions at the four corners of the lot. The entrance buildings are also two-storied. Figure 115, showing the entrance on Bredgade, gives a small but dignified glimpse of the large and noble hospital, the first in Denmark and one of the first in Europe to be built specifically for curable patients and teaching purposes. To the right of the entrance was the medical doctor's residence, with rooms upstairs for the surgeon and assistant doctors; obviously the surgeon ranked well below the medico. The great kitchen was to the left. The wards, down both long sides of the square, were all of one story. Operating rooms were placed at the northwest and northeast corners of the square simply because there the light could come in from two sides. Six- and seven-bed wards for operated patients lay adjacent to them. At the southeast corner, across the corridor from one

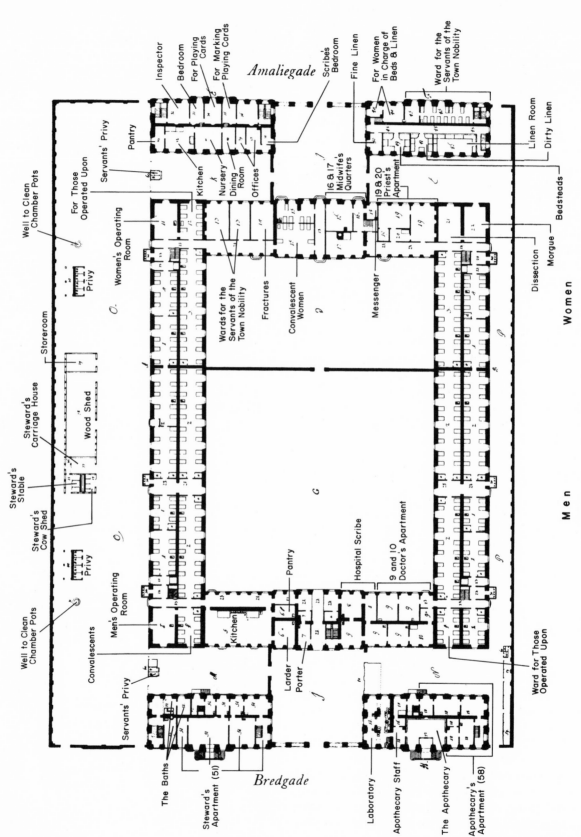

Fig. 114. Ground-floor plan of Frederiks Hospital, Copenhagen (1758). All rooms with a single dot in them are those where the watchers had their beds. A row of dots indicates a privy. Numbers indicate rooms, lettering indicates courts. 1, 2, 3, and 4 are wards; 23, corridors or vestibules.

of the wards, were the morgue and a dissection room.

John Howard reports that patients were divided both as to service (in 1794, 158 medical, 69 surgical) and sex (142 men, 85 women).[49] Separate wards were given to each service. The two operating rooms indicate that the sexes were divided front and rear, not left and right as might be expected in a symmetrical building; indeed, a separating wall without a single door in it was erected two-thirds of the way back and clear across the court garden after the hospital was finished.[50] The authorities were trying to ward off a problem—one-sixth of the male beds were reserved for soldiers (not free beds, by the way; a single soldier donated full pay, married one-half pay). In this connection we may allude to the situation at the beginning of the eighteenth century at Haslar, the English Naval Hospital. The men could not be kept in or the women out, and the route for both was the same, namely through the bog house (privy) and the main drain.[51] However, once the wall was up at Frederiks, the staff was faced with an even bigger problem: how to get through to the women's wards in the rear. Eventually they cut doors in the wall and when that seemed to work out without incident, they removed the wall.

Passages into the courtyard ran through the center of the front and rear buildings, and three of them crossed the wards to the courtyard on either long side, but there was no way to traverse the length of the side buildings indoors without using the center aisles between the beds. A transverse wall divided the long wings into parallel wards (without connecting passages such as those of the London Hospital); thus half the wards faced south and received the sun, but the other half never. In the corner of each ward a space the width of two beds was walled off as living space for the day nurse, just big enough for her bed, chair, and commode (Gotfredsen, p. 34). Privies for each ward were placed off the transverse corridors.

Of the four 2-story pavilions, one was the apothecary's shop and house, one the steward's, one the inspector's, and the fourth, called the washhouse, contained linen and bed storage and twelve pay beds for the female servants of Copenhagen aristocrats. On the top floor of the steward's house were the "noble rooms"—private rooms for those who could pay for privacy plus a few two-room suites that came equipped with private attendant (p. 23).

With the above exceptions, beds were free—and the king stressed that this hospital was built from royal funds not tax moneys. It was dedicated "to the glory of God and the abandoned, poor, helpless and suffering sick: for teaching, alleviation, help and shelter." (Note: teaching is put first.) Contagious, syphilitic, chronic, and insane cases were excluded,

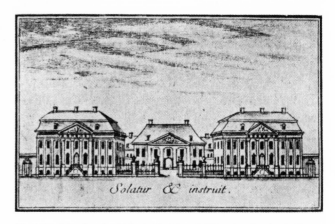

Fig. 115. The facade of Frederiks Hospital fronting Bredgade Street.

as well as all who were not citizens of Copenhagen with the exception of certain major surgical cases arranged for and payable in advance. Before admission the indigence of the patient had to be testified to by the tax collector, his landlord, and if possible his pastor. The medical urgency of the case was then ascertained by a house visit from one of the assistant doctors, and if the patient passed both tests, the hospital portchaise was sent for him—the sedan chair if he could sit up (fig. 116), the stretcher if he must lie down (pp. 37–38).

Patients paid no deposit upon admission and were given hospital clothing for their stay. By day they were tended by the "room woman," who lived in the cubicle at the end of the ward and whose working hours were from 6:00 A.M. to 10:00 P.M. (She was helped with the cleaning by a "day woman" and relieved at night by a watcher.) The patients were given two meals a day, dinner at eleven, supper at six. Fixed

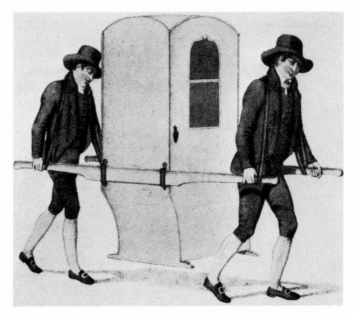

Fig. 116. Frederiks Hospital's portchaise ambulance with bearers.

menus for both hung in the ward. Meat and bread were weighed out carefully, and the weights and measures were kept in the ward so the patients would be sure they got what was coming to them (p. 33). Although on a given day of the week dinner was always the same, compared with English hospital fare of the same century the diet was rather fancy and astonishingly rich in green vegetables.[52]

The drink was tea, beer, or ale for a very simple reason: Frederiks Hospital had an unspeakable water supply. The buildings were erected on filled land, over seawater, and although permission was received to tap the city water supply, no one could foretell what would come through the water pumps. Gotfredsen says this lake water, brought into the city through underground pipes of hollowed-out Pomeranian fir-tree trunks, "was rich in organic matter and it was matter you could take hold of and feel, such as mosquito larvae, toads, leeches and small fishes, not to mention eels." It also had an annoying overtone of rotten fish.[53] And this was but a grace note in the orchestra of smells at Frederiks Hospital. To save money the wards had been built without basement on the damp fill. By the time they were ready for occupancy they stank, and so did the privies the workmen had been using for three years. The boards were relaid, they were laid double, the ground beneath them was filled in with pressed clay; the king would still not release money for cellars. Privies were built and rebuilt according to every system then known: pit, tank, bucket. An expert was called in who claimed a new odorless invention, which did not work; he tried again, it failed again. To avoid diluting privy accumulations, sawed-off wine barrels were set up in the courtyard with funnels to receive urine from the night pots. Frederiks Hospital unquestionably had a certain air about it.

But stench was nothing new in hospitals. What is significant is the changing attitude toward the chapel in the eighteenth century. True, the first staff appointee at Frederiks Hospital was the pastor, who prayed with patients in the wards and prepared surgical cases for an ordeal always incredibly painful and often fatal. Also, the room women were supposed to be Lutherans and know how to read, that is, how to read a service. But the chapel for the ambulatory was on the second floor of the entrance building to the rear, up a steep flight of stairs. In 1771 the great physician, prime minister, and reformer Struensee converted it to a ward for venereal diseases.[54] People professed themselves scandalized, yet when Struensee fell from power two years later the room did not revert to its original purpose but was converted to an operating room with amphitheater, and was thenceforth used for services only on Sundays (Gotfredsen, p. 22).

We have mentioned a large theater in the attic of the Edinburgh Royal Infirmary, where it was said (1778) that "upwards of 200 students can, at once, see operations; and the same serves the purposes of a chapel."[55] At King's College Hospital, London (1839), chapel and operating room, side by side and of equal size, shared a wing of the second floor.[56] A plan of the Liverpool General Infirmary (1749) shows "the Hall, where the general Courts of Governors are held, which likewise serves as a Chapel to the Hospital."[57] The chapel of the new Hôtel-Dieu of Paris (1878) came to be used as a linen room.[58] And the central chapel of St. Luke's Hospital, New York City, was proudly exhibited (1857) as "an immense reservoir of pure air for the wards."[59] We conclude this partial list of ways the hospital chapel was put to secular use with a footnote from Enlart: "In 1616 the poor patients hospitalized at Montepezat adopted the hospital chapel to satisfy their needs; only in 1624 was it decided to build them two *privés*, after complaints from the neighbors."[60]

Very nearly the whole of the extensive building complex of the Allgemeines Krankenhaus, the General Hospital of Vienna (figs. 117–119), was erected in the seventeenth century as an imperial and palatial almshouse for soldiers and the poor, similar in intent and extent to the Hôpital Général of Paris. The scale of the building is baroque and is intended to astonish; at the time it was built Prince Karl-Eusebius von Lichtenstein was asserting that the longer a building is, the more pleasing it becomes. He recommended an extended facade with a great many windows and "advised his fellow peers to make the magnificence of their palaces a point of honor amongst themselves."[61] An emperor who dedicated an enormous palace to the poor was doing himself honor twice over.

Only the circular Narrenturm and the hollow square of the maternity hospital were newly built for the Emperor Joseph II when he had the immense existing structure adapted in 1784 to his expressed purpose of founding the most scientific hospital possible for curable cases. There was something baroque in his insistence upon using the grand old poorhouse as a hospital for all the sick of Vienna rather than dividing patients among smaller, separate, and more specialized institutions for sanitary reasons. European hospital theorists of the late eighteenth century, horrified by wholesale infections and deaths at the mammoth Hôtel-Dieu of Paris, were thinking entirely in terms of subdivision, and so were the emperor's own architects.[62] But Joseph had his way and the opposite took place: a dozen ancient assorted charitable foundations were dissolved so that their endowments might be reallocated to provide running expenses for the central hospital. To build and furnish it, Joseph II also reached into his own pocket; like Frederik V he was averse to using public tax moneys. Further, he exploited the strong desire of certain landowners to be elevated to a title: the price for promoting a count to a prince ran very high while Joseph was trying to finance his favorite project.[63]

However, in many ways Joseph II was a man of the late eighteenth century or even ahead of his time. Medicine had already sufficiently advanced beyond the almost absolute nadir of previous centuries for doctors to feel, "Now we can really treat some patients!" To differentiate between curable and hopeless cases became essential. Joseph II earmarked his new hospital for the so-called curable and consigned chronic and senile patients to the secularized monasteries. From the outset he viewed the Allgemeines Krankenhaus as a teaching institution, where doctors of any nationality would be welcome to attend ward rounds or operations. He demanded of his architects that they retain the massive skeleton of the poorhouse–palace while at the same time redesigning the interior as a new, modern, sanitary hospital for 2,000 curable patients.

Corridors were done away with to give the wards windows on both sides. The windows began 6–8 feet from the floor so that cross ventilation might be accomplished well above the patients' heads, and there were also ventilators over the doors, under the ovens, even under the beds. Thus patients were protected whether prevalent theory declared that noxious vapors rise or fall.[64] A rule of one patient to one bed was strictly adhered to. The bed, without curtains, stood at least 3 feet from other beds with its head to the window wall. Beside it stood a small table to hold medicine, drinking utensils, a leaden dish for blood, phlegm, mucous, and other substances, and a urine glass. A blackboard above the patient's head identified him and his bed by number and gave information as to his treatment, disease, and diet. The night stools, stored in niches in the walls (or beside the beds of the weakest patients), were very carefully guarded against odors. The lower half of a long table in the middle of each ward was divided into containers for each patient's necessities. Above one door to the ward was a clock ("which shows seconds and minutes") and above the opposite door were two night lamps, glasses full of hardened tallow with a wick. An oven of glazed brick was fueled from outside the room. In each ward was a large copper wash basin with a dipper kept constantly filled with fresh water. It was said by a contemporary that in this hospital cleanliness was stressed to the highest degree and that it was particularly noticeable since all furniture and paraphernalia were brand new.[65]

But they poured new wine into defective bottles because the arrangement of the wards was less than satisfactory. Supposedly between every two wards, upstairs and down, there would be a separate entryway, and on both stories at the top of the stair was a kitchen with fireplace (and woodpile) for warming dressings, dinners, and drinks for the patients, as well as toilets connecting with underground drains installed throughout the hospital at great expense. However, the room pattern is not entirely regular, and sometimes between two wards served by stairs a third ward was inserted that could be reached only by the timeworn walkway between the patients' beds. This arrangement has caused considerable inconvenience to all generations including our own. The wards range wildly in size from huge ones for syphilitics (90 and 94 beds each) to single rooms for first-class paying maternity patients. Normal wards had 18, 20, or 22 beds, but in some there were 40 or 50.[66]

Another device adopted to avoid the pitfalls encountered at the Hôtel-Dieu, where every sort of sickness was tumbled together pell-mell, was to organize the 2,000-bed Allgemeines Krankenhaus as though it were five separate hospitals: (1) for the sick, both men and women; (2) for maternity cases; (3) for the insane (the Narrenturm); (4) for senile and chronic cases, who went to the secularized monasteries; and (5) for foundlings. Sick infants were cared for at the headquarters of the foundling house in Vienna, whereas healthy ones were put to nurse in foster homes in the surrounding countryside. This service was one of the amenities of the maternity house. The thought was to discourage child murder, a crime for which the mother was condemned to be beheaded,[67] but its practical implementation left something to be desired. Despite the best intentions of the founder and all kinds of rules about inspecting foster homes at intervals, as late as 1867 three foundlings could die under the care of the same foster mother and she could still receive a fourth child to care for. The problem was that payment was higher for a child in its first year than in succeeding years. These women became "experts at turning out little angels."[68]

All reforms were inspired by the desire of Joseph II to increase the population and thus the potential wealth of his state in every practical way. Franz Xavier Fauken, physician and chief designer of the transformation of the poorhouse into a hospital, expressed his ruler's intent as follows:

The state loses nothing through the expenditure [i.e., for the hospital]; the products of the land will be used for it, and the small amount of money which will go out of the land every year for medicines which must be imported will be generously recompensed, through the preservation of so

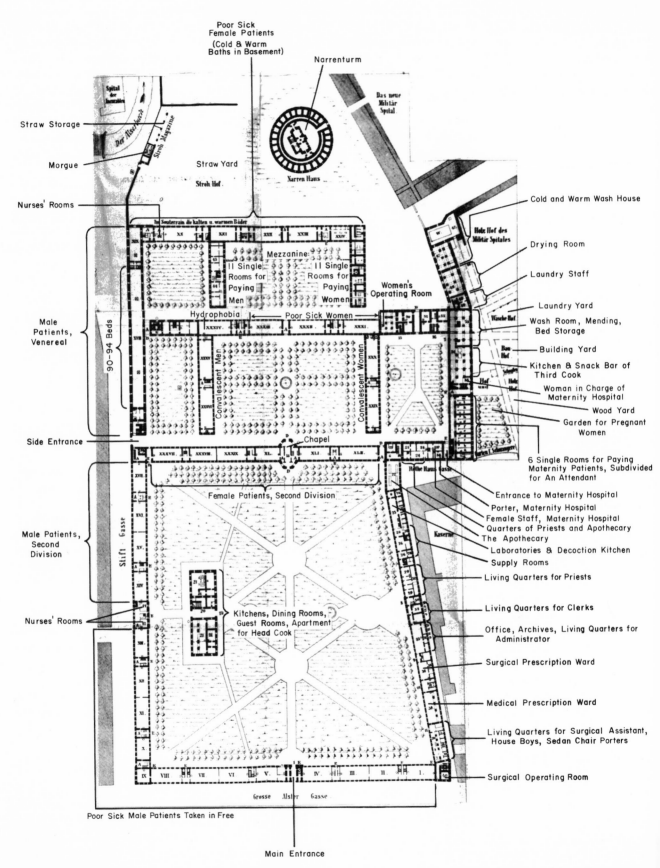

Poor Sick
Female Patients
(Cold & Warm
Baths in Basement)

Narrenturm

Das neue
Militär
Spital.

Spital der
Unruhigen

Straw Storage

Der Alserbach

Stroh Magazine

Morgue

Straw Yard

Stroh Hof.

Narren Haus

Nurses' Rooms

Im Souterrain die kalten u. warmen Bäder

Cold and Warm Wash House

Holz Hof des
Militär Spitales

Drying Room

Mezzanine:

Laundry Staff

II Single
Rooms for
Paying
Men

II Single
Rooms for
Paying
Women

Laundry Yard

Wäsche Hof

Women's
Operating Room

Wash Room, Mending,
Bed Storage

Male
Patients,
Venereal

90-94 Beds

Hydrophobia

Poor Sick Women

Building Yard

Bau
Hof

Kitchen & Snack Bar of
Third Cook

Convalescent Men

Convalescent Women

Holz
Hof

Holz Hof

Woman in Charge of
Maternity Hospital

Wood Yard

Garden for Pregnant
Women

Side Entrance

Chapel

6 Single Rooms for Paying
Maternity Patients, Subdivided
for An Attendant

Female Patients, Second Division

Rothe Haus Gasse

Entrance to Maternity Hospital
Porter, Maternity Hospital
Female Staff, Maternity Hospital
Quarters of Priests and Apothecary
The Apothecary

Male Patients,
Second
Division

Stift - Gasse

Kaserne

Laboratories & Decoction Kitchen

Supply Rooms

Living Quarters for Priests

Living Quarters for Clerks

Nurses' Rooms

Kitchens, Dining Rooms,
Guest Rooms, Apartment
for Head Cook

Office, Archives, Living Quarters for
Administrator

Surgical Prescription Ward

Medical Prescription Ward

Living Quarters for Surgical Assistant,
House Boys, Sedan Chair Porters

Surgical Operating Room

Grosse Alster Gasse

Poor Sick Male Patients Taken in Free

Main Entrance

Fig. 117. Ground-floor plan of the Allegemeines Krankenhaus, Vienna, 1784. (A) Stairs, vestibules, kitchens, privies; (E) entrances to the wards.

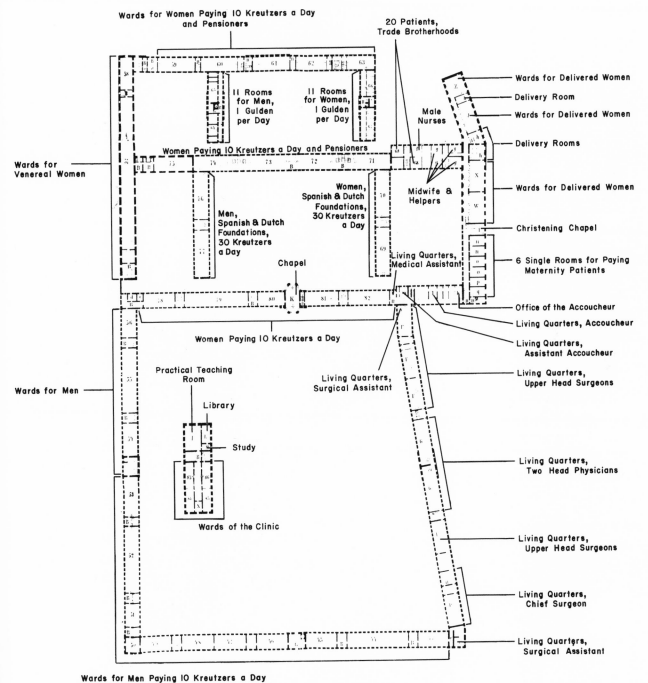

Narrenturm

Wards for Women Paying 10 Kreutzers a Day and Pensioners

20 Patients, Trade Brotherhoods

11 Rooms for Men, 1 Gulden per Day

11 Rooms for Women, 1 Gulden per Day

Male Nurses

Women Paying 10 Kreutzers a Day and Pensioners

Wards for Venereal Women

Men, Spanish & Dutch Foundations, 30 Kreutzers a Day

Women, Spanish & Dutch Foundations, 30 Kreutzers a Day

Midwife & Helpers

Chapel

Living Quarters, Medical Assistant

Wards for Delivered Women

Delivery Room

Wards for Delivered Women

Delivery Rooms

Wards for Delivered Women

Christening Chapel

6 Single Rooms for Paying Maternity Patients

Office of the Accoucheur

Living Quarters, Accoucheur

Living Quarters, Assistant Accoucheur

Women Paying 10 Kreutzers a Day

Practical Teaching Room

Living Quarters, Surgical Assistant

Living Quarters, Upper Head Surgeons

Wards for Men

Library

Study

Living Quarters, Two Head Physicians

Wards of the Clinic

Living Quarters, Upper Head Surgeons

Living Quarters, Chief Surgeon

Living Quarters, Surgical Assistant

Wards for Men Paying 10 Kreutzers a Day and Pensioners

Fig. 118. Second-floor plan, Allegemeines Krankenhaus. (B) Stairs, vestibules, kitchens, privies.

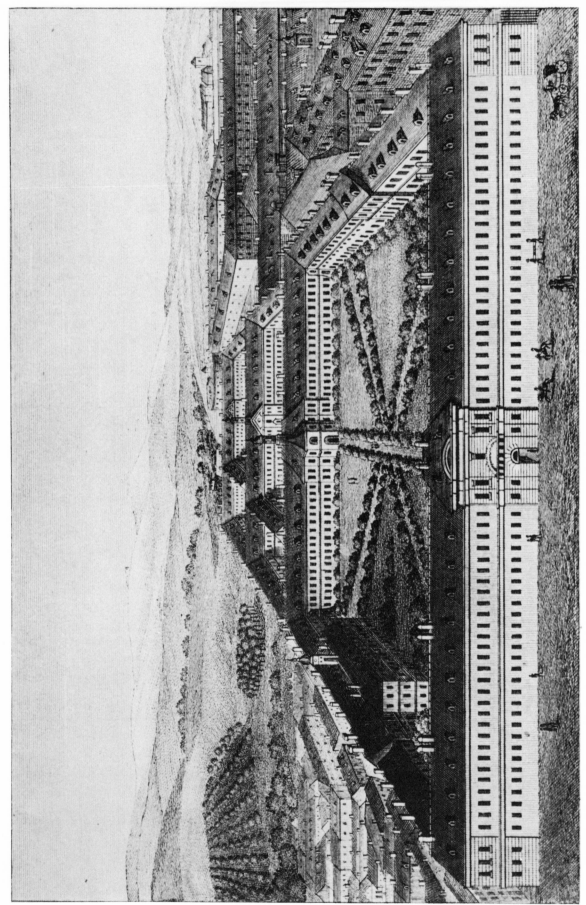

Fig. 119. Allegemeines Krankenhaus, Vienna. The gate to the right leads to the maternity division. Erna Lesky dates this print about 1834.

many citizens who would otherwise perhaps have been lost or made permanently ill, and of whom one can never have too many . . . since it is customary to draw conclusions concerning the wealth of the state from the number of useful inhabitants.[69]

This is an expression of the orthodox Cameralist doctrine (as the mercantile theory of the state was called in German principalities).

Hence the emphasis on a maternity house. The previous such institution for unwed mothers in Vienna was opened daily to every curious person and on certain days to the rabble; street urchins and common prostitutes were permitted or encouraged to come in to jeer at these unfortunates. By deliberate contrast, the entrance to the courtyard of the new maternity buildings of the Allgemeines Krankenhaus was approached by a private alleyway between them and the military barracks, it was kept locked and guarded, mothers were allowed to arrive "wearing masks, veiled, or made unrecognizable in any manner that they wished," and identified themselves only by a sealed piece of paper bearing their names in case of death. When they left, the paper was returned unopened. They could keep the baby, find private nurses for it, or leave it forever in the foundling house. The personnel were bound to strictest secrecy, and proof of a stay in the maternity house could not be accepted as legal proof in the courts.[70] One is reminded of a maternity house in Göttingen (1785) where the cab delivering an unwed mother could enter on the median axis, halt under a roofed rondel three stories high and surrounded by columns, and there let its passenger dismount unseen.[71]

In 1789, 72 of the 86 wards of the Allgemeines Krankenhaus had been made ready to receive patients. Inmates were classified according to disease: "those with hot illnesses are placed together, as are the cold fever patients, the dropsical patients, patients with crabs, or scabies, or dysentery;" there was even a ward for "those bitten by mad dogs."[72] Convalescents were completely separated from other patients, and venereal diseases were segregated "where no stranger will ever be allowed to come."[73] Within disease classifications patients were divided by sex. One more division runs through the whole hospital, an innovation rather shocking to a public long accustomed to thinking of the hospital as the abode of charity. Patients were strictly divided by ability to pay. This comes as no surprise in a hospital where—as we have seen—a leading preoccupation was economy in every detail.

The first class patients paid 1 gulden a day and received a private room. Naturally there were few of them, 40 to be exact. To the left of the rear court

can be found the rooms for men, to the right those for women, and in the right lower corner of the maternity hospital were 12 narrow rooms, each with its window, for wealthy erring women—"twelve neat rooms," as John Howard described them in 1791, "with every thing in them proper for *lying-in women*— a bed—drawers with white child-bed linen—a toilet —tea things—and a bed for the nurse."[74] The 6 rooms on the ground floor were partitioned down the center for an attendant, the 6 on the upper floor were all one room. It was assumed that patients buying privacy would bring their own servants.[75] Payment was by the week, one week in advance.

Second-class patients paid half as much, were lodged five or six to a room (Howard reports), and also paid one week in advance. They were separated by sex, but all ailments were accepted save chronic and incurable ones. First-class beds had curtains, second class none; otherwise bedding was the same: a straw sack with cushions underneath, a horsehair mattress with cushions over it, two fine bedsheets, and a smaller pillow for the head; in winter there was some kind of comforter, in summer a counterpane. Patients of both upper classes ate off pewter and were supplied with fine napkins and hand towels. Both classes had to bring their own underwear, bathrobes, and slippers and to pay for laundry. In the matter of food, those on an invalid diet were fed no differently from the charity patients, but those on the "full diet" got a great deal more meat, beef, stew, or roast, and, for first-class patients, chicken when it was to be had, green vegetables, plums or cherries or other fruit, and wine, at the patient's expense. One measure of wine cost a first-class patient 16 kreutzer, a second-class patient 10 kreutzer; our source does not say whether it was the same vintage.[76]

A third-class patient paid for a room per day a bit less than a first-class patient paid for a measure of wine: 15 kreutzers. For this he received a bed in a ward with anything from 18 to 90 patients in it, a straw sack with cushions, two bedsheets, and a horsehair pillow. An extra pillow was allowed when necessary. The hospital provided nightshirts, sleeping caps, stockings, bedroom slippers, and handkerchiefs plus daytime apparel according to sex. All items were of better quality than those given to patients in class four, who paid 10 kreutzers a day or nothing. Their full diet stressed such dishes as tripe, chopped lung, ground lunch cheese, or lung strudel. If patients of the two lower classes wanted bread, rolls cost a kreutzer apiece, and beer or wine 8 kreutzers, "by order and permission of the doctor."

A fourth-class patient had to bring a certificate of indigence from the pastor of his parish and the beadle in charge of alms. All on relief or pensions of any

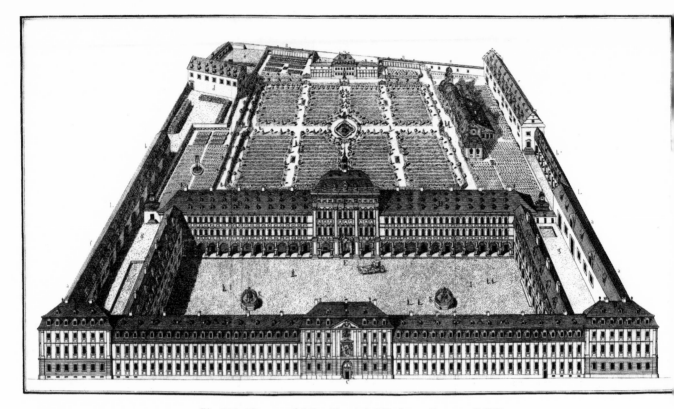

Fig. 120. The second Julius Hospital, Würzburg, Germany (1798).

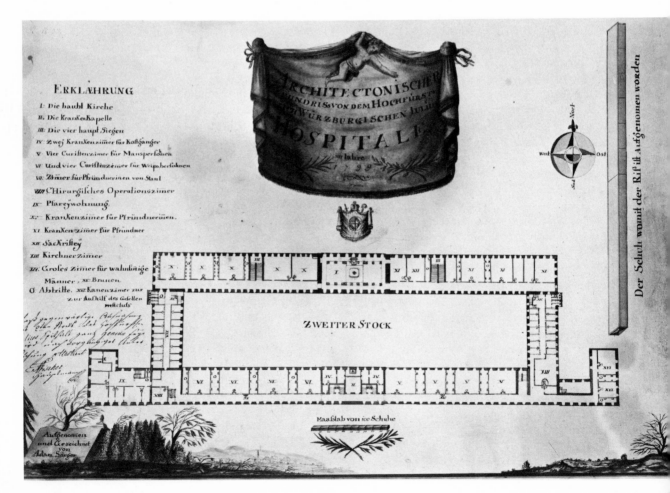

Fig. 121. Plan of the third floor, second Julius Hospital, Würzburg. Privy corridors run between multiple-bed rooms (see fig. 122); t
single rooms in the short wings were for pensioners.

kind had to assign that amount to the hospital while they were inpatients, which usually admitted them to the third class. Foreigners belonging to hospital insurance associations generally went into second class, the fees being paid by the organization. Servants were paid for their masters at the third-class rate of 10 kreutzers a day, save where the master brought testimony via pastor and beadle of *his* inability to meet the charges or keep the servant in his home, in which case the servant was accepted free. A similar schedule of prices applied in the Narrenturm and the orphanage.

On leaving the Allgemeines Krankenhaus, we may point out the chapel, a projecting steepled structure over the passage between the first and second courtyard. None of the sources referred to seem to have much to say about it. As Hempel puts it, "Faith was demonstrated in a rational way—a contradiction of its very essence."[77]

A German hospital complex comparable in layout to Frederiks Hospital in Denmark or the Allgemeines Krankenhaus in Austria is the second Julius Hospital of Würzburg, Germany (figs. 120 and 121). It is interesting to compare the eighteenth-century wings around this fountained court with the original structures that had one foot in the Renaissance and one still in the Middle Ages (fig. 82). In 1788 the rear wing, for pensioners, was rebuilt and its centrally located court hall became a church. The front wing for acute cases was added about 1789–93 after the old one burned down. The whole square complex was divided symmetrically by sex, women left, men right.[78]

It was an important building (destroyed in World War II and rebuilt with the same exterior facades but modernized interior arrangement). Here it is more to the point to discuss, by way of an eighteenth-century German hospital, the Krankenspital of Bamberg (fig. 122), dedicated in 1789, the year the cornerstone was laid for the southern (front) wing at Würzburg. The same prince–bishop, Franz Ludwig von Erthal, was responsible for both institutions. "The sovereign is for the people's sake, not the people for the sovereign's," he proclaimed at the Bamberg dedication. "His whole effort can be said to be to make his people as happy as possible." The new hospital was called a "temple dedicated to charity and medicine." As Jetter points out, the name of the Deity, significantly, was omitted.[79]

The main block of the hospital, facing east, was joined to two preexisting buildings that became its rear wings. The corridor omitted in Denmark and abolished in Austria was reinstated here, along the western wall, and 10-bed wards open into it in a fashion extremely influential for all "corridor hospitals" thereafter built on the European continent. Beds lie parallel to the windows, five on a side. Intriguing to contemporaries and likewise much imitated were the privy passages between wards, where closestools were kept when not in use. There was one privy stool per patient (a real sanitary improvement) and also one door per person to the privy corridor. The relationship of doors to beds cannot help but remind one of Milan.[80] An inner route from ward to ward at Bamberg cut across the privy passages along the window wall and served a double purpose. The central chapel was out of sight for all bedridden patients in this hospital, but the sound of the Mass could be conveyed to the women's wards on one side and men's wards on the other via the privy-passage doors. And at night the closestools could be emptied without bearing them through any patient rooms by way of the door from the privy passage to the corridor—a very useful planning device (no wonder it was copied widely and at Würzburg as well).

Wards for men and women, and for medical and surgical patients, were built on one standard pattern at Bamberg. Where they wanted a 5-bed ward they had only to run a wall down the middle of a 10-bed ward. They also inserted privy passages between 3-bed wards for contagious patients in the wings. A maternity house was added later to this teaching hospital, and an insane asylum was projected but probably never built across the rear garden. The symmetrical, classical facade recalls country estate models of Europe and America. The oculus in the pediment of the front elevation is above the chapel altar, but one cannot tell from the facade exactly where the chapel leaves off and the wards begin, though the sacred room is still marked on the roof by a slim tower.

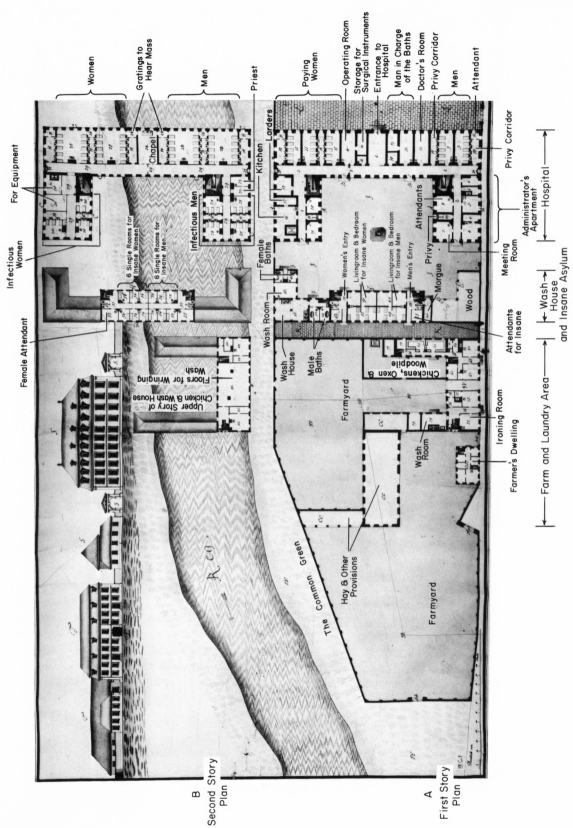

Fig. 122. Plans and elevations of the Krankenspital of Bamberg (1788). Figure 122b follows to the right of 122a, so that the areas read, from left to right: farm and laundry area; washhouse and insane asylum; then follows the hospital, all three stories of which are spread out; in front of the entrance to the hospital lies the botanical garden, which contains an anatomical theater (above) and the gardener's house (below); the site tapers off in a vegetable garden. A, First-story plan; B, second-story plan; C, third-story plan; D, gardens and anatomical the-

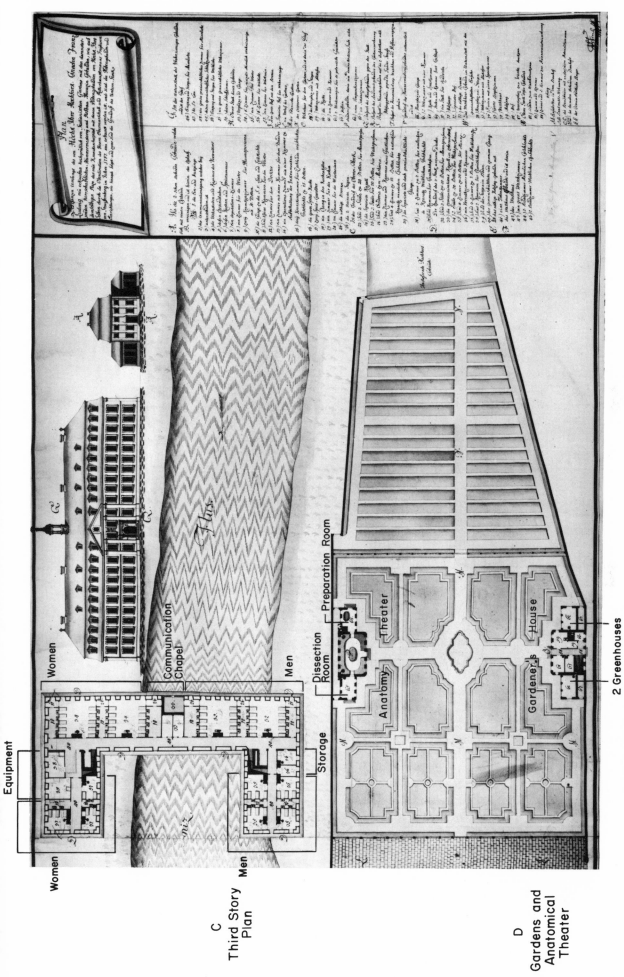

Women

Equipment

Women

C
Third Story
Plan

Communication

Chapel

Men

Men

Storage

Preparation Room

Dissection Room

Theater

Anatomy

Gardener's House

2 Greenhouses

D
Gardens and
Anatomical
Theater

Botanical Garden

Vegetable Garden

CHAPTER 5

The Pavilion Hospital: A Designed Plan

The Hôtel-Dieu of Paris and How It Grew

Wards of the derived hospital plans discussed in the foregoing chapter might have been rendered more sanitary by careful supervision, but they were not designed primarily to serve sanitary ends. The pavilion, however, when used for wards is a sanitary code embodied in a building. Pavilion in this sense means an open ward, but of limited extent; ventilated on both long sides by windows, on both short sides by doors; connected to a corridor that serves similar pavilions, but self-contained with its own service rooms. This type of ward came into use in the middle of the nineteenth century and the last examples are only vanishing now. For a hundred years the pavilion was the dominant ward form.

The pavilion hospital derived from the most dangerous hospital in Europe, the Hôtel-Dieu of Paris. Planners tried to guarantee that, whatever the Hôtel-Dieu had become in the eighteenth century, the pavilion hospital would be the opposite. One generally thinks of a shadow as being cast by light, but the pavilion form may be said to be a light cast by the shadow of the Hôtel-Dieu.

The Hôtel-Dieu was not intended to be horrible. Indeed, its guiding principle was the medieval and laudably Christian intent to relieve all who sought succor there. As the pavilion was shaped by sanitary convictions, so the Hôtel-Dieu was shaped by a dream of indiscriminate, boundless charity and clung to this principle long after smaller institutions discarded it as unworkable. With this one idea in its little head, the hospital body grew as immense as that of a dinosaur. It is amazing how long the Hôtel-Dieu managed to survive by adhering blindly to the extinct principle of receiving all who came, while other institutions of its species had either evolved or been wiped out. A brief review of its building history is not irrelevant for us, who also dream about universal medical relief of uniformly high caliber for an entire population.[1]

In the heart of Paris, then and today, is the Ile de la Cité, an island formed by a fork in the Seine. There are indeed two islands, the Ile de la Cité and the Ile St. Louis, since a small branch of the river flows between the two behind Notre Dame Cathedral. The old Hôtel-Dieu stood in front of and south of the cathedral, between it and the river. If one stands on the site today there seems to be no room for a great hospital on that quai: the space the buildings occupied was until recently filled by a quite small park and statue of Charlemagne. How the hospital fitted in, how it spilled across two bridges to the southern bank of the small arm of the river, may be seen on a late eighteenth-century map (fig. 123). It must be remembered that all plans of the Hôtel-Dieu henceforth presented will be topsy-turvy to our way of thinking—north is down and south is up. Thus on this map we must speak of the Hôtel-Dieu as having expanded from the Ile de la Cité on the northern or right bank of the little arm of the Seine toward the south and across the river to the Left Bank of Paris on the mainland.

As early as the eighth century there was a hospital on this site. Coyecque believes it took over a basilica that had been used as the first cathedral of Paris when the second cathedral was finished.[2] The Notre Dame we know is the third cathedral to stand here. Begun at the apse end in the last years of the eleventh century, this great edifice necessitated the relocation of the hospital, for the last two bays and western portal overlapped the site of the basilica, which had to be destroyed; not, however, before an entry chapel on the Parvis (the open space before the western portal of Notre Dame) and a first ward, the Salle St. Denis, were completed about 1195, so that patients could be moved in (fig. 124).

More space was needed immediately. The Salle St. Thomas was built at right angles to the first ward around 1210. The Salle de l'Infirmerie, in a straight line westward from St. Denis, followed in 1225-50 and ten years later the Salle Neuve was added with a chapel at the end of it, bringing construction up against the street called Marché Pâlu, which led to the little bridge across the small arm of the Seine, the Petit Pont. There westward expansion was checked. The area was already built up and at the time even the Petit Pont was lined with houses on both sides (Coyecque, p. 159).

The wards were large open medieval ones, two naves separated by a row of pillars, with altars included on

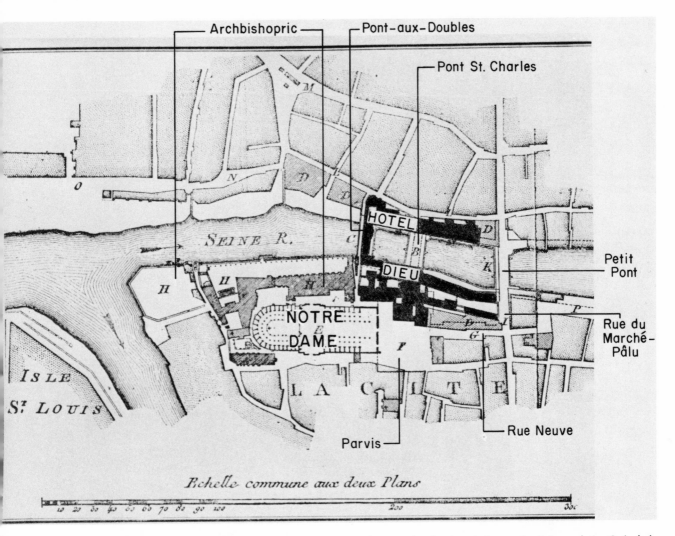

Fig. 123. Plan of the Hôtel-Dieu of Paris by Poyet, end of the eighteenth century, showing its relation to the Seine and the Cathedral of Notre Dame.

chapels attached. The Infirmerie was used for the sick and dying of both sexes, St. Denis for the curable, St. Thomas for convalescents from both these wards, and the Salle Neuve for women (pp. 63–64). Maternity cases were sent to the basement of the Salle Neuve because secrecy was desired for these women above all. Not until the sixteenth century did it occur to anyone to wonder whether someday the level of the Seine in flood might *not* stop a foot below the level of the windowsills (pp. 70–71). Windows were set high in the walls; although water did not actually pour in, the ward must have been extraordinarily dank.

There was no more building for nearly 300 years; the existing structures were simply patched and restored. In 1531 a new ward was built parallel to the Salle Neuve with a beautiful Renaissance portal on the Rue Marché Pâlu. This was for a hundred contagious cases, particularly plague victims.[3] The Hôtel-Dieu always had a problem with contagion and tried at least to draw the line at syphilis, which was prob-

ably introduced to Europe after the first voyage of Columbus and was immediately recognized as infectious. By 1495 there were a great number of syphilitics at the Hôtel-Dieu. A special farm outside Paris was bought for them and the patients were expelled from the Hôtel-Dieu. To the terror of the canons, they retired to the lands behind Notre Dame. Thence they were conveyed to the farm and a parish subsidy was mobilized, but one year later they were back at the Hôtel-Dieu in great numbers, and the farm was abandoned. Twelve years later special hospitals were decided upon, one for men, the other for women. No one would support them, and the Hôtel-Dieu received syphilitics for another thirty years—only one of many occasions when with infinite elasticity the Hôtel-Dieu of Paris returned to the status quo.[4]

A detail from the Turgot plan (1739; fig. 125) shows the hospital after the houses on the Petit Pont burned down in 1718: on the right bank of the Seine, from left to right, a row of private houses along the Rue

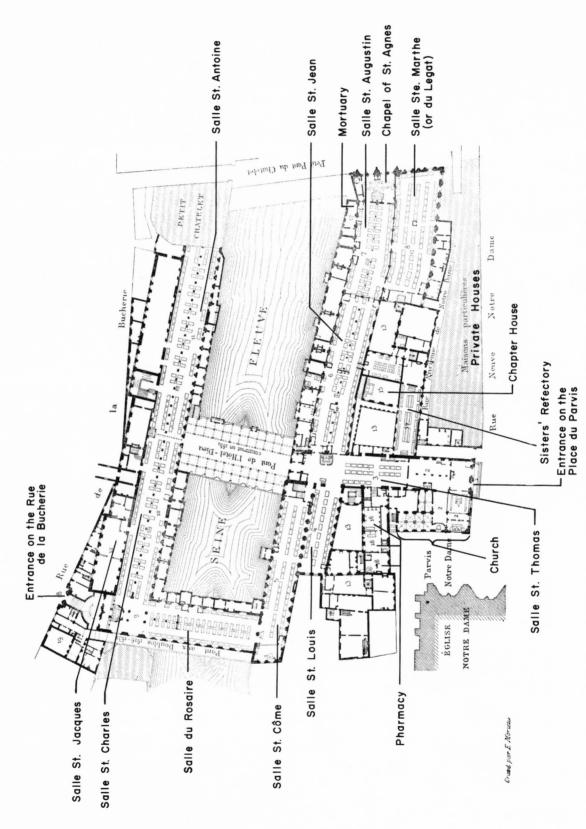

Entrance on the Rue
de la Bucherie

Salle St. Jacques

Salle St. Charles

Salle du Rosaire

Salle St. Côme

Salle St. Louis

Pharmacy

Church

Salle St. Thomas

Salle St. Antoine

Salle St. Jean

Mortuary

Salle St. Augustin

Chapel of St. Agnes

Salle Ste. Marthe
(or du Legat)

Chapter House

Sisters' Refectory

Entrance on the
Place du Parvis

Private Houses

Gravé par E.Morieu

Fig. 124. Plan of bed areas on the ground floor of the Hôtel-Dieu of Paris before the fire of 1772. All courts are numbered 13.

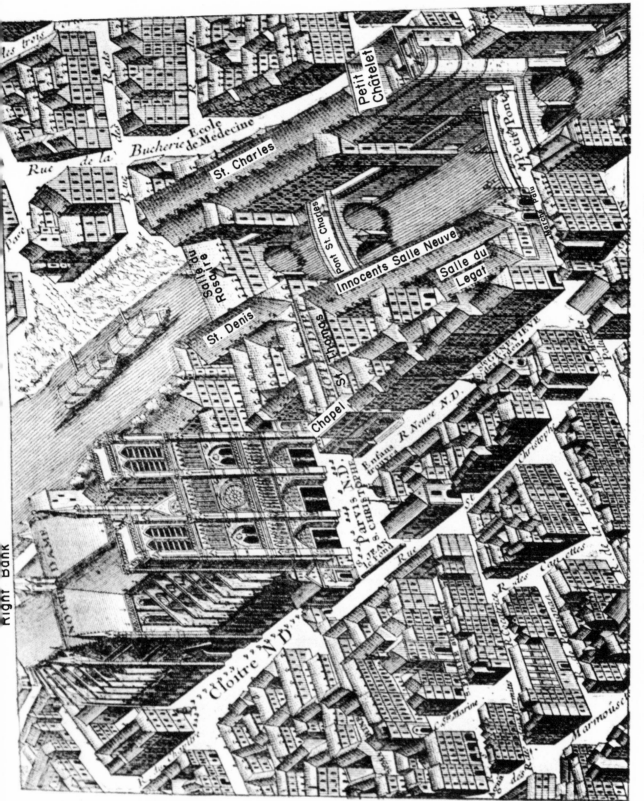

Right Bank

Cloître N.D.

Petit Châtelet

Ecole
Bucherie de Medecine

St. Charles

Rue de la

Rue

Pont St. Charles

le Petit Pon

Marche Palu

Salle du Rosaire

St. Denis

HOTEL Thomas

Chapel St. Thomas

Innocents Salle Neuve

Salle du Legat

R. Neuve N.D.

Enfans

Parvis N.D.

S. CHRISTOPHE

JEAN le fond

Rue

S. Martin

Ruë

Marmousc

Fig. 125. A comprehensive view of the Hôtel-Dieu, from the Turgot plan of Paris, 1739.

Neuve, the shorter Salle du Legat with its elegant portal, and parallel to it, along the river, the earlier series of three long wards that terminate at the near end in the chapel on the Marché Pâlu. Of these buildings, the Salle Neuve and Salle des Innocents lie under one unbroken roof, the Salle St. Thomas follows at right angles, and behind it the original ward, the Salle St. Denis. When there was no more room to expand on the right bank, the hospital received permission to throw a bridge across the river, called the Pont au Double because when a two-story ward for lying-in women was built on this bridge in 1626 (Salle du Rosaire), a toll foot-path ran alongside it that charged a small coin, called a "double," for crossing. Once the hospital had a foothold on the left bank of the Seine, expansion proceeded at a rapid rate. The St. Charles building along the Rue de la Bucherie went up between 1646 and 1651 and was then connected by an open bridge, the Pont St. Charles, to the original structures on the right bank that were more and more used as service areas and housing for personnel. By the early eighteenth century, patients were mainly kept in the new wards on the left bank. These wards were enlarged to extend clear to the Petit Châtelet, a small prison given over to the Hôtel-Dieu by Louis XIV in 1684, of which the Hôtel-Dieu made full use until its demolition in 1782.

By the end of the eighteenth century there were 2,627 patients in 20 wards on 4 stories (and possibly the attic floor as well) of the St. Charles building. Only 589 were left in the old buildings on the right bank, 202 in the wards on the Pont au Double.[5] Beneath the wards on both sides of the river were the *combles,* an institution unique to the Hôtel-Dieu that, like the hospital as a whole, "just growed." The wards along the river had been built out over the river to gain ground, but because there was a fear of narrowing the river at flood time, the extensions were propped up on stone piers among which the water could meander freely. Boats could thus still travel the river beneath the wards of the hospital and supplies could be brought by boat to the very doors of the cellars. As more and more storage space was required, the space between piers was vaulted and the floors filled in to form intricate, irregular, extemporized cellars for the laundries (all washing was done in the river, of course), storage of provisions, wine, coal, lamp oil, and so forth, butchering, candlemaking, and other functions.

How things stood at the Hôtel-Dieu at the end of the eighteenth century can be conveyed almost without comment by the floor plan of the ground floor of the St. Charles building in 1788 (fig. 126). The Pont St. Charles—sole promenade ground for convalescents in the hospital and also one of the few open spaces

for hanging out sheets to dry[6]—leads into the Salle St. Charles, with 110 *grands lits* and 9 *petits lits.* A grand lit held anything from three to six patients lying crosswise in the bed with the feet of one patient between the heads of the two on either side. When the hospital was really crowded, as during a pestilence, as many patients again were sometimes placed in an upper berth formed by the canopy of the bed. In the case of the St. Charles ward in 1788, the 110 grands lits held 404 fever patients (male) plus the 9 patients lying alone in the petits lits. The St. Antoine ward, also for male fever patients, had 29 grands lits for 116 patients and 29 petits lits. The St. Roch ward for boys from 3 to 14 years of age had 35 grands lits for 150 patients and 3 petits lits.

The only possible charitable comment on such a bed arrangement was made in 1666 by an English visitor to Paris: "Must charitie be blamed because she has a latitude of hearte?—to suffer all, to solace all, to do good to all? Must they be blamed for choosing rather to save the lives of two in one bedd, than to suffer one of them to die on a dunghill or in a ditch?"[7]

Each ward is a complete hospital, a bed space surrounded by services. Little rooms snuggled up against the outside walls to the height of the windowsills. These side rooms were used for nursing offices and nurses' lodgings, for the storage and distribution of food, bread, wine, water, straw, and coal, for linen storage, featherbed storage, dirty linen, and of course for latrines. There were separate latrines for the patients and the nursing sisters. Tenon reports filth backed up clear to the door of the passage to the patients' latrines (*Memoires,* pp. 207–08). Most patients used *chaises percées,* emptied each day right in the ward into a larger vessel (p. 171). The solid straw of the mattresses for the incontinent was dumped into the middle of the ward floor before being carted away (p. 209).

Over the service rooms, which were only on the ground floor (on upper stories service space had to be taken from the width of the floor itself) ran an uncovered walk, which was used for clotheslines. The same use was made of any vacant court, bridge, or walkway in this huge hospital on an insufficient site in the center of Paris. As Tenon pointed out, each ward had windows only on one long wall and thus all light or air from the windows was filtered through wet sheets (pp. 141–43).

There were two staircases in the center of the building, only 7½ fathoms apart (about 45′), in a building 65 fathoms (390′) long (p. 147). They operated as open wells to draw the air of the fever wards on the ground floor up to the surgical wards and operation room on the second floor. The third floor was shared by rooms for pregnant women, the ward for mad-

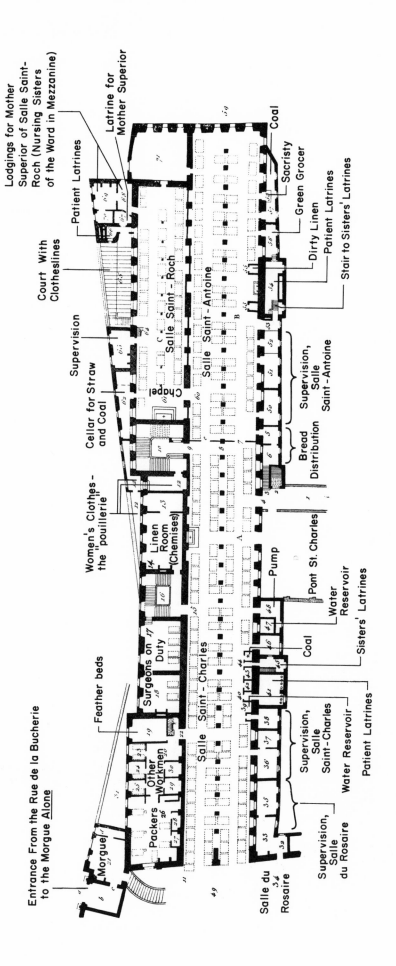

Entrance From the Rue de la Bucherie
to the Morgue Alone

Lodgings for Mother
Superior of Salle Saint-
Roch (Nursing Sisters
of the Ward in Mezzanine)

Latrine for
Mother Superior

Patient Latrines

Court With
Clotheslines

Supervision

Cellar for Straw
and Coal

Women's Clothes -
the "pouillerie"

Linen
Room
(Chemises)

Chapel

Salle
Saint - Roch

Salle Saint - Antoine

Coal

Sacristy

Green Grocer

Dirty Linen

Patient Latrines

Stair to Sisters' Latrines

Supervision,
Salle
Saint - Antoine

Bread
Distribution

Surgeons on
Duty

Feather beds

Salle
Saint - Charles

Morgue

Packers

Other
Workmen

Pump

Pont St. Charles

Water
Reservoir

Sisters' Latrines

Coal

Supervision,
Salle
Saint-Charles

Water Reservoir

Patient Latrines

Salle
du Rosaire

Supervision,
Salle
du Rosaire

20 Toises

Fig. 126. Ground-floor plan of beds and services, St. Charles building, Hôtel-Dieu of Paris, 1788.

women, and a crèche for children, while the same open staircases led up to the fourth floor to men and women with fevers and smallpox, the anatomical theater, a depot for bodies and, needless to say, a rich variety of miscellaneous services and rooms for staff. Services as well as beds were impulsively tucked into the St. Charles building wherever they would fit. Another aspect of the staircases to consider is that there were no other exits. If fire breaking out anywhere from the cellar to the attic found the airwells of the stairs, the patients were lost. Only one flight of one of the stairs (between the first and second stories) was made of stone (p. 146). The same stairs descended to the subterranean regions, where were stored 6,000 *voies* of wood, not to mention, in the depths of this incredible hospital, ample supplies of tallow, unguents, gums, resins, and oil kept not in barrels that might be easily rolled out but in vast leaden reservoirs.[8]

The stairs themselves of the St. Charles building, in their double function as spreaders of infections and of fires, account for many features of the subsequent pavilion plan: separate buildings no more than two stories high for separate illnesses, with no communication between their air supplies, with exits at both ends, with all inflammable stores kept at a great distance from the patient wards, across a court if possible and in individual sheds. It was stupidity, stubbornness, and sheer good luck that kept the Hôtel-Dieu mostly all in one piece on the same site until the middle of the nineteenth century, when it was finally demolished after a new Hôtel-Dieu was built close by in pavilion form.

There were fires throughout the eighteenth century. In 1718 the Petit Pont and all the houses on it burned down. The hospital took this as a solemn warning. All the buildings were visited, an overall fire-preven-

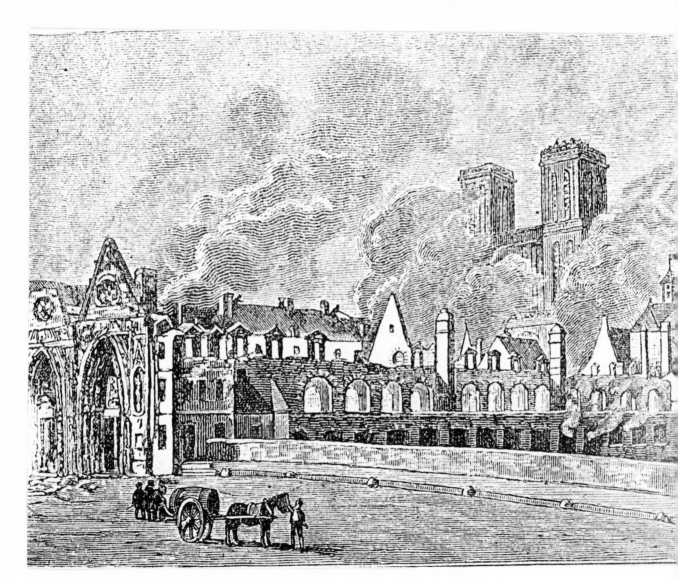

Fig. 127. Firemen to the rescue during the Hôtel-Dieu fire of 1772.

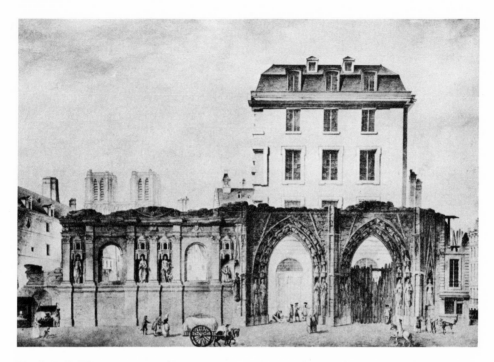

Fig. 128. Building the new Hôtel-Dieu within the shell of the old one after the fire of 1772.

tion plan was drawn up, firefighting equipment was furnished to all the wards, smoking was forbidden, and so on; this program was never carried through. But the houses on the Petit Pont were at least not rebuilt, thus affording the wards a new draft of free air that, it was estimated, saved 400 patient lives a year. The dean of the Chapter of Notre Dame supplied this figure, so it must be accurate (Fosseyeux, p. 258). In 1737 a fire broke out at night that the nurses thought they could handle themselves, and they shut the doors; by the time help was summoned there was general desolation in the wards and the patient population had to be moved to the cathedral. Services were held for the dead and a commission was named to investigate ways of preventing accidents from fire (p. 259).

The fire of 1742 inspired a general inspection and repair of chimneys and stoves that were to be repeated every three months. New rules were issued. Candles were forbidden on the shelves at the heads of the beds. "Rockets and fireworks were not to be let off within the house or in nearby areas by officers, surgeons, or servants, even on the eve or the day of St. John" (p. 261). One does not know if these rules were observed, but surely real reform should have followed the fire of December 30, 1772. It broke out in the tallow stores in the basement of the older buildings on the right bank and consumed the Infirmerie, the Salle du Legat—all the wards parallel to the river at that end (fig. 127). This time twelve patients died in the cathedral and a frightful turmoil broke

out in the press. Concrete proposals were made for relocating the Hôtel-Dieu on the outskirts of Paris; plans were drawn up. But the archbishop and Chapter of Notre Dame did not want to lose their hospital, and the prioress of the Hôtel-Dieu referred to the innovators as "perpetrators of projects inaugurated by a desire for profit." She vowed that "twenty-five millions would not be sufficient to make the new Hôtel-Dieu as commodious and vast as the old one, where all the buildings should be as perfectly distributed" (p. 266). She had to appear before Parliament and eat her words because Louis XV decreed in 1773 that the hospital population be divided in half, one half to be relocated, whereas for the other half all the present structures should be razed and rebuilt on the same site. But Parliament was really on the side of the conservators and by evading the issue for several years managed in 1781 to guarantee rebuilding of the burnt-out wards just where they were before (fig. 128).

Projects for Rebuilding the Hôtel-Dieu: Cross Wards

Plans for a new Hôtel-Dieu of a different size and shape on a different site must thus be viewed against a background of political frustration, hygienic outrage, and humanitarian indignation at the imminent danger to the poor of Paris, who supposedly had been gathered into the arms of an all-embracing Christian charity. The inscription over one portal of the hospital took on sardonic overtones: "Here is the House of God, and the Door to Heaven."

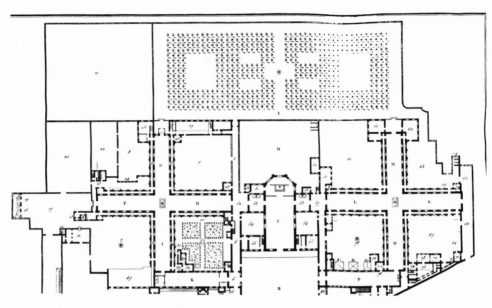

Fig. 129. Plan of the Hôpital des Incurables, Paris (1635–49).

As early as 1737, the suggestion was made to relocate the Hôtel-Dieu lock, stock, and barrel on the Ile des Cygnes (where the Eiffel Tower now stands).[9] They were still thinking in terms of a single monumental new structure for the approximately 5,000 patients. A year after the great fire of 1772, Jacques François Blondel, a practicing architect who conducted a professional architectural school in Paris, stated his preference for several hospitals to replace the very large one: "The sick would be better cared for, there would be less confusion, it would be easier to maintain them, the administrators would be more attentive; finally, the rich and fashionable would more willingly frequent the sites of these hospitals to succour the poor with their superfluous wealth."[10] In 1777 the king appointed a commission of the Académie Royale des Sciences to look into the problem, and during the next decade the leading scientific minds of the nation were involved as never before or since with the design of hospitals and with the health of the nation. The majority opinion was that the hospital in the center of Paris should be demolished and replaced by a mere first aid station on the island in the Seine and that four hospitals of a thousand patients each should be built on the outskirts of town, distributed as evenly as possible to serve the four quarters. What was demanded from the planners at this point, therefore, was the best and most hygienic plan for a thousand-bed hospital.

The outcome of all this eighteenth-century planning was the creation of the pavilion ward, which for a hundred years, from the early nineteenth to the early twentieth century, was the unchallenged inpatient accommodation. In a masterly essay, Dieter Jetter relates the triumph of the pavilion to the disappear-

ance of derivatives of the cross-shaped ward.[11] We shall accordingly first discuss further refinements of the cross-ward plan and afterward trace the evolution of the pavilion ward. As Jetter observes in this essay, although the architects almost never referred to one another, French hospital projects seem to an observer today but different stages of a single developing phenomenon (p. 155).

An early French cross plan was that of the Hôpital des Incurables of Paris (1635–49; fig. 129). The four wards in the cross to the left were for men, four in that to the right for women; the two great buildings were connected by a central church. This plan had the disadvantage for a city hospital of taking up a great deal of ground space, and furthermore, since a separate altar was required for each cross, two priests had to be on duty constantly. At the end of the seventeenth century Antoine Desgodet proposed a plan that would fit on a smaller site, that could be tended by only one priest, and yet that quadrupled the patient population of a single cross building. *Eight* wings —each two stories high—were to radiate from a central altar. The dome of the central chapel was consciously designed for the collection and expulsion of foul air from all wards opening into it (Jetter, p. 150).

In 1765, summarizing all thinking to date on the appropriate form for a new Hôtel-Dieu (which he took it for granted would be moved upriver from the present site), Marc Antoine Laugier suggested a similar form: eight radial structures three stories high with a domed church in the center (p. 152). The plan by Pierre Panseron for the Ile de Cygnes (1773; fig. 130) was more complicated: at the very center was a pump (worked by horsepower) instead of an altar, communication corridors that contained latrines radiated from it, and four-winged wards in the form of hollow squares were placed at the four corners, the bottom two joined by a cross-shaped church and the top two by a cross-shaped kitchen. Each ward contained 44 patients in four rows. Since the wards were on the second floor, the inner courts were filled in to second floor level to spare the patients climbing stairs. Buildings around the edges of the site were intended for staff, and semicircular lines represent gardens (p. 153).

In 1774 Antoine Petit proposed a huge six-winged radial structure around a central church (fig. 131), but one can confidently assert that he was much less interested in patients hearing and seeing the Mass than in hygienic measures. The hospital is a machine for ventilation. The church has a conical dome (fig. 132), which was not only to siphon off foul air from the wards but also to serve as an exhaust for the kitchen, apothecary, bakery, and laundry surrounding it at the hub of the wheel. The wards were to be great open pipes, and the beds are ranged along both long sides in four stories. The beds of the upper three stories were placed on balconies one above another so that a free wind might sweep the vitiated air along the open central nave into what Jetter calls the "cloaca maxima" over the central church (p. 154). How nurses were to ascend to those balconies to care for the sick was of secondary importance. "The principle of ventilation took priority over everything else. If poisonous gases could kill, if pestilential exhalations could bring about diseases, then getting rid of the pathogenic agents should be looked upon as the chief mission of hospital architecture" (p. 155). Jetter presents two other ward plans in which the most evident concern is effective ventilation. The one by Duhamel de Monceau (1752; fig. 133) was to have cylindrical apertures for ventilation at fixed intervals along a flat ceiling and extending above the roof. They could be opened and shut, depending on the weather, and on windy days an oven built into the pipe would set the whole chimney mechanism working (p. 151). The utopian plan of Maret for Dijon (1783; fig. 134) is shaped like a blimp and streamlined: no projections or indentations on the walls or ceilings, circular windows flush with the walls. The ward swells in the middle and narrows in funnel-shaped windows at both ends that are intended to capture the west wind. What happens if the wind blows north or south (p. 159)?

A plan for the ultimate in radial hospitals, utilizing every foot of the plot, was published in 1785 by Bernard Poyet (figs. 135 and 136). This wheel-shaped hospital for the Ile des Cygnes was to contain 5,200 beds, hopefully all single. Sixteen spokes represent the wards, three stories high, each ward containing 84 beds. In the center is the church, surrounded by

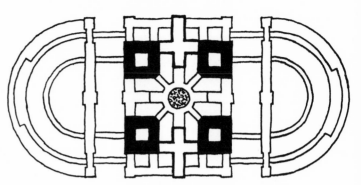

Fig. 130. Project for a Hôtel-Dieu by Pierre Panseron, 1773.

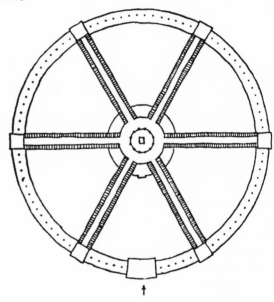

Fig. 131. Project for a hospital by Antoine Petit, 1774.

a circular court and open on all sides—a convention rather than a convenience since only ambulatory patients could watch the Mass there from the wards and few could hear it. Hygienic measures were allowed for: the hospital is surrounded by an isolation space and separated by a man-made canal from the mainland, a sewer runs under the building, and the wards are separated from one another by triangular grassy courts. Following a long tradition, privy passages for the emptying of closestools are allowed for between the heads of the beds and the long walls. Service stairs are on the inner circumference (which would save steps) close to storage and service rooms.

In the rim of the wheel are smaller 12-bed patient rooms inserted, one feels, rather to fill out the splendid architectural circle than to divide patients into medically manageable groups. It would have been wiser to leave open the space between the spokes, for what this hospital outstandingly lacks is a free draft of air in the central court and the grassy courts

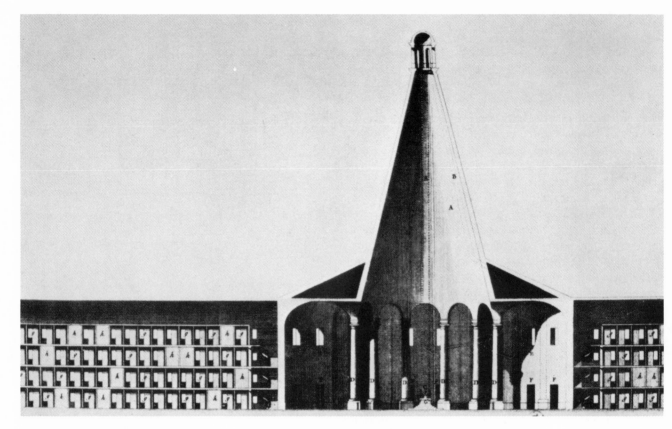

Fig. 132. Cross section of Petit's hospital project.

between wards. And, of course, in a circular hospital there can be no question of prevailing breezes or orientation to the sun. However, not hygienic considerations or economy in the utilization of land or convenience in the relationships among its parts is the overriding preoccupation of this plan. It aspires to grandeur, as is at once evident in the elevation and cross section (fig. 137). This proposal for a Parisian Coliseum was so enthusiastically received that Louis XVI was obliged to appoint a committee of the Academie des Sciences to evaluate it. The members pondered a long time before rejecting it.

With this decision by so august a body, Jetter believes, imaginative developments of cross-shaped plans over more than a century were arbitrarily brought to a halt (pp. 166–67). The cross-shaped hospital, characterized by John Howard around 1790 as the "usual form of hospitals in many Roman Catholic countries," almost completely disappeared, to be replaced everywhere by pavilion wards.

Projects for Rebuilding the Hôtel-Dieu: Pavilions

Pavilion plans continued to appear and moved steadily toward the final classic solution evolved by members of the committee of the Academie des Sciences. Before examining these plans, a disgression might

be useful concerning the evolution of the word *pavilion.* A dictionary of architecture defines pavilion as "an ornamental building, lightly constructed, often used as a pleasurehouse or summerhouse in a garden . . . also a projecting subdivision of some larger building, usually square and often domed, forming an angle feature on the main facades or terminating the wings."[12] Pavilions terminated the wings at Bethlem, for example (fig. 72). Pavilions in the playful sense of pleasure houses were constructed at Marly, Louis XIV's retreat from Versailles, a modest country house for his personal use that cost the nation 11 million francs (fig. 138).[13] The king's conceit was to feature himself as the sun inhabiting the central palace at the head of the plan and surrounded by twelve planets (i.e. courtiers), who were to dwell in six perfectly square two-story pavilions for men on one side of a large reflecting pool with fountains, and in six similar ones for women on the other.[14] Later, one of the pavilions was turned into a bathhouse and all the accessories of the baths were decorated with English lace.[15] A far cry from pavilion wards! But the separation principle was at work in the Marly pavilions, which were eagerly imitated at Bouchefort in Brussels, Nyphenburg in Munich (1702, single pavilions along a semicircle), and Clemenswerth in Westphalia (1736–50, eight pa-

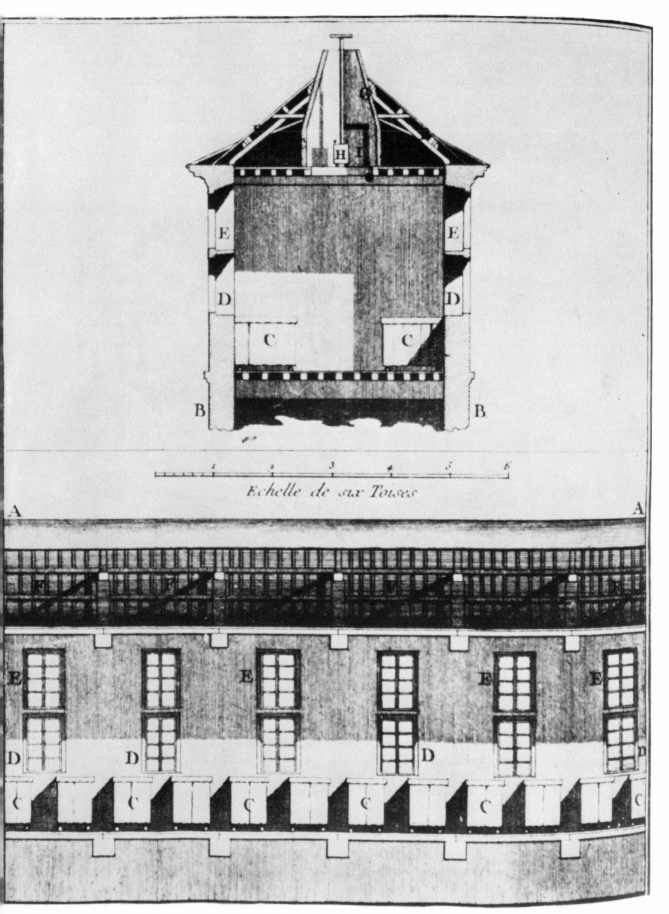

Echelle de six Toises

Fig. 133. Transverse and longitudinal sections through a ward projected by Duhamel de Monceau, 1752.

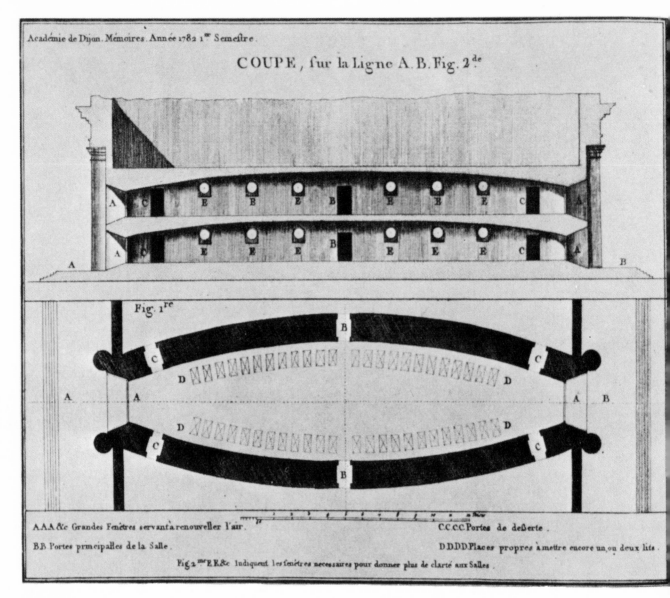

Fig. 134. Longitudinal section and floor plan of Maret's projected ward, 1783.

vilions around a central block).[16] Pavilions were thus in style in court architecture, which sets the fashion for lowlier forms.

The pavilion ward in its definitive form consisted of a long open hall for patients terminating in a square connected block for services, often of a different width or height—to which the first definition of pavilion can correctly be applied. The term for the part extended to the whole, and this application was probably reinforced by the concept of separateness that had adhered to the pavilion when it was thought of as a pleasure house.

Radial cross-wards are likewise composed of separate units, and if they are detached, placed side by side, and connected by some kind of communication building or corridor, they form a pavilion hos-

pital.[17] In 1773 Julien David Le Roy conceived of doing just that (for the first time in history, he believed), and, ranging twenty-two gigantic parallel Greek temples in two rows on either side of a central court "like tents in an army camp or like the pavilions of the garden of Marly," he put every square foot of the site to use as intensively as Poyet had done in his coliseum (fig. 139). The court architect Charles François Viel, in his drawings of this concept for presentation to the academy in 1777, tried to inject some variety by adding square courts for the administration and services at the entry and a semicircular court before the central church. Fifty-eight beds are shown in the plan as "a part" of one immense ward unit (fig. 140). Here is another wind tunnel: in addition to the free draft from one narrow end of the ward to the other

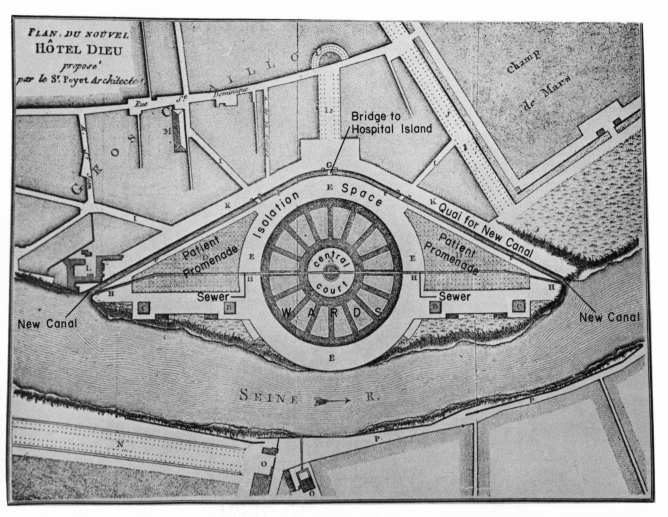

Fig. 135. Site plan of the circular hospital project of Poyet, 1785. The new canal was "to isolate the site of the new Hôtel-Dieu." B—B, "symmetrical pavilions for pumps to serve the house" (probably fire pumps); C—C, "identical pavilions that might be used as lazarets for contagious diseases."

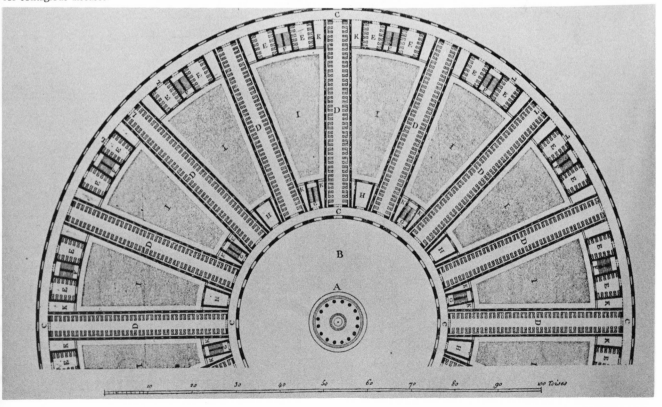

Fig. 136. Plan of the wards of Poyet's circular hospital project. A, Chapel; B, central court; C, corridors serving all rooms on the inside and outside of the circle; D, 84-bed wards with a corridor between the heads of the beds and the wall for closestools; F, main stairs; G, service stairs; H, service rooms; I, grassy courts.

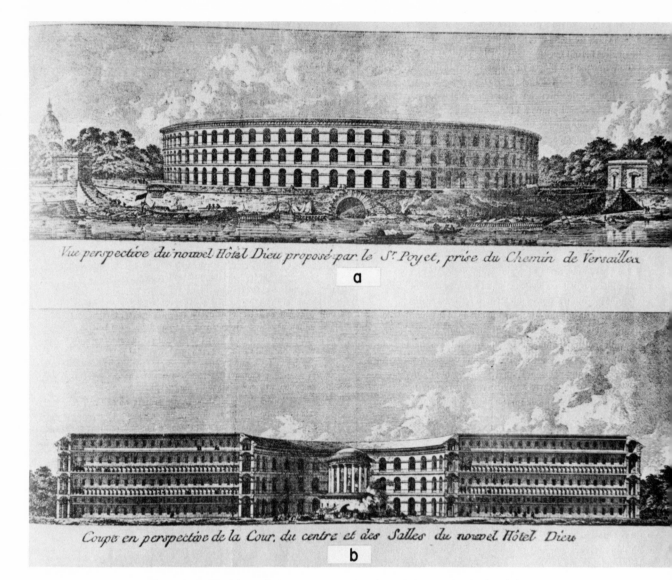

Fig. 137. (*a*) Elevation and (*b*) transverse section through Poyet's circular hospital project.

air is introduced by ducts from the ground floor and expelled through a row of domes in the ceiling, each of which terminates in an exhaust pipe and flag-shaped mobile extension that could turn with the wind (Jetter, pp. 157–58).

There are canopy-high partitions around each bed and two privy niches per patient. The ward buildings are porticoed on all four sides, which means that the connecting corridor from building to building would be open to the elements where it crossed the grand entrance to each ward. The entry vestibule recalls Tenon, who recommended such a room (which he said he never found in any hospital) to keep the ward warmed, serve as a distribution point for all supplies, and protect the distributors from contact with the patients. It was also to be used as a winter promenade and as a room for visiting to keep the ward quieter.[18]

Figure 141 shows Tenon's own detailed and much more practical plans for a single ward with its necessary service rooms. (Tenon had been for many years a physician of the Hôtel-Dieu.) The two square service rooms at the top of the page are supposed to be attached to either of the wards depicted below them. The ward of Tenon's figure 3 is for noncontagious patients and his figure 4 is for smallpox patients. The difference between the two lies mainly in the partitions 6 feet high and open on top for smallpox patients, thus sequestering them two by two—not to prevent them from spreading a disease all of them already have but to keep them from wandering off and harming themselves while in a state of delirium. The necessary vestibule is added to prevent contact between the patients and service personnel from outside the hospital. For better ventilation, small-

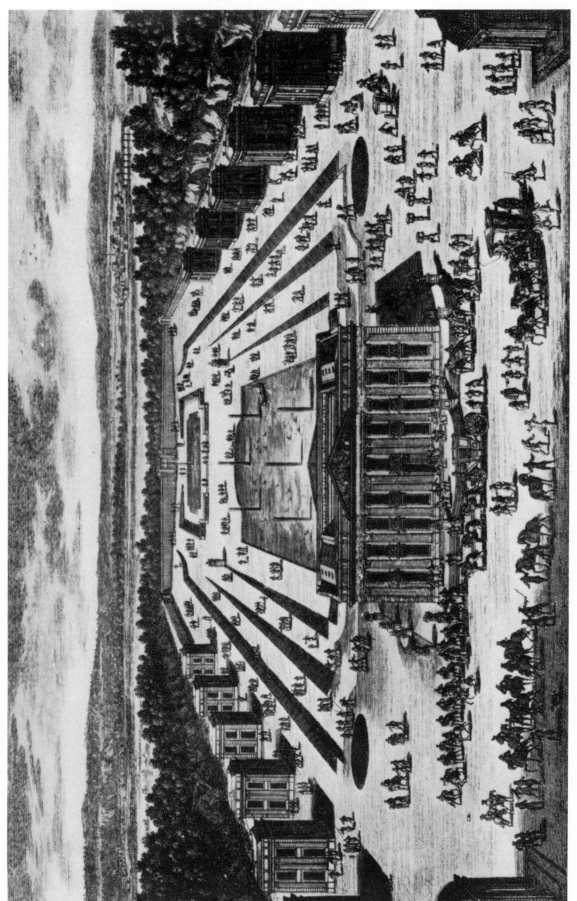

Fig. 138. Pavilions of Marly, 1695.

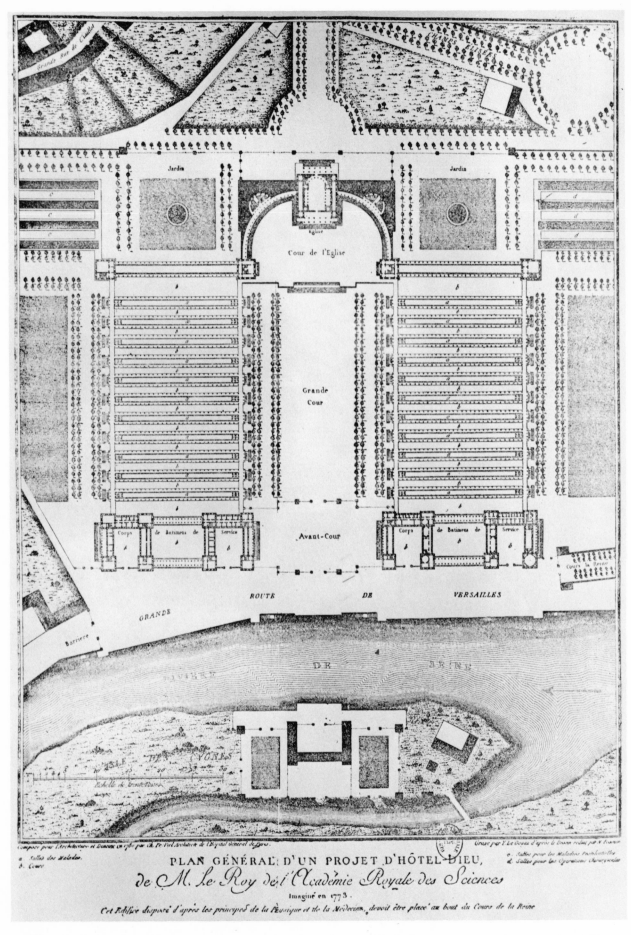

Fig. 139. Project for a Hôtel-Dieu by Le Roy and Viel, 1773–77. a, Wards; b, courts; c, contagious cases (top left); d, surgical wards (top right).

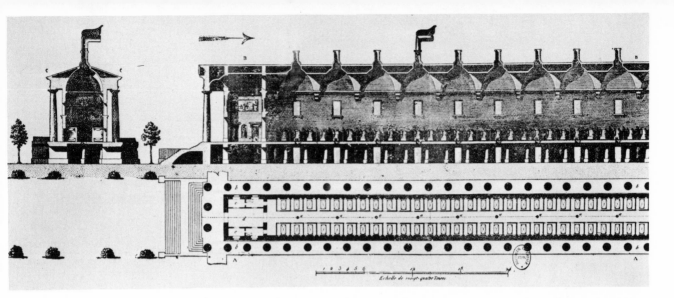

Fig. 140. Transverse section, longitudinal section, and floor plan of one ward of the project for a Hôtel-Dieu by Le Roy and Viel. a, Air intakes; b, service gallery; c, offices; d, vestibule.

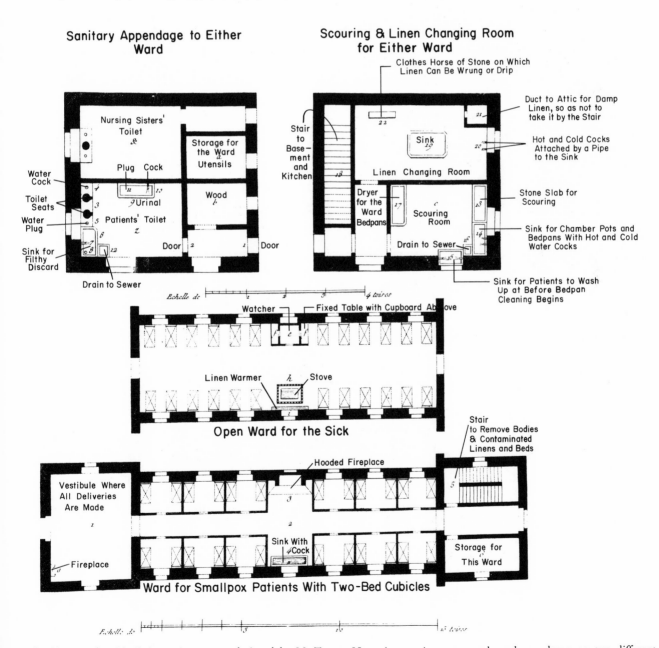

Sanitary Appendage to Either Ward

Nursing Sisters' Toilet

Storage for the Ward Utensils

Water Cock

Plug   Cock

Toilet Seats

Urinal

Wood

Water Plug

Patients' Toilet

Sink for Filthy Discard

Door   Door

Drain to Sewer

Scouring & Linen Changing Room for Either Ward

Clothes Horse of Stone on Which Linen Can Be Wrung or Drip

Duct to Attic for Damp Linen, so as not to take it by the Stair

Stair to Basement and Kitchen

Sink

Hot and Cold Cocks Attached by a Pipe to the Sink

Linen Changing Room

Dryer for the Ward Bedpans

Stone Slab for Scouring

Scouring Room

Sink for Chamber Pots and Bedpans With Hot and Cold Water Cocks

Drain to Sewer

Sink for Patients to Wash Up at Before Bedpan Cleaning Begins

Echelle de

Watcher   Fixed Table with Cupboard Above

Linen Warmer   Stove

Open Ward for the Sick

Stair to Remove Bodies & Contaminated Linens and Beds

Hooded Fireplace

Vestibule Where All Deliveries Are Made

Fireplace

Sink With Cock

Storage for This Ward

Ward for Smallpox Patients With Two-Bed Cubicles

Echelle de

Fig. 141. Two wards with their service rooms, designed by M. Tenon. Note that service rooms and wards are drawn on two different scales; both service rooms joined by a corridor would be only a bit wider than the narrow end of the ward (see fig. 142).

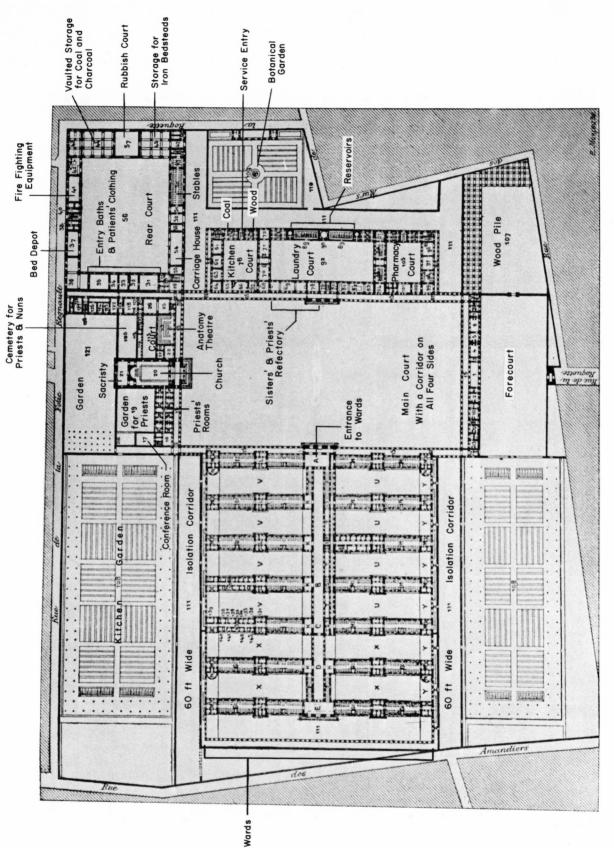

Fire Fighting
Equipment

Bed Depot

Cemetery for
Priests & Nuns

Vaulted Storage
for Coal and
Charcoal

Rubbish Court

Storage for
Iron Bedsteads

Service Entry

Botanical
Garden

Reservoirs

Entry Baths
& Patients' Clothing
56

Rear Court

Stables

Carriage House

Coal

Wood

Kitchen
Court

Laundry
Court

Pharmacy
Court

Wood Pile
107

Garden
121

Sacristy

Court

Anatomy
Theatre

Church

Sisters' & Priests'
Refectory

Entrance
to Wards

Main Court
With a Corridor on
All Four Sides

Forecourt

Garden
for Priests

Priests'
Rooms

Conference Room

Kitchen Garden

Isolation Corridor

60 ft Wide

Isolation Corridor

60 ft Wide

Wards

Fig. 142. Plan for a hospital of 1,200 beds for the sick and maternity cases, by Tenon and Poyet, 1787.

pox patients are given a hooded fireplace whereas the merely sick patients have a stove; this is sensible, but, oddly, a centrally located nursing station in the ward for the sick is replaced in the smallpox ward by a sink.

The most interesting aspect of both ward plans is that the nearly unlimited number of beds in one room at the Hôtel-Dieu (up to 100) is reduced to 24. Tenon says he would never place more in his largest wards, so as not to assemble too many patients in the same place, and in order to keep their number proportionate to the reasonable usage of the nurses' time and strength while giving the wards the requisite heat and volume of air.[19] He calculated that to avoid wards too high and cold or too low, warm, and fetid, their dimensions should be about 90 feet long, 15 feet wide, and 16 feet high for the sick or 15 for convalescents.

Now how shall these wards for a limited number of patients be joined together to form a general hospital of approximately 1,000 beds? (Tenon too was preparing a plan for one of the four new hospitals in the four quarters of Paris.) Tenon presented in his *Memoires,* as the *pièce de résistance* of his planning efforts, a hospital of 1,200 beds: 472 sick men, 310 sick women, and 422 maternity cases. He enlisted the services of Poyet, who embodied the sanitary conception in an architectural format and fitted the plan to the very site this branch of the Hotel-Dieu was supposed to occupy. The wards for the sick assume a pavilion form (fig. 142).

The plan is startlingly asymmetrical. Pavilions and services have been very carefully separated by the huge central court, which is closed below by a line of offices for the reception of patients. Opposite, in its traditional location, is the church, with appendages religious and scientific: priests' lodgings to the left and to the right an anatomy amphitheater, dissection rooms, and morgue. Lower court buildings still farther to the right are entirely given over to services: storage for the patients' hospital clothing and disinfection and storage of the clothes they came in with, bed disinfection (the iron beds were deloused with flaming torches) and bed storage, and the principal charcoal and coal supplies, vaulted for fireproofing, and separated from them by the dung heap, the stables and carriage houses. The oblong grouping of three courts to the right of the Main Court is for kitchen, laundry, and pharmacy. Service buildings and wards are surrounded by a service road 60 feet wide. Useful green areas include two large kitchen gardens, a botanical garden, and a garden behind the church area for the anatomical service!

Asymmetry prevails in the allocation of wards. The central gallery is not used to divide men from women but might contain an altar from which Mass could be heard upon opening the doors from all the wards (Tenon, *Memoires,* p. 371). Four men's wards at the rear open off both sides of the gallery and have their own entrance. Their section of the gallery is emphatically closed off, after which the front two-thirds of the gallery serves the women's wards: medical and surgical on one side, maternity on the other, with a separate women's entrance. Exercise grounds between the maternity pavilions are covered for secrecy's sake. The five wards are linked by an interior corridor (fig. 143) so that a maternity patient need only be seen twice in the public gallery: once upon arriving and again when discharged. The four beds for contagious patients at the head of each maternity pavilion, wedged between the two corridors, are given no windows whatever on the wider one.

Each pavilion is made up of Tenon's component parts: two 24-bed wards for noncontagious patients, practically unaltered, attached to a central service section made up of the individual elements of the service rooms in figure 141. Privies and wood storage are on one side of the corridor, linen changing and scouring rooms on the other. The service section, which is wider than the bed space, is what Tenon calls a pavilion.[20] The word had still not expanded to include the entire structure. Three of the bed areas are to be entirely given over to services and form the men's and women's baths and the reception rooms of the maternity section. Each building for the sick has its own vestibule.

Tenon's own project had neither the logic nor the classic simplicity of the plan submitted by the Hospital Commission and eventually approved by the Academy of Sciences (fig. 144). This too appeared in 1788 and also embodied the ideas of Tenon, one of the commission's most active members. Three reports were presented to the academy, in 1786, 1787, and 1788. The first was written after visits to a number of the hospitals of Paris, but members were refused admission to the Hôtel-Dieu, principal object of their concern. They had to rely on Tenon's many years of experience there and on his figures, which were sufficiently damning. In the second report they note that two of their members have been sent abroad to investigate foreign hospitals; travel being exceedingly difficult, the two commission members (Tenon being one) actually visited only certain hospitals in England. The third report presents a plan for a model hospital approved by all nine members of the commission and again translated into architectural terms by the king's architect, Poyet.

The final formula resembled Le Roy's plan as much as Tenon's—but Le Roy's plan redone on a sensible scale. (English influences will be discussed below.) Seven pavilions of limited size have been disposed

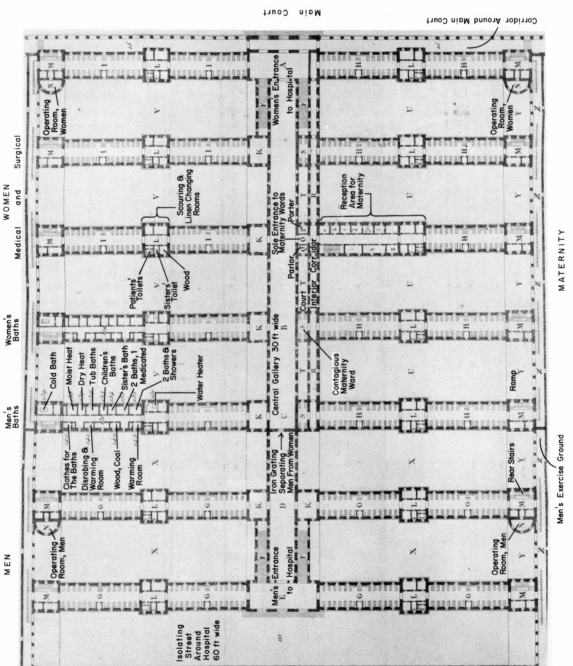

Fig. 143. Detail of wards, project of 1787 by Tenon and Poyet for a 1,200-bed hospital. G, Men's wards; H, maternity wards; I, women's surgical and fever wards; K, vestibules, L, service rooms for wards (for detail, see fig. 141); M, rear stairs for corpses and infected goods; S, 4-bed rooms for contagious maternity patients; U, exercise grounds for maternity (covered for secrecy); X, exercise grounds for men uncovered

to either side of a huge central court, and the services, to which Tenon had given courts of their own, are lined up along the top and bottom of the plan. The church with its attendant scientific and funereal-religious appendages is flanked by men's and women's laundries and drying sheds. The design is absolutely symmetrical: women left, men right. Patients' baths, storage, and disinfection of clothing are joined to the admission service in a long row of buildings at the entrance. Exceptions to the symmetry can be found in the middle pavilions on either side: the one to the left is for the kitchen and on the two floors above it are refectories and sleeping quarters for the female staff; the one to the right is for the pharmacy on the second floor, with male staff above. The planners had second thoughts about this location for the service pavilions and in a footnote suggested that it might save steps if the pharmacy and kitchen were located in the center of the court and the number of pavilions were reduced to twelve.[21]

The pavilions are separated from one another by large airing grounds for convalescents, who are completely cut off from one another to avoid contagion. The pavilions are joined by an access corridor on the ground floor only; in each building a staircase at the corridor end leads to the upper stories. In the *Third Report* of the commissioners, the word *pavilion* is used both specifically and generically: in the key to the plan it refers to the square service sections at either end of the open wards[22] while in the text it is used to refer to the building block as a whole.[23]

The wards have no more than 36 beds; the commissioners would have preferred 30. They were also strongly convinced that only a building one or two stories high can be kept truly sanitary, yet in the end they proposed three stories with an attic for the servants—but no basements save in the kitchen and pharmacy pavilions. One thousand two hundred patients in two-story ward buildings with only 36 patients to a ward would have covered too much ground.

All plans have their necessary limitations. . . . In order not to add a third floor, it would be necessary to increase the number of pavilions, to make 20 instead of 14, or to extend their length. In either case the overall arrangement would be made larger, it would occupy more land, more buildings must be built, service would become more difficult and exhausting. Economy of expenditure and the convenience of those who serve are important, necessary considerations; economy is a present necessity, ease of service a necessity all the time. Had we increased the number of pavilions, those at the ends would have been too far away from the kitchen and pharmacy, which

make up the service center; had the pavilions been extended in length, 50 patients would have had to be placed on each floor.[24]

The *Third Report* continues in words that are as relevant today: "Please note that the construction of a hospital for 1,200 patients depends upon a great number of components (*elements*): they must be modified, they must all be brought into harmony in order to combine them. One cannot accomplish each detail the very best way; one must keep in view the general result; it is above all necessary to be content with what is good, and to take away from the perfection of each part in order to make up the perfection of the whole." The planners conclude that "an isolated building intended for a hundred patients, divided in three floors or wards of 34 beds each, is healthful enough."[25]

Academy endorsement rendered this plan definitive. Building sites were cleared and the hospital was not built only because the French Revolution intervened. In 1821 a Bordeaux hospital, Saint André, was constructed along these lines, but the pavilions were poorly oriented, placed too close together, and the ward ventilation was defective.[26] The plan was used again in 1848 for the hospital of St. Jean in Brussels, described by a contemporary as "a stone pile possessing undeniable artistic qualities, a courtyard not without character, giving a certain impression of grandeur. . . . Unfortunately the architect did not take into account that, in a construction of this nature, ornament is secondary, and purity of line must be subordinated to the proper juxtaposition of its parts for hygienic and practical purposes."[27] Hygienic thinking had progressed beyond the best pre-Revolutionary theory. Nevertheless, simultaneously the plan was used in Paris for the first time, for the Hôpital Lariboisière (1846–54; fig. 145), and it was used literally because "too much care had gone into its devising for anything to be changed. It was rigorously respected."[28]

It is interesting to note the changes made in the face of this reverent conservatism. First of all, they built a smaller hospital. One no longer needed precisely four hospitals of 1,200 beds each for the four quarters of Paris; the Lariboisière had half the number of beds in three patient pavilions to a side instead of six. The height remains three stories and its relationship to the width of the intervening courtyards is about the same (the higher the pavilion, the wider the courtyard must be to get any sun). The service pavilions are relocated (fortunately not to the middle of the court): kitchen and pharmacy occupy, respectively, the left and right pavilions at the bottom of the plan to either side of the entrance. Dining rooms, later turned into drying rooms, have been added behind a communica-

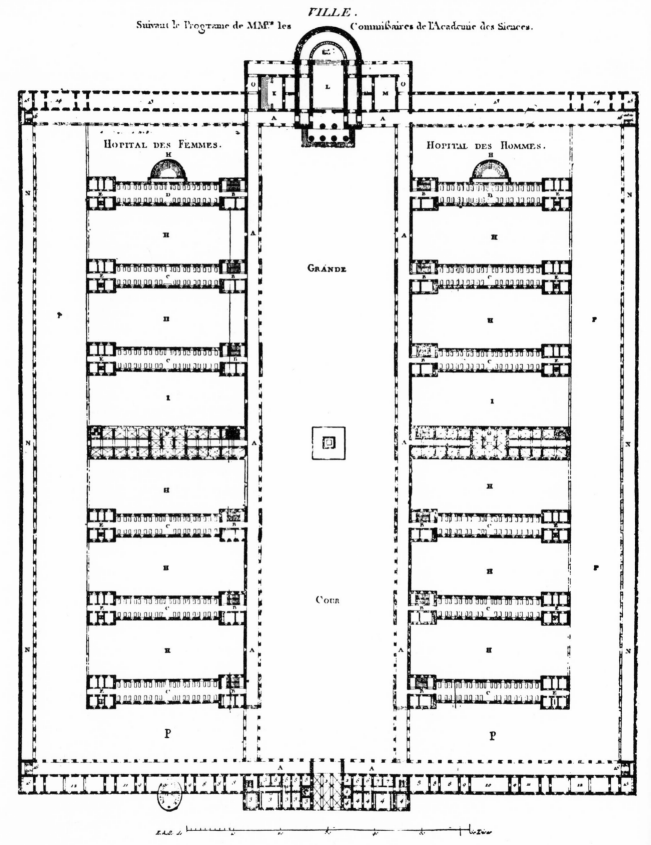

Fig. 144. Plan of the Third Report of the Hospital Commission to the Academy of Sciences, 1788.

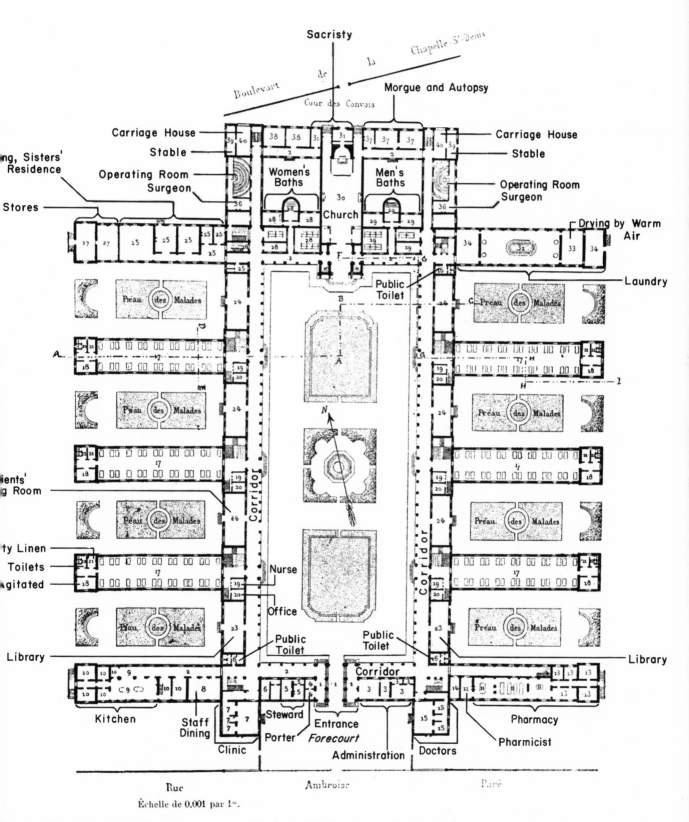

ig. 145. Plan of the Hopital Lariboisiere, Paris (1846–54). 17, Wards; 18, room for disturbed patients; 19, nurse; 20, office; 21, dirty nen; 22, patients' toilets; 24, patient dining rooms.

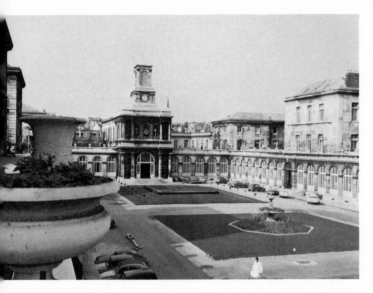

Fig. 146. Central court, Hôpital Lariboisière, in 1967.

tion corridor and are, like it, one story in height. A court has grown up around the chapel to accommodate male and female baths, and two laundries differentiated by sex are no longer thought necessary. Nevertheless, the layout is very much like the original plan. The hospital was oriented to the sun and the width of its courts prevented dampness; it was built of stone and brick and consequently fireproof; it was not too large for a single administration, was conveniently laid out, and was centrally located in the heart of Paris (fig. 146).[29] Surgeons of that preantiseptic age were saddened to discover that this model edifice proved no better, from the point of view of salubrity, then the other hospitals of Paris, "and they were reputed to be the worst in Europe."[30]

The Royal Naval Hospital of Plymouth, England

When in 1787 the two representatives of the French royal commission to investigate foreign hospitals departed from London, where all doors had been opened to them, and headed toward Plymouth, they were not traveling at random in the English provinces but making their pilgrimage to a hospital known to be "the most up to date in Europe, if not in the world,"[31] the Royal Naval Hospital at Stonehouse near Plymouth, completed 1764–65. John Wesley, who visited twenty years after it was finished, reported enthusiastically, "I never saw anything of the kind so complete; every part so convenient, and so admirably neat."[32] John Howard, visiting in 1782, described the layout in detail and reproduced in *The State of the Prisons in England and Wales* both a plan and an elevation but omitted in the latter the two front ward buildings he considered improperly placed.[33] One did not have to be a hospital expert to appreciate

the advantages of this hospital for sick seamen: sick soldiers were known to desert to the naval hospital and more than once had to be evicted from the wards.[3]

Tenon and his confrere Coulomb admired the cleanliness and efficient administration of the hospital, to be sure, but what they responded to with rapture was the fact that this hospital was the very embodiment of their pavilion principle. There stood, and had been standing for twenty-four years, stone buildings incredibly resembling the theoretical projects that existed in France only as architects' plans.

Although reason alone, without any experience whatever, were a sufficient assurance that parallel buildings, isolated pavilions, would be a healthful and salubrious building arrangement, it was still very satisfactory to find this experiment already carried out, and on a grand scale. The hospitals of Portsmouth and Plymouth, destined for sailors and the navy, the one containing 2,000 the other 1,200 or 1,400 patients, *are* laid out in parallel lines, and in isolated pavilions; with the distinction, that the Portsmouth hospital offers parallel buildings which are separated from one another by streets only 18 feet wide, where the air cannot circulate freely enough; while that of Plymouth, also made up of isolated pavilions arranged around a very vast court, has a layout almost like that we had already expressed a preference for. The hospital at Plymouth is known to be very healthful.[35]

The capacity of Plymouth, that magic number of 1,250 patients, must particularly have enchanted the commissioners. It was just what they were looking for. The patients were accommodated in five ward buildings on either side of the site, each of three stories (figs. 147 and 148) with two wards on a floor— that is, one square ward partitioned down the middle in the English manner with doors at either end of the partition. The wards, designed for 25 beds apiece were being used with only 20, and all were single beds. Only in pavilion 8 were there patients in the basement in two wards of 25 beds each, but these were reserved for the slightly ill. Most of the pavilions had no cellars at all. The cellars of pavilions 7 and 9 were used for the storage of beer and coal and for the mason's and carpenter's workshops.[36] The central building at the top of the plan was for the church, as one would expect, plus staff apartments and a dispensary. There was no pharmacy, because medications for this hospital were received from a central pharmaceutical supply house in London.[37] There were four smaller one-story service buildings, two on either side, between the ward pavilions. One was

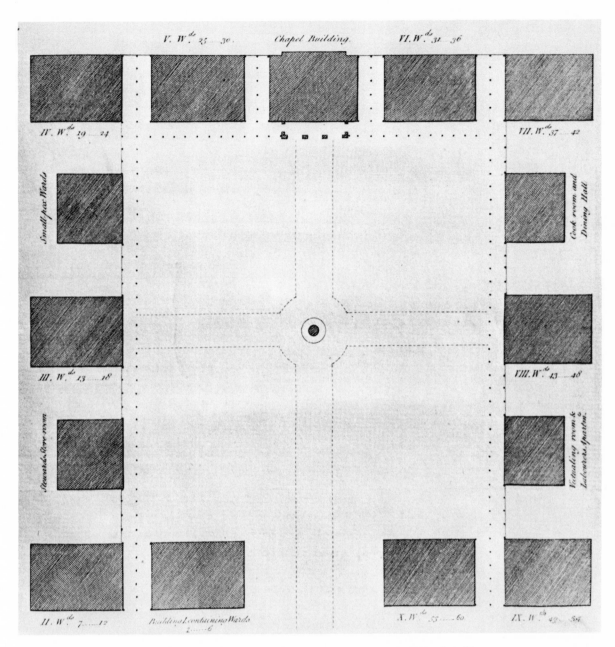

V. W.^{do} 25 . . 30 .   *Chapel Building.*   *VI. W.^{do} 31 . 36*

IV. W.^{do} 19 . . 24   *VII. W.^{do} 37 . . 42*

Small pox Wards

Cook room and Dining Hall

III. W.^{do} 13 . . 18   *VIII. W.^{do} 43 . . 48*

Stewards Store room

Victualling room & Labourers Apartm.^{ts}

II. W.^{do} 7 . . 12   *Building containing Wards 1 . . . 6*   *X. W.^{do} 55 . . 60*   *IX. W.^{do} 49 . . 54*

Fig. 147. Plan of the Royal Naval Hospital of Plymouth, England (1765).

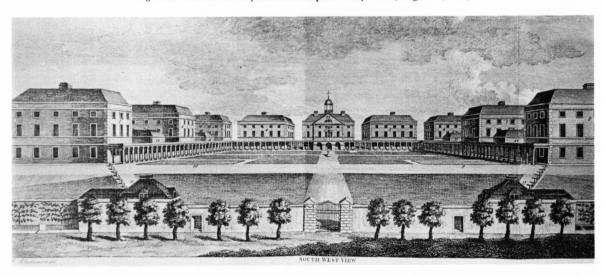

SOUTH WEST VIEW

Fig. 148. Elevation of the Royal Naval Hospital, Plymouth.

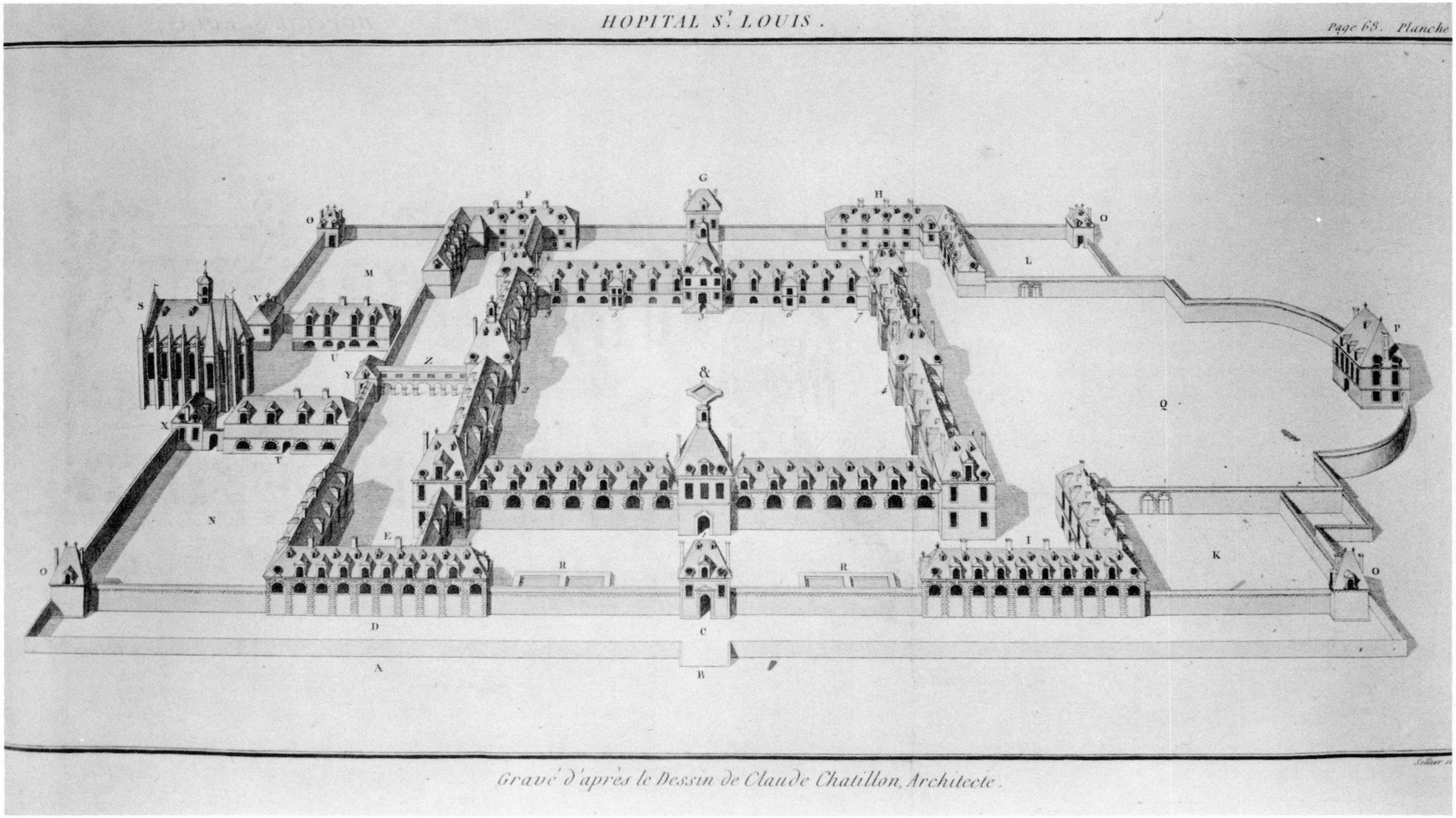
HOPITAL S.t LOUIS.
Page 68. Planche
Gravé d'après le Dessin de Claude Chatillon, Architecte.

Fig. 149. Elevation of the Hôpital St. Louis, Paris (1608).

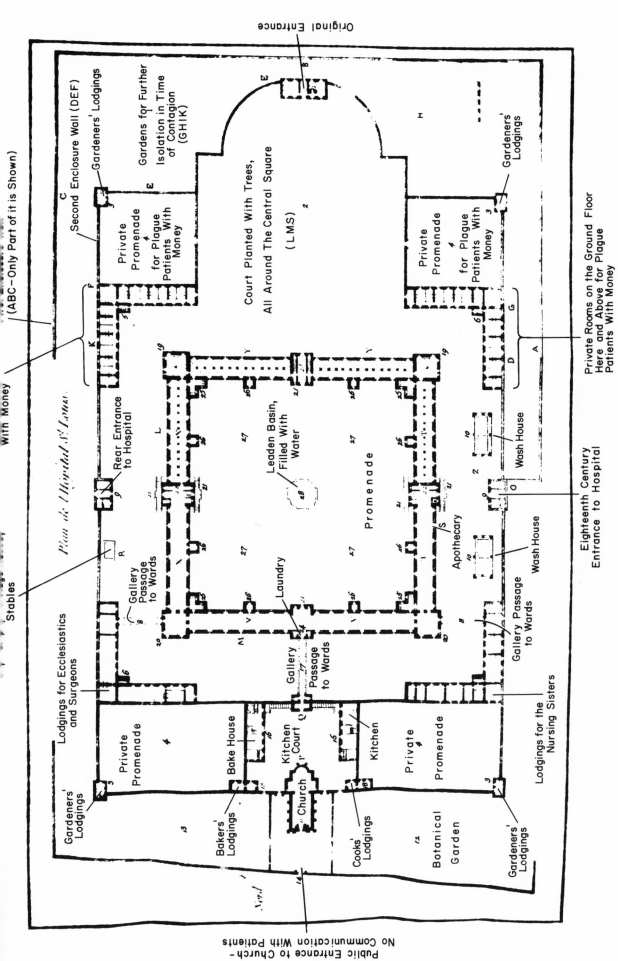

Fig. 150. Plan of the Hôpital St. Louis, Paris. The right half is a ground-floor plan, the left half a second-story plan. At the time, pavilions XX and VV were used for men, TT for women, YY half and half. Q, The crucial double pavilion for kitchen and bakehouse deliveries where the ward personnel called for the food; 19 and 20, warming rooms and chapels, two of each diagonally across from one another; 21, four structures in which were placed the baths, sweating rooms, and showers (three bathtubs each for men and women); 25, corner privies; 26, ward kitchens.

The following labels appear within the plan:

Original Entrance

Public Entrance to Church—
No Communication With Patients

Gardeners' Lodgings

Second Enclosure Wall (DEF)
(ABC—Only Part of it is Shown)

Gardens for Further
Isolation in Time
of Contagion (GHIK)

Private Promenade
for Plague Patients With
Money

Court Planted With Trees,
All Around The Central Square
(LMS)

Gardeners' Lodgings

Private Promenade
for Plague Patients With
Money

Private Rooms on the Ground Floor
Here and Above for Plague
Patients With Money

Rear Entrance
to Hospital

Gallery
Passage
to Wards

Leaden Basin,
Filled With Water

Wash House

Wash House

Eighteenth Century
Entrance to Hospital

Promenade

Laundry

Apothecary

Gallery Passage
to Wards

Lodgings for Ecclesiastics
and Surgeons

Gallery Passage
to Wards

Lodgings for the
Nursing Sisters

Private
Promenade

Gardeners'
Lodgings

Bakers'
Lodgings

Bake House

Kitchen
Court

Church

Kitchen

Cooks'
Lodgings

Private
Promenade

Gardeners'
Lodgings

Botanical
Garden

Stables

Plan de l'Hôpital St. Louis.

used for smallpox wards that very properly were one
storied with no other patients above them; the other
three were for the steward's storeroom, the kitchen
and dining hall, and a "victualing room" (the latter had
four one-room cells on the roof for the insane). Insane and maniacal patients would only be put up
temporarily until they could be shipped to Bethlem
in London.[38] Ward and service pavilions were linked
by a connecting corridor one story high with a flat
roof covered by lead, which served as an airing ground
for convalescents in bad weather.[39]

The French commissioners could not but approve.
All this was unique in its time. "In not one of the
hospitals of France and England, we would say in
the whole of Europe, except the Plymouth hospital,"
they reported, "are the individual buildings destined
to receive patients as well ventilated and as completely isolated."[40] They particularly approved of
the dimensions of the open spaces surrounding the
hospital: the immense central court (720' × 128'),
the promenades between pavilions (168' × 72'), and
the isolating street (72' wide) surrounding the institution.

But they reluctantly concluded that they could not
use the plan of Plymouth unaltered for a thousand-
bed general hospital to replace the Hôtel-Dieu. They
had stood long in the court of the Naval Hospital
trying to project upon the structures around them
the requirements for each class of patient they were
under obligation to provide for. Plymouth was a hospital meant for patients of one sex with a limited range
of illnesses and as such could not be more perfectly
designed. But for certain categories of patients it
would not do at all. In hospitals for both men and
women one must guard against the sexes mingling in
the communicating corridors. In hospitals taking
in children, one must make sure they do not run
away (Tenon, Memoires, p. 386). Maternity hospitals
could not provide the indispensable secrecy if all
patients were allowed to mingle in a common corridor. The maternity division must have its own services so patients may not be seen going to and from
them (pp. 387–88). The insane must absolutely be
treated in single cells, which could never be arranged
in any orderly way in parallel pavilions (p. 393).[41]
And pavilions used for the contagious would require
the addition of individual service rooms for the collection and cleaning of patients' mattresses, linen,
and clothing—at least as much to be feared as the
contagious patients themselves (p. 407).

However, there were elements of Plymouth in the
final plan approved by the Academy of Sciences. How
that French plan with an English antecedent recrossed
the channel seventy years later will be discussed in
the section of the chapter on Florence Nightingale.

Forerunners of the Pavilion Plan

Thus a trend toward separation operating on both
sides of the English Channel expressed itself in a
gradual evolution toward detached wards—for of
course the pavilion form did not spring fully formed
from the traditional rectangular, hollow, or three-
sided block in England any more than it did in France.
Two ward plans in the process of detachment may
now be examined in some detail, one French, one
English.

The Hôpital St. Louis was built in 1607–12 on the
outskirts of Paris as (finally!) an annex for contagious
diseases of the Hôtel-Dieu. Dieter Jetter says of
this complex that "the principles of its form deviate
to such an extent from anything up to then that it is
not possible to point to any predecessors."[42] Apart
from certain ventilation ideas that were imitated, it
had no followers.

At St. Louis they went to extraordinary lengths
to separate the patient wards from the outside world.
One passed through an outer wall, an inner wall, and
yet another space deliberately made too wide for a
patient to be able to throw anything from the hospital
wards over the inner wall, before coming to the wards
themselves, which were arranged around a square
courtyard (fig. 149). True, the planners were a little
inconsistent, and in two of the four L-shaped buildings at the corners of the inner wall (fig. 150) they
kept "personnes de distinction"—who suffered from
the plague. These rich and noble patients were pre-
dictably given single rooms and private promenades.
The other two L-shaped corner buildings were used
as living quarters for nursing and ecclesiastical staff
and for surgeons. The church to the north of the plan
could be attended by outsiders, who entered by a
special door in the wall and did not come into contact with the patients. It could even be used by personnel of the kitchen and bakery—but not by nurses,
because service into the hospital was planned to go
one way only. Food was taken from the kitchen and
bakery to a little building with a partition across it
and there placed on a turntable; personnel from the
infected areas collected it on the other side of the
dividing wall and carried it across a little bridge into
the central pavilion of one of the large wards.[43]

This central pavilion, into which both halves of the
long wing open and which is repeated on all four
sides of the quadrangle, was not only entry and service area and isolation area between the large wards
on either side, but it also ventilated those wards in a
manner unique when this hospital was built but afterward widely imitated (fig. 151). The earlier method
of ventilation was through a central dome, usually of
the chapel. At St. Louis, a wide opening was made

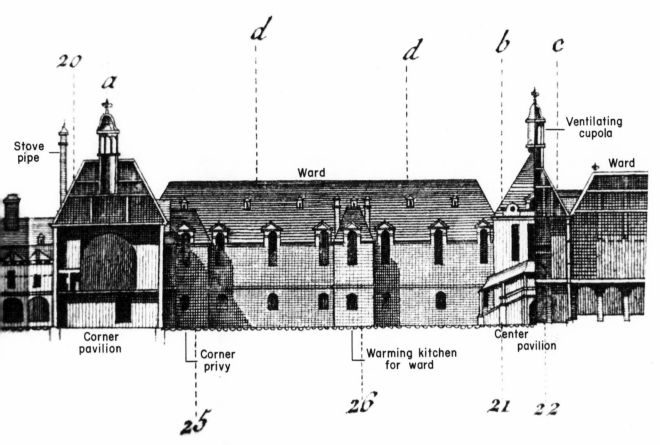

Fig. 151. Hôpital St. Louis; transverse section, elevation, and longitudinal section of the buildings comprising the top left half of the main square in the plan (fig. 150) and similarly numbered.

in the wooden barrel vault of the center pavilions, leading to a chimney that vented through a small cupola or open lantern above the roofs. Into the center pavilions the wards on each side opened widely by means of a very large arch. The four main wards were on the second floor, and Jetter suggests that the ground-floor halls, only half as high and divided by a row of central pillars, may have been intended not for the patients afterward lodged there but entirely as an intake for air, which was to be drawn up through holes in the floors of the main wards to supplement the supply from six casement windows opposite each other on the two long walls.[44]

Ventilation and the separation principle commonly go hand in hand in hospital planning. This hospital, by ingenious use of the four corner pavilions where the wings join at right angles, could be divided between men and women or between two different kinds of contagious diseases, or half could be shut up entirely when the plague abated. The system was simple: the two corner pavilions diagonally across from each other were used as altar rooms (though not architecturally differentiated in any way) while the two others were made into warming rooms by the addition

of huge open fireplaces—the only heat for the wards at the beginning; later three stoves were added in each ward, one at each end and one in the middle.[45] Thus the hospital could be divided in half diagonally, or even in quarters, and still each wing would have its altar and its warming room. In the corner angles on the court side were four privies nicely venting into a shaft that opened at roof level. They too were divided by a diagonal partition to serve the wards on both sides of them. Each ward had its own warming kitchen projecting into the court so that utensils belonging to patients with different diseases would not get mixed up.

The Hôpital St. Louis may thus be described as a large hollow square composed of four wings, each of which was made up of two completely separate ward buildings. The smaller hollow square created in 1729 by James Gibbs for St. Bartholomew's Hospital, London, had four separate ward blocks, one to a side (figs. 152 and 153). In both cases the plague was the innovative factor. There is nothing like a plague to make one think how to avoid it. It is not irrelevant to the new building at Bart's (which until then occupied an irregular medieval complex including a long open ward

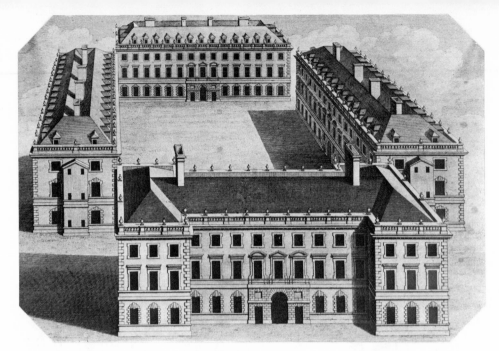

Fig. 152. The buildings by James Gibbs for St. Bartholomew's Hospital, London (1729).

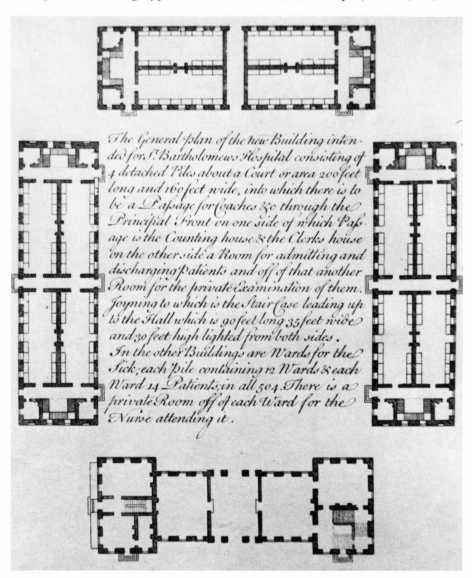

The General plan of the new Building intended for St Bartholomews Hospital consisting of
4 detached Piles about a Court or area 200 feet
long and 160 feet wide, into which there is to
be a Passage for Coaches &c through the
Principal Front on one side of which Passage is the Counting house & the Clerks house
on the other side a Room for admitting and
discharging Patients and off of that another
Room for the private Examination of them.
Joyning to which is the Stair Case leading up
to the Hall which is 90 feet long 35 feet wide
and 30 feet high lighted from both sides.
In the other Buildings are Wards for the
Sick; each Pile containing 12 Wards & each
Ward 14 Patients; in all 504. There is a
private Room off of each Ward for the
Nurse attending it.

Fig. 153. Floor plan of the four ward blocks of the James Gibbs buildings, St. Bartholomew's Hospital.

and auxiliary cloisters) that in 1719 the plague had broken out in Marseilles with especial violence.

The foreground block was for administrative offices, the treasurer's house, admission, examination, and discharge of patients, and the Great Hall, 90 feet long, 35 feet wide, and 30 feet high and lighted from both sides. In contrast, the wards in the other three blocks were lit from one side only. Ventilation was assisted by an open fireplace to either side of a dividing wall. The staircases were at the ends of the building with a private room for the nurse. When the buildings had to be enlarged, an attic floor was added to all but the administration block.[46]

In view of these early attempts to separate ward structures, it is startling to come upon a plan for Greenwich Hospital executed by Christopher Wren some thirty years before Gibbs's plan for Bart's (between 1696 and 1702; fig. 154).[47] It is in all essential respects a real pavilion plan—and was even intended as a naval hospital for retired sailors half a century before Plymouth. How familiar the courtyard looks: the colonnaded communication corridor, the row of oblong pavilions issuing from it comblike! The proportions adhere to much later dimensions, the cubicles or cabins for the sailors being narrower than the service rooms at the ends. The courtyards between pavilions are of a proper width. At the head of the plan, instead of a church, is Inigo Jones's Queen Anne's House, which still stands on the spot and which Wren was not permitted to demolish. The non-pavilion aspects of this plan were accepted and modified by Wren's successors at Greenwich: the hollow oblong approach buildings very roughly correspond to the Queen Anne and King Charles blocks, the two domed halls to the present Chapel and the Painted Hall. But the pavilions vanished. They had to be reconstructed step by step for hospital use on logical principles and from other predecessors. And Christopher Wren, after tossing off this bit of prophecy, dropped his connection with the Greenwich project and went on to build St. Paul's Cathedral.

Barracks

When the plague broke out in Marseilles it caused great anxiety in England, for the plague year of 1666 was only too well remembered. A leading medical practitioner of London, Richard Mead, was asked by the government for his opinion as to whether plague was caused by contagion and could therefore be excluded by quarantine, or whether it arose spontaneously from some quality of the air and was thus beyond human control. Mead replied with *A Discourse on the Plague* (1721), in which he combined the thinking of classical authors on the causes of infection with his own clinical observations. Winslow reminds us that the mystification of the best physicians of the time before the phenomenon of contagion was natural because there was not enough scientific information to permit them to make a more accurate diagnosis until the beginnings of our own century.[48] The general public could see that there was an element of contagion, but physicians could not accept a simple contagion theory of disease spread by contact between persons or through formites (clothing or other infected objects), because they knew cases where no such contact occurred. Such cases could not be explained until germs were regarded as living things (Mead thought of them as chemical entities) and the role played by rodent and insect vectors in spreading diseases was understood.

Mead reasoned his way through the five causes of epidemics proposed in the Hippocratic writings: the wrath of the gods; the epidemic constitution of the atmosphere; local miasmatic conditions due to climate, season, and organic decomposition; contagion; and variations in individual vital resistance (Winslow, p. 181). The first was not taken seriously after the Middle Ages, the fifth applied only in exceptional cases. What relative importance should be assigned to the other three? Mead came to the conclusion that both contagion and a predisposition of the atmosphere were in operation, that "a corrupted State of Air is without doubt necessary to give these Contagious Atoms their full Force," but on the other hand "it is evident, that *Infection* is not received from the Air itself, however predisposed, without the Concurrence of something emitted from Infected Persons" (pp. 186–87).

In the 1850s John Snow came to the same conclusion. His thinking ran as follows:

> No mere emanation arising from evolution of foul smelling gases can, per se . . . originate a specific disease, such as small-pox or scarlet fever; as well expect that the evolution of such gases should plant a plain with oaks or a garden with crocuses. The small-pox may occur over a cesspool as an oak may spring up through a manure heap; but the small-pox would never appear over the cesspool in the absence of its specific poison; nor the oak rise from the manure heap in the absence of the acorn which seeded it.[49]

In 1750 the British army physician John Pringle presented his *Observations on the Nature and Cure of Hospital and Jayl-Fevers* in the form of an open letter to Dr. Mead. This little volume went through numerous editions and was widely quoted and of great influence in England and the United States. It bluntly attributed contagion to "a corruption of the air, pent up and deprived of its elastic parts by the respiration of a multitude, or more particularly vitiated with the

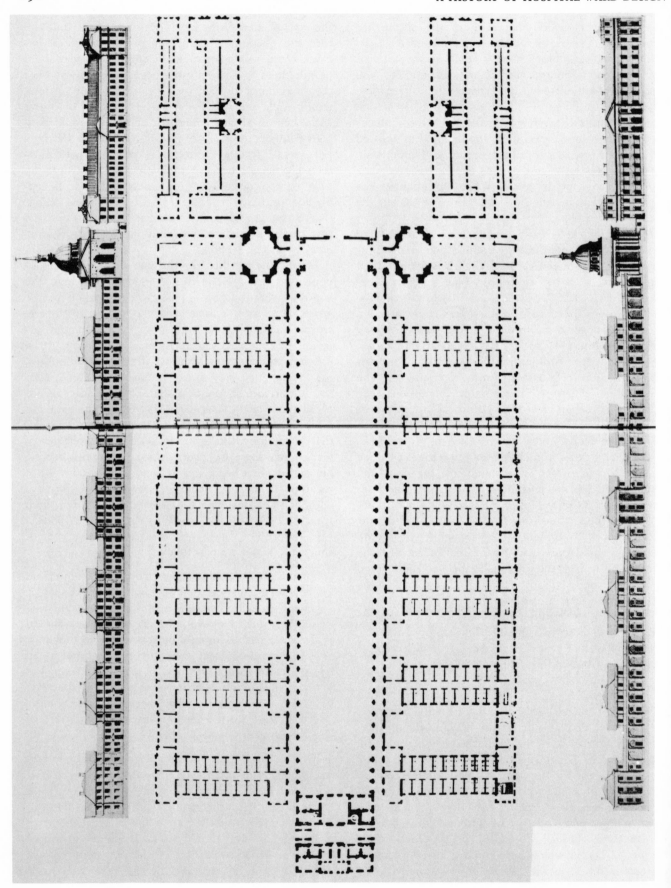

perspirable matter, which, as it is the most volatile part of the humours, is also the most putrescent."[50] Pringle concluded that "upon this account, jayls and military hospitals, are most obnoxious to this kind of pestilential infection; as the first are kept in a constant state of filth and impurity; and the last are so much filled with the poisonous *effluvia* of sores, mortifications, dysenteric and other putrid excrements" (p. 8).

Pringle relates a hair-raising experience with a fever that seized all the patients of a crowded military hospital in Germany during one of the English campaigns in that country. Although what the patients had been hospitalized for was dysentery, half of them died of the fever (probably typhus), all the attendants caught it, and some died. Furthermore, the inhabitants of a nearby village fell prey either to the dysentery or the fever and between the two were almost utterly destroyed (p. 11).

An American army doctor, James Tilton, quoted Pringle's experience in Germany and topped it with one of his own during the Revolutionary War:

> At Bethlehem [Pa.] was another hospital, and I found it convenient to rest there a day or two. During my stay, it was natural to enquire into the state of their hospital. The method I took was to propose a competition, not whose hospital had done the most good, but whose hospital had done the most mischief. I was requested to give an account of Princeton hospital; I stated with all the exaggeration I could with truth, not only an affecting mortality among the sick and wounded soldiers, but that the orderly men, nurses and other attendants on the hospital were liable to the infection; that I had myself narrowly escaped death; and that five other surgeons and mates had afterwards been seized. I was answered that the malignancy and mortality of Princeton hospital bore no comparison with theirs; that at Bethlehem not an orderly man or nurse escaped, and but few of the surgeons. . . . One of the surgeons asked me if I were acquainted with that fine volunteer regiment of Virginia. . . . Forty of that regiment had come to their hospital, and then asked me how many I supposed would ever join the regiment? I guessed a third or a fourth part. He declared solemnly that not three would ever return, that one man had joined his regiment; that another was convalescent and might possibly recover; but that the only remaining one besides, was in the last stage of the colliquative flux [dysentery] and must soon die.[51]

The problem that arose in military hospitals was equally acute in civilian hospitals. A solution was discovered by the military almost by chance. Armies

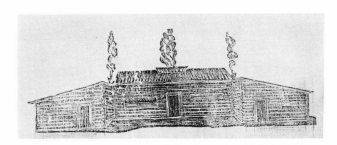

Fig. 155. Elevation of James Tilton's Indian Hut, 1779.

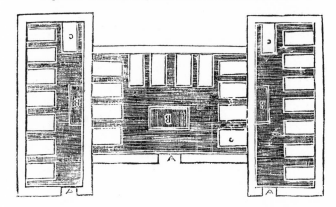

Fig. 156. Floor plan of Tilton's Indian hut. A, Doorways; B, fireplaces; C, beds.

are often forced to improvise lodgings, both for sick soldiers and well, and it might often happen that the hospitals of an occupied town would be filled to overflowing while casualties were still being brought in. They had to be put somewhere; they were piled in barns or deposited on haylofts. The astonishing thing was that the patients in the hospitals died and the patients in the barns, exposed to cold and inadequately attended, were the ones who recovered.

Pringle advises that "the sick should not be sent to one common hospital. . . . Barns, granaries, and the like places, will allow the steams to disperse. . . . It is common to look out for close and warm houses, and therefore to prefer a peasant's house to his barn; but experience has convinced us, that air more than warmth is requisite."[52] During the Revolutionary War, John Jones reports, "by the judicious advice of Dr. Rush . . . the patients were carried out every day and placed under apple trees, where they recovered with astonishing rapidity."[53] James Tilton, from his experiences during that war, recommended tents, "common horseman's tents, and long tents formed like the roof of an house prepared expressly for hospital purposes."[54] For cold climates and the winter season he designed a kind of log cabin, which he called an "Indian hut," affirming that it was the best hospital he ever contrived (figs. 155 and 156).

The fire was built in the midst of the ward, without any chimney, and the smoke circulating round

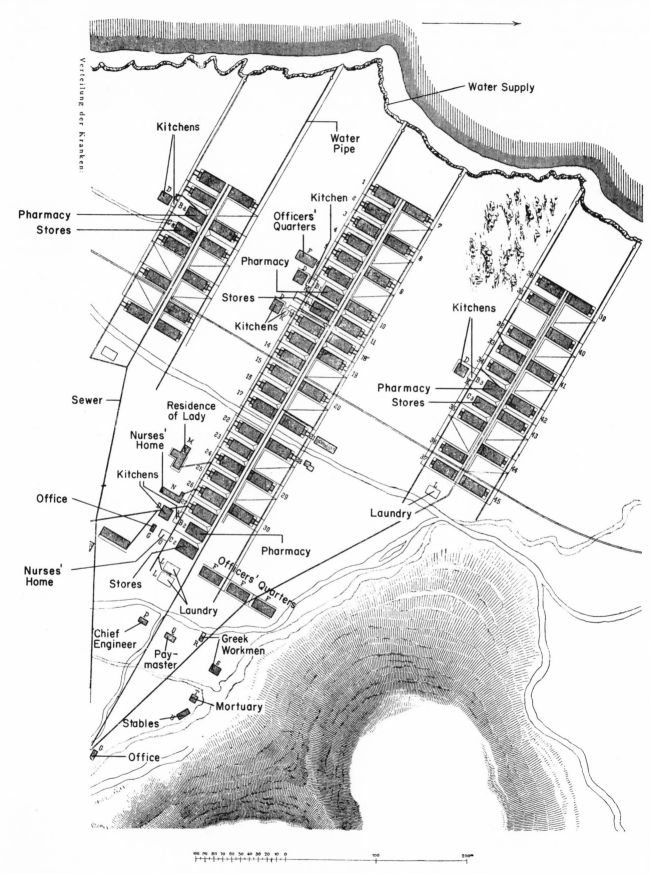

Verteilung der Kranken:

Water Supply

Kitchens

Water Pipe

Pharmacy
Stores

Officers'
Quarters

Kitchen

Pharmacy

Stores

Kitchens

Kitchens

Sewer

Pharmacy
Stores

Residence
of Lady

Nurses'
Home

Kitchens

Office

Laundry

Nurses'
Home

Stores

Laundry

Pharmacy

Officers' Quarters

Chief
Engineer

Pay-
master

Greek
Workmen

Mortuary

Stables

Office

Fig. 157. Site of the British barracks hospital at Renkioi, Turkey, 1855.

about, passed off thro' an opening about four inches wide in the ridge of the roof. The common surface of the earth served for the floor. The patients laid with their heads to the wall round about, and their feet were all turned to the fire. The wards were thus completely ventilated. The smoke contributed to combat infection, without giving the least offence to the patients: for it always rose above their heads, before it spread abroad in the ward. And more patients could be crowded with impunity in such wards, than in any others I have seen tried. This was the expedient I employed in the hard winter of 79, 80, when the army was hutted near Morris Town, and I was well satisfied with the experiment. . . . The smoke passes off through funnels elevated above the roof . . . one window is open and the others shut . . . all the air and light are let in from the south front. . . . It should be noted also that the walls of this hut were built of rough logs, without hewing; that the chinks were daubed with mortar made of common clay and water only; that the middle or main ward 31 1.2 feet by 19 1.2 in the clear was assigned to febrile patients; and the smaller end wards 35 1.2 by 16 feet clear were occupied by the wounded and other cases of topical affection.[55]

This is only one instance when a decisive step forward in the building of hospitals was accomplished by the military. It will be remembered that Plymouth was a naval hospital, and one suspects that its contemporary reputation owed as much to the orderliness with which it was administered as to the architectural form in which it was built. Not surprisingly, major improvements were achieved during wars, under extraordinary pressure to get the job done efficiently and cheaply. Economy, efficiency, ease of supervision, and intense concern for a sanitary environment are all to be found in the design by Isambard Brunel for a barracks hospital for British troops during the Crimean War. (Note: he was not an architect but a civil engineer.) The hospital was erected in 1855 near the small Turkish village of Renkioi, a site deliberately selected for its gradual slope seaward, light, porous, sandy soil, and proximity to the sea in front for water transport and sewage disposal, and to ample springs at the rear. (fig. 157).[56]

Renkioi was a prefabricated hospital whose basic unit for 50 patients was a wooden hut of the lightest, cheapest construction possible. An experimental model was set up on the premises of the Great Western Railway at Paddington and carefully criticized. It had to be self-sufficient—two ward rooms, one nurse's room (orderlies' bedroom), a small storeroom, a bath-room, surgery (medical officer's room), water closets, and lavatories (fig. 158)—because it was to be shipped a very great distance, and other parts of the hospital might not arrive at the same time. For the same reason, it must be built of lightweight materials: wood covered by extremely thin and highly polished tin to insulate from the heat. Also, every bit of woodwork not covered by tin was to be whitewashed inside and out. In winter, insulation from cold could be achieved by an internal lining of boards, the interstices to be filled with a nonconductor. The wooden sections were made weatherproof in all seasons by the expedient of insisting on only English workmen to put them together. It had to be cheap: each hut must be small enough to lie on almost any kind of terrain without the expense of digging a basement. Its ventilation must be superb, and to this end there were openings under the eaves along the full length of each unit and opposite narrow windows on the long walls. Even the shutters to protect from sun were so designed that they let in air. Other openings were inserted immediately beneath the roof at the two gables, and in addition artificial ventilation was arranged for in an input system by means of a rotary air pump for each hut, whose mechanism was capable of being worked by a single man. This could force a thousand cubic feet of air per minute through shafts under the floors and into the wards. The vents were located under the tables between the rows of beds. (The healthfulness of the Lariboisière, originally designed for natural ventilation, was ruined by the superimposition of artificial ventilation and heating on an extract system, which promoted airborne cross-infection.)[57]

Finally, the units had to be infinitely and easily repeatable to allow for expansion in any direction. Work began at Renkioi on May 21, 1855. The hospital was ready to receive 300 patients on July 12, 500 on August 11, 1,000 on December 4, 1,500 in January 1856, and 2,200 by the end of March—at which point peace was declared, one suspects to the planners' considerable regret, for in only three months more "this immense establishment for 3,000 sick could have been finished and in full activity."

The double row of huts down the middle of the site was constructed first; the other two rows followed in the free space above and below it and some sections were never used. The center row alone held 1,500 men. The huts opened upon a central corridor 22 feet wide, which served as an exercise ground for the patients because it was absolutely level with the ward. In winter the north side of the corridor was boarded up and it could still be used. When peace was declared, plans were being made for a railroad track along this corridor to deposit an incoming patient at the very door to his ward.

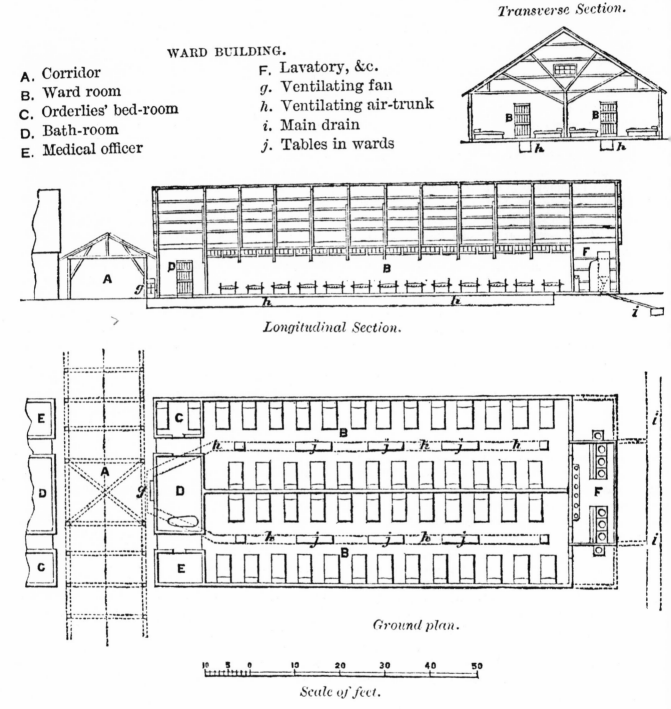

Transverse Section.

WARD BUILDING.

A. Corridor
B. Ward room
C. Orderlies' bed-room
D. Bath-room
E. Medical officer

F. Lavatory, &c.
g. Ventilating fan
h. Ventilating air-trunk
i. Main drain
j. Tables in wards

Longitudinal Section.

Ground plan.

Scale of feet.

Fig. 158. Transverse section, longitudinal section, and plan of one of the barracks huts at Renkioi.

Huts for the administration and nursing staff were similarly built and sited strategically; from the officers' quarters one had a clear view up the third-of-a-mile corridor and could supervise the convalescents to some degree and also the men who worked the air pumps. (It turned out that pumps were never needed in the climate of the Dardanelles.) Laundries were down by the water and for every 500 patients there was a separate kitchen. These were the only iron buildings, the only ones where fire was allowed. Heating in the wards was done in a small boiler over candles, and lighting was by candles too, in specially constructed lamps and lanterns.

Sanitary facilities were at the rear of each ward on a main sewer. The nearby springs proved completely adequate; at no time was pumping needed for the

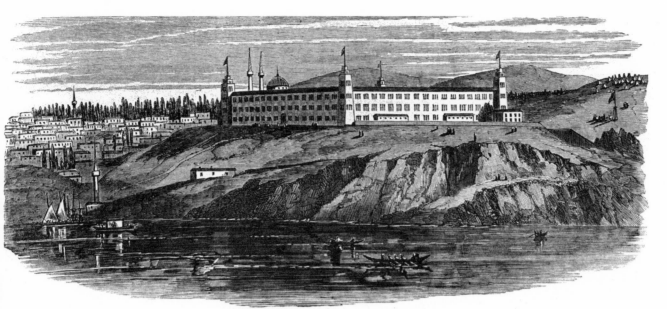

Fig. 159. The converted Turkish barracks at Scutari.

water pipes or drainage. Separated barracks assured isolation of diseases. Of 1,331 total admissions to the hospital at Renkioi, 961 were discharged cured, 320 were invalided, and there were 50 deaths.

The Nightingale Ward

Now compare the hut hospital at Renkioi with 2,200 patients and a mortality rate of 3 percent to the British army hospital at Scutari, a converted Turkish barracks, with 2,500 patients and a mortality of 42.7 percent (fig. 159). Such popular indignation was felt in London when Florence Nightingale's reports about Scutari were received that a government fell on its account. Brunel's huts were designed and shipped to Renkioi in record time but too late to make much difference for the Crimean War. However, other wars in other countries were not slow to present themselves, and design principles of the huts at Renkioi were extensively applied, as we shall see in the next chapter.

The hospital at Scutari was Florence Nightingale's Hôtel-Dieu. Its effect upon her is comparable to that of the Paris monstrosity upon Tenon. All her life she referred to her experiences there in great detail, and she actively sought out hospital wards the very opposite of those in which *her sick*—the common soldiers of the British army—had been bedded in long rows, had become infected by hospital fevers, and had suffered and died as a result. At one point during the Crimean War there were 12,000 men in hospital and only 11,000 in the military encampment.[58]

Florence Nightingale came to the Crimea with 38 nurses under her command to make a point: that female nurses were competent to nurse men. If

under such conditions she could succeed, never again would women as nurses be despised (Woodham-Smith, p. 89). But a more demanding mission was thrust upon her in default of adequate management under abominable circumstances—that of single-handedly administering and purveying the hospital. From public funds entrusted to her and from her own pocket she bought the most elementary necessities because the army had provided nothing; she was the one who kept this vast, filthy, rat-ridden and infected barracks functioning, which (as was presently discovered when "hospital fever" and dysentery ravaged the wards) was floating on a sea of dung from sewers underneath the building that had completely rotted away (fig. 160). The hospital's water supply, meager at best, was found to have been flowing through the decaying carcass of a dead horse (p. 140).

Of Florence Nightingale, Lytton Strachey observed, "No doubt . . . if her experience had lain, not among cholera cases at Scutari but among yellow-fever cases in Panama, she would have declared fresh air a fetish, and would have maintained to her dying day that the only really effective way of dealing with disease was by the destruction of mosquitoes."[59] But she experienced Scutari and for the rest of her life manifested the most passionate and single-minded concern for cleanliness, efficiency, and the proper disposition of the drains.

Upon returning to England she conveyed her concern in a popular volume, *Notes on Hospitals* (1858), which together with *Notes on Nursing* (1859) brought her directly into contact with a general public that already idolized her for her role in the Crimea. Here

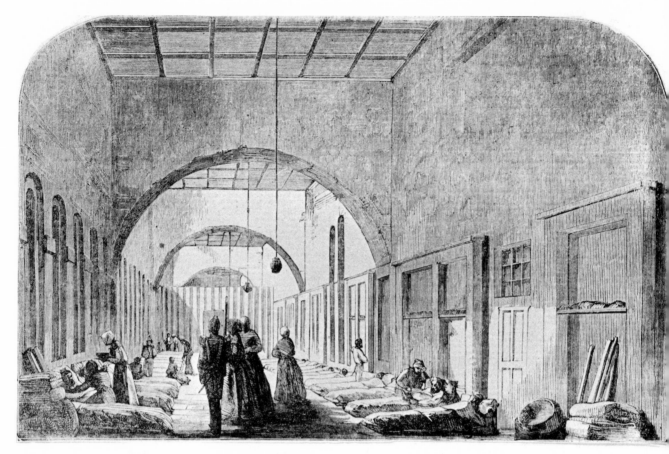

Fig. 160. An improvised ward in the barracks hospital of Scutari, 1854.

again at the outset her ambition was limited. She hoped only to direct public interest to the construction of proper housing for the British soldier—whose image, as Cecil Woodham-Smith says, she transformed from that of a drunken brute and scum of the earth to a symbol of courage, loyalty, and endurance, just as she transformed the nurse from a tipsy, promiscuous harridan to a noble professional, a nurse after her own image (p. 179). But with her vast knowledge of hospital conditions, Miss Nightingale could not be permitted to limit herself to military constructions, and soon she was advising the rulers of England on how general hospitals ought to be built. She operated through gentlemen of influence, keeping herself well hidden, for she wished her opinions to be taken seriously and knew she could get no solid work done if she were thought of simply as a heroine—in that age before the emancipation of women. However, she speaks up in her own voice in the *Notes on Hospitals* with clarity and eloquence.

Her requirements for a working ward were based on personal experience. By her own account, in thirteen years Florence Nightingale had visited "all the hospitals in London, Dublin and Edinburgh, many county

hospitals, some of the naval and military hospital in England; all the hospitals in Paris . . . the hospital at Berlin, and many others in Germany, at Lyons Rome, Alexandria, Constantinople, Brussels; also the war hospitals of the French and Sardinians."[6] Of these we may mention three she particularly admired: the barracks at Renkioi, "magnificent huts,"[6] the Lariboisière, "finest hospital in the world,"[62] and the Vincennes Military Hospital, a derivative of Tenon's twin wards sharing a central service section (fig. 161).

For its negative influence one other hospital plan may be added, that of the Royal Victoria Hospital at Netley, cited in *Notes on Hospitals* as a horrid example (fig. 162). It was in the process of being built when Florence Nightingale returned from the Crimea. She tried to halt construction but it was too far along and she could only effect the most minor sanitary improvements. Bitterly she contrasted the plan of this newest of English hospitals with the new pavilion in France (*Notes on Hospitals,* p. 8). Netley was simply a corridor hospital, much like the one at Bamberg with beds in rows parallel to the windows and privy constructions between every two wards.

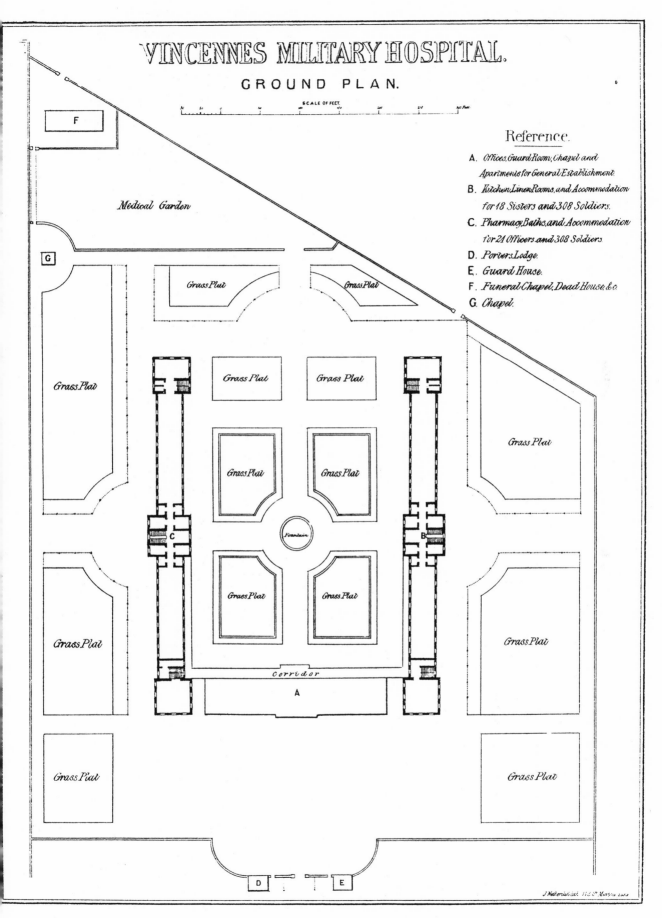

Fig. 161. Ground plan of Vincennes (France) Military Hospital (637 beds).

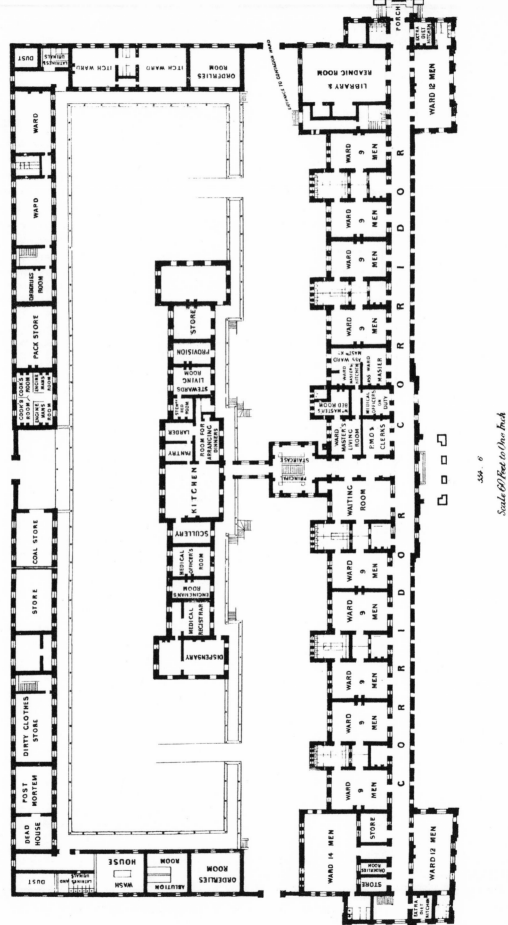

Scale 60 Feet to One Inch

The new ideas about a sanitary environment and ease of nursing supervision meant rejecting the eighteenth-century corridor plan, an advanced idea in its day. Double wards, back to back, were objectionable on every account. Truly, from the nurse's point of view, they prevent her from being able to observe all her patients at one time. When the windows are open, the effluvia must blow over all the intervening beds before escaping. The dead wall at the foot of the beds and the wall along the corridor directly interfere with the natural ventilation of the ward. Worst of all, joining all ward doors and windows on one side by means of a corridor must cause foul air from the wards to pass into the corridor, "and hence, without extraordinary precautions, such as are not usually nor likely to be bestowed on such matters, these corridors are the certain means of engendering a hospital atmosphere." (pp. 14-15)

The Nightingale ward may be called an edifice built up out of pure air. Some aspects of the theory behind it hark back to the Hippocratic *On Airs, Waters and Places*. This miasma theory of disease took on a practical vitality during the fifth decade of the nineteenth century, and an empirical recognition of the relation between filth and disease was close enough to the truth to lead to real sanitary reform before germs were understood.[63] Florence Nightingale was a thoroughgoing miasmatist for whom germs did not exist. She believed that the human body even in health is constantly exhaling from the lungs and skin, awake or asleep, watery vapor and organic matter "ready to enter into the putrefactive condition." How much more so the sick body, "the exhalations from whom are always highly morbid and dangerous." These morbid exhalations must be instantly and perpetually carried off by ventilation (p. 11). To deprive the sick of pure air "is nothing but manslaughter under the garb of benevolence" (pp. 90–91). Every hospital should have either a concrete foundation in dry ground or an arched basement unconnected to the wards by staircases. There shall be no enclosed courts with high walls, for they stagnate the air. And "all closed courts, narrow culs de sac, high adjacent walls, closed angles, overshadowing trees, and other obstructions to outer ventilation should be sedulously avoided, at whatever cost" (p. 96).

The sick must be subdivided among a number of separate buildings not more than two stories in height. Building walls must not be so high as to interfere with the sunlight and ventilation of neighboring pavilions. "It is little else than a breach of trust to build great lofty architectural structures merely to flatter the bad taste of committees or governors" (p. 95). This means spreading patients over a wider area. The central court and the space between pavilions should be laid out as gardens for convalescents, and there must be sheltered exercise grounds besides (p. 99). No offices should be duplicated; a central kitchen should lie convenient to all wards, yet not below any; the laundry should be kept at a distance, administrative offices close by for efficient supervision (p. 95).

The suggested inpatient unit, which became known as a Nightingale ward, was not a concept originating with Miss Nightingale but rather the embodiment of sanitary insights of the nineteenth and earlier centuries. Miss Nightingale endorsed an oblong ward with windows on both sides (p. 96). To patient space should be added, at the entrance, a head nurse's room with one window commanding the ward and the other opening outdoors, and opposite that room a scullery; at the far end of the ward, behind a partition and independently ventilated, should be a bathroom and a lavatory on one side of the corridor and water closets on the other. And that is all. No dining rooms, no smaller patient rooms (p. 102).

> Every unneeded closet, scullery, sink, lobby and staircase represents both a place which must be cleaned, which must take hands and time to clean, and a hiding or skulking place for patients or servants disposed to do wrong. And of such no hospital will ever be free. Every five minutes wasted upon cleaning what had better not have been there to be cleaned, is something taken from and lost by the sick (p. 16).

As for the dimensions of an ideal ward, the width should be 30 feet: "It does not appear as if the air could be thoroughly changed, if a distance of more than thirty feet intervenes between opposite windows" (pp. 13–14). If you overextend a 30-foot-wide ward, you form a tunnel like the barracks at Scutari that is fatal to good ventilation. If you cut it too short, "you multiply corners in a greater ratio than you multiply sick;" air has been shown to move three or four times faster at the center than in the corners of a ward. For 32 patients the length should be at least 111½ feet; 128 feet would be better (p. 104). How high should the ward be? If only 10 or 12 feet high, it cannot be properly ventilated, and the same is true if a very great height is left above the windows. How many patients? Let us assume 30 to 32 to a ward, not too many to be supervised by one head nurse and also a good-sized unit for sanitary reasons (p. 17). A room long enough for that number of beds, allowing each a "territory to itself" at least 8 feet by 12 feet (p. 10), can be well ventilated with a ceiling 16 to 17 feet high if the windows reach to within 1 foot of the ceiling—otherwise the top of the ward becomes a reservoir for foul air (p. 13).

Rather a ward too light than a ward too dark; window

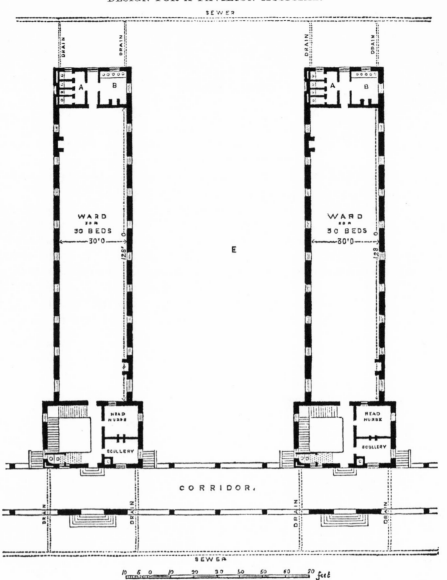

DESIGN FOR A PAVILION HOSPITAL.

A. Ward Closets.
B. Bath and Lavatory.
C. Lift in Scullery.

D. Private Closet.
E. Ornamental Ground.
Ward Windows to be 4 ft. 8 in. in the clear.

Fig. 163. Plan of the Nightingale ward. The "closet" is a WC, the scullery "lift" a dumb-waiter. The "private closet" is hidden in the stair opposite the scullery.

shades can always be pulled down but the gloom of a dark ward is irremediable (p. 12). For the sake of sun at all hours of the day, the axis of the ward should be as nearly as possible north and south, and the windows should take up one-third of the wall space. There should be at least one window to every two beds, and it should descend to within 2 or 3 feet of the floor. Your safest warmer and ventilator is an open fireplace; Miss Nightingale would be glad to see one in the center of the ward rather than on a side wall for more efficient and even heat (p. 13). The planning goes down to the last detail: lacquered oak floors,

walls of pure, white, polished, nonabsorbent cement (p. 15) or the palest possible pink.[64] Dishes should be glass or earthenware; true, they break, but tin on the other hand smells (*Notes on Hospitals,* p. 16). And finally, "the bright colors of flowers. . . . It is generally said that the effect is upon the mind. Perhaps so, but it is no less so upon the body on that account" (p. 12).

The ward designed on these principles is shown in figure 163. It is a ward that only now is vanishing in the United States, while some in Britain still favor it for its ease of supervision. At St. Thomas's Hospital

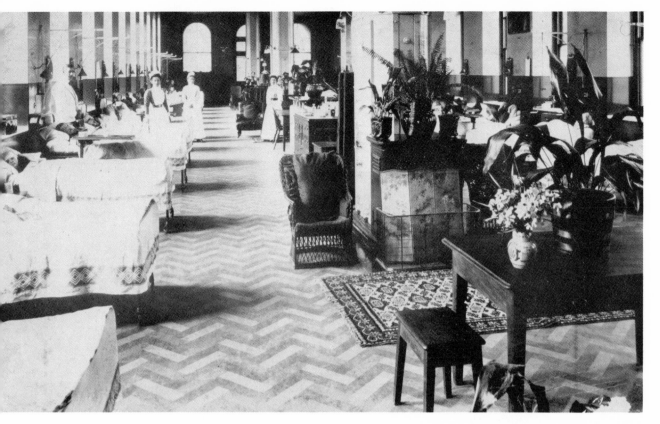

Fig. 164. Interior of a ward at St. Thomas's Hospital, London, at the beginning of this century.

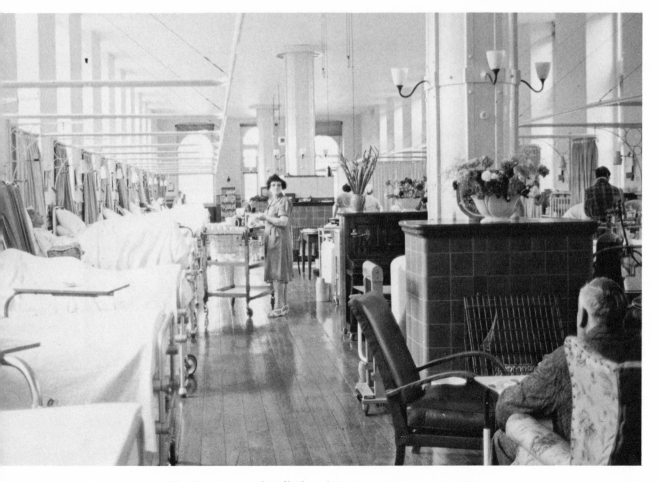

Fig. 165. Interior of Nuffield ward, St. Thomas's Hospital, in 1966.

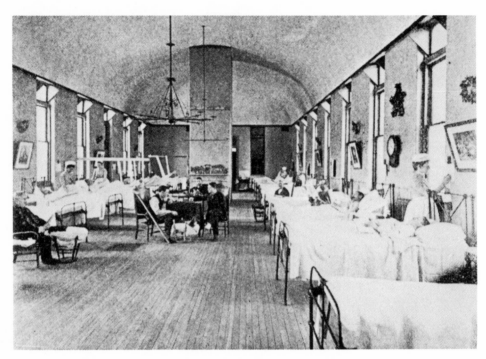

Fig. 166. Interior of Marquand Pavilion, Bellevue Hospital, New York City, about 1893.

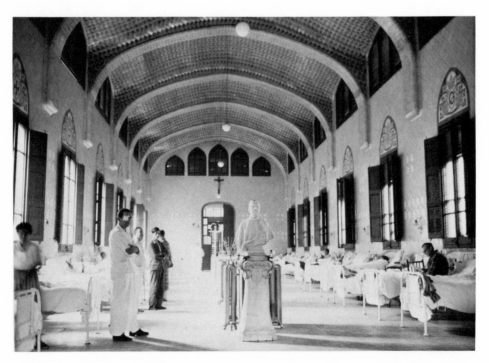

Fig. 167. Ward interior, Hospital de la Santa Cruz y San Pablo, Barcelona, Spain (1905–10) in 1968.

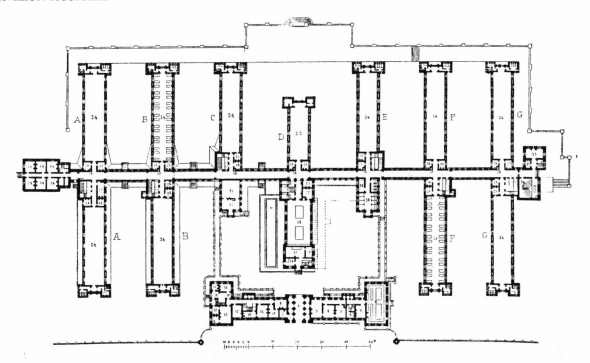

Fig. 168. Plan of Herbert Hospital, Woolwich, England (1859–64). 1, Entrance; 2, porter; 3, waiting room; 4, examination room; 5, surgery; 6, nurse's laundry; 7, mending laundry; 8, clean linen; 9, director; 10, clerk; 11, chief physician; 12, registry; 13, captain of orderlies; 14, sergeant major; 15, paymaster; 16, chief cook; 17, steward; 18, clerk; 19, library; 20, librarian; 21, porter; 22, dayroom; 23, officer's dwelling; 24, ward; 25, nurse; 26, pantry; 27, washroom; 28, elevator; 29, dressing room; 30, bath; 31, pharmacy; 32, drugs, 33, operating room; 34; amphitheater.

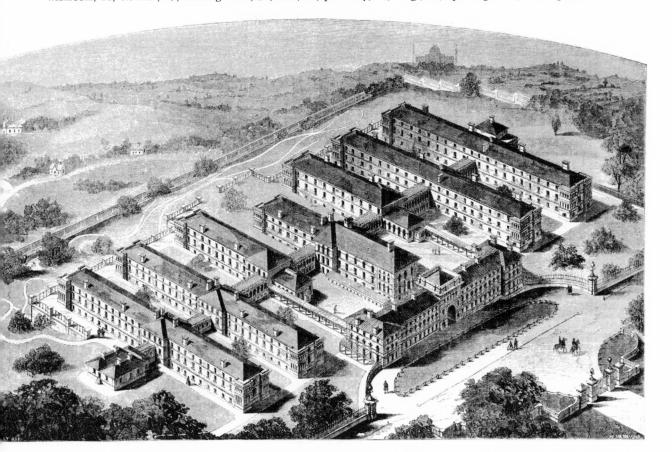

Fig. 169. Elevation of Herbert Hospital.

164

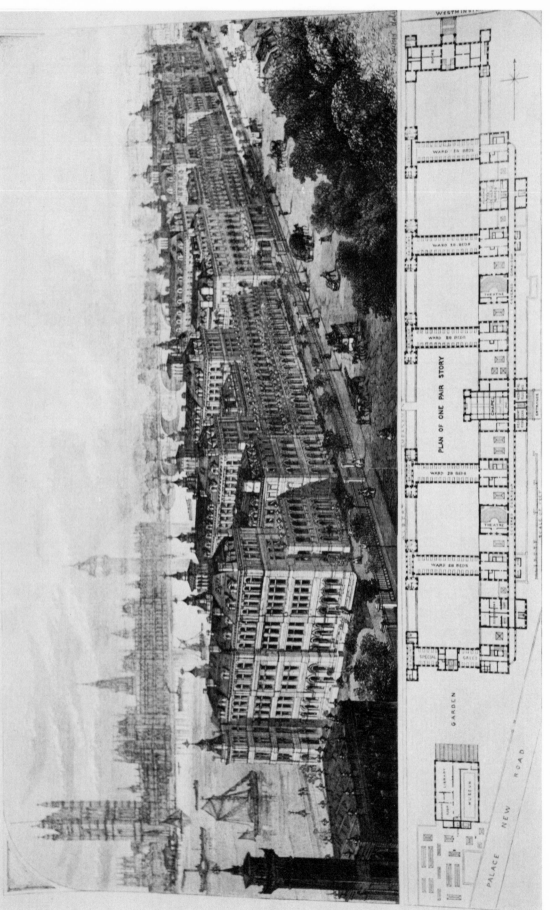

Fig. 170. (a) Elevation and plan of St. Thomas's Hospital, London from the street side (eastern facade).

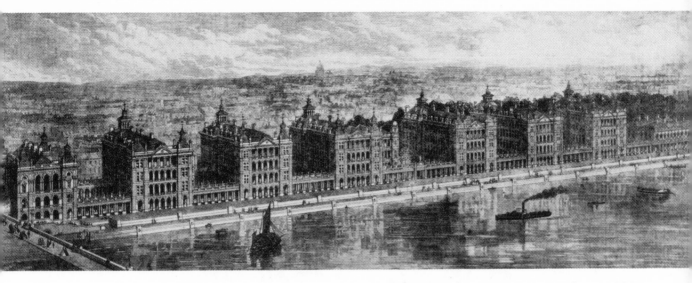

Fig. 170 (b) Elevation of St. Thomas's Hospital from the Thames (western facade), 1871.

London, the interior of these wards has changed very little since the beginning of the century (figs. 164 and 165). An American interior from Bellevue Hospital, New York, about 1893 (fig. 166) may be matched in countless photographs of hospital interiors from all over the world. A ward of the hospital of Santa Cruz y San Pablo of Barcelona (1905–10; fig. 167) shows the basic sanitary arrangements as embellished by a pupil of the eccentric Spanish architect Antonio Gaudi. There was always space down the center of these 30-foot-wide rooms for radiators, armchairs, statuary, altars, flowers, tables for all purposes, and—in the ward at St. Thomas's—a piano for Sunday services. The median line serves as a kind of recreation center and has ever been the site of incessant activity. But in the beds is felt a military immobility. One pictures them as so many soldiers lined up for inspection, sheets very tightly drawn, pillows immaculate, chair tucked neatly under foot or side. Florence Nightingale was trained by the army. Her wards reveal, both architecturally and administratively, the barracks influence.

Nightingale Hospitals

How Florence Nightingale would fit together three (not two!) stories of 26-bed wards to form a hospital of 658 beds is shown in the plan and elevation of the first hospital to be built entirely under her supervision, Herbert Hospital (1859–64; figs. 168 and 169). The pavilions were connected by a central corridor that was kept to one story so as not to cast unnecessary shadows on the ground.[65] The administration building is recognizable from French forms, though the pavilions were turned another way from those of the much-admired Lariboisière. At St. Thomas's (fig. 170a) the central entrance at the rear used in recent years was given over to physicians' apartments, and patients were actually admitted at the first pavilion along the river closest to the bridge, a convenience for whose sake perfect symmetry was set slightly

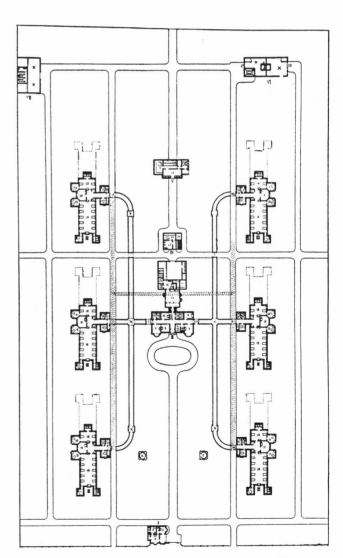

Fig. 171. Plan of a city hospital for contagious diseases at Newcastle-upon-Tyne (1884), 84 beds.

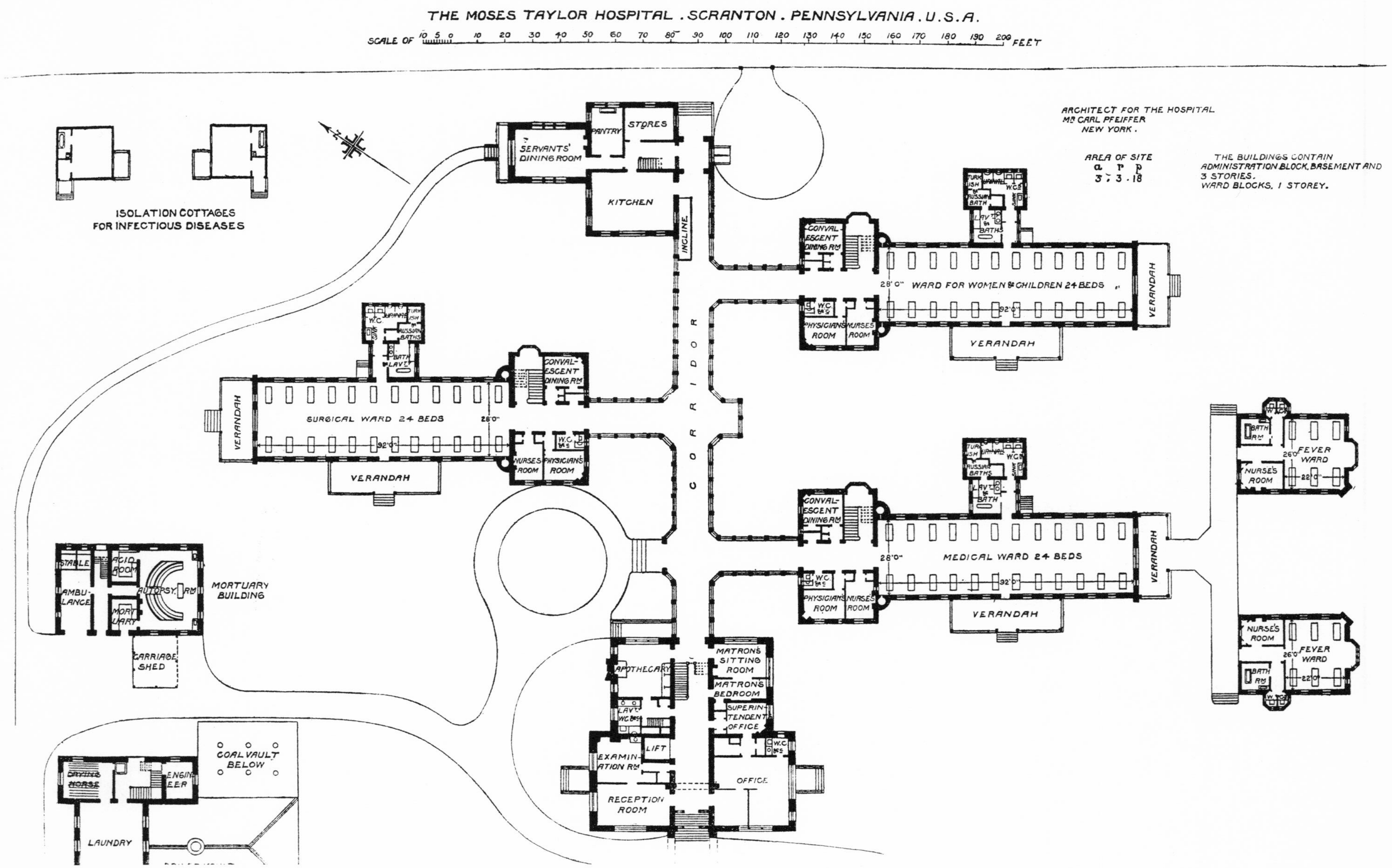

Fig. 172. Plan of Moses Taylor Hospital, Scranton, Pa.

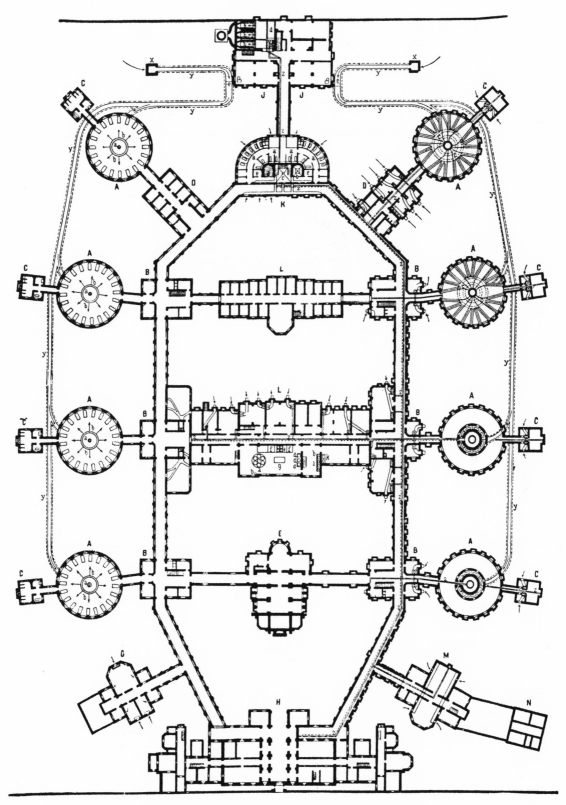

Fig. 173. Plan of the Civil Hospital, Antwerp (1878), 388 beds.

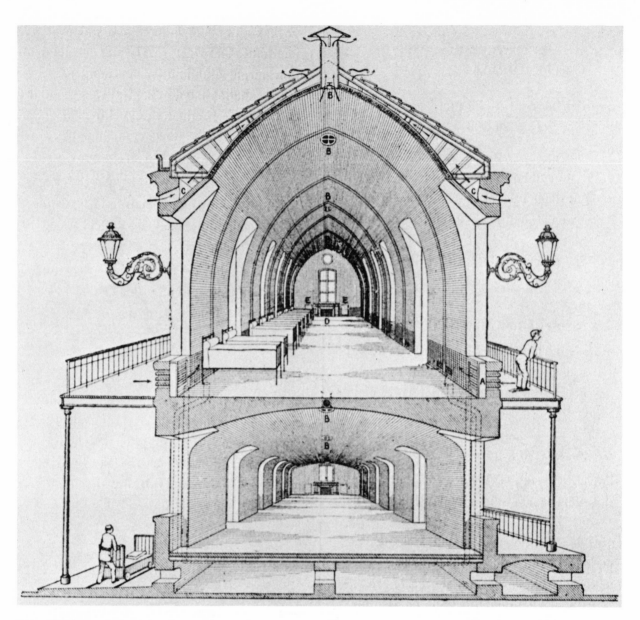

Fig. 174. Transverse section of the Toilet ward at the Civil and Military Hospital, Montpellier, France, 1884. A, Pure air intake; B, ceiling vents, upstairs and down, for the vitiated air; C, a mass of ventilating air caught between the vaulting and the roof (arrows indicate the direction of its flow); D, intakes at the two extremities of the ward; E, vents of vitiated air activated by the chimney flues.

askew. These fine pavilions on the banks of the Thames (fig. 170b) face the Houses of Parliament; from the windows of the bathrooms and water closets at the end of each pavilion could be had one of the noblest views in London.

Architecture in the neo-Gothic style was employed as the skin for Miss Nightingale's sanitary conceptions to a far greater extent at St. Thomas's than at Herbert Hospital. After 1835, Gothic was accepted as the official style of England. This form of architecture, long despised, was thought of in the expansive, prosperous decades after Waterloo as natively English and

a reminder of what was supposed to have been the Golden Age.[66] The Gothic format came in handy for utilitarian structures; like the medieval architecture of which it was the derivative, it freed their component parts. Each function occupied a segment to itself.[67] An oriel for a water closet may seem incongruous, but it permitted placing that water closet at the outer end of a ward, where sanitary exigencies required it to be. When long passages aired from both sides were stipulated to isolate the water closets from the ward, the Gothic proved capable of disguising them as well. Behind a Gothic exterior, architects played with the components of the Nightingale hospital, lavishing on the relationship of long ward to sanitary conveniences as much ingenuity as in an earlier age had been devoted to the relationship of long ward and chapel.

Thus, in an overall view, only three moves were made in hospital architecture from the early Middle Ages to the beginning of the twentieth century: from medieval forms where every function expressed itself straightforwardly in a fitting structure visible from the outside, to classical forms where all functions were hidden behind a relentlessly uniform and symmetrical exterior, to nineteenth-century Gothic forms where again one might guess at the component parts of the building however ornately concealed, as one might guess at the naked woman under the bustle and the lacy bust.

Under the most ornate plans of the next quarter of a century may similarly be perceived the Nightingale idea. In Newcastle-upon-Tyne (fig. 171), Scranton, Pennsylvania (fig. 172), Antwerp (fig. 173), and in countless other cities of Europe, the United States, and even India, variations were played upon the theme. It is interesting to observe that in Antwerp the basic plan was blown out like a balloon. Note the date—1878.

Some suppose that circular wards are a phenomenon of our own day.

Meanwhile in France, where the pavilion style began, the engineer Casimir Tollet was manipulating Tenon's double pavilion and produced a version he proudly named the "Tollet ward" (fig. 174). The site plan is roughly that of the French Academy and the ward is Tenon's, with the addition of a veranda on both long sides and jutting two-bed rooms for isolation or paying patients at the far ends. The greater part of the ground floor was used for ventilation[68] and as covered recreation ground for convalescents; at its ends were the convalescent dormitories and dining halls. Air was introduced into the ward by pipes that led up through its floor from the basement and bypassed the ground floor. A ceiling with a pointed arch supposedly encouraged upward drafts. At intervals along the ridgepole, covered chimneys drew air straight upward from the ward in the manner of the ventilators of the French projects, and air brought in under the eaves escaped at the peak of the roof. Burdett reports that the very great care brought by Tollet to hospital problems revolutionized their construction in France. He also mentions that the attention of Tollet was first drawn to the subject of ventilation during his army service.[69]

CHAPTER 6

From Pavilions to Skyscrapers

Civil War Barracks, United States

Notes on Hospitals was published in 1859, and in 1861 the American Civil War broke out. An American Sanitary Commission was formed upon the English model—a sort of cross between the U.S.O. and the Red Cross, George Rosen calls it. Its members insisted on inspecting existing government military hospitals in Washington, however unwelcome the intervention was to all sectors of the military—"the fifth wheel of the coach," was President Lincoln's term for it. In the first year of the war the commission issued a report describing five hospitals in and around Washington, four of which were converted buildings. The Union Hotel Hospital in Georgetown was typical:

> The building is old, out of repair, and cut up into a number of small rooms, with windows too small and few in number to afford good ventilation. Its halls and passages, are narrow, tortuous, and abrupt, and in many instances with carpets still unremoved from their floors, and walls covered with paper. There are no provisions for bathing, the water-closets and sinks are insufficient and defective, and there is no dead-house. The wards are many of them over-crowded, and destitute of arrangements for artificial ventilation. The cellars and area are damp and undrained, and much of the wood work is actively decaying.[1]

"The scaly walls and cracked wood-work of old buildings present innumerable lurking places for foul air," the inspection committee continues (U.S. Sanitary Commission *Report*, p. 4). The case is cited of a soldier whose arm was amputated above the elbow on the field after the Battle of Bull Run; he walked all the way to the hospital in Washington in safety, but "it is much to be regretted that he has since died from erysipelas in the Hospital on E street" (p. 5). The final recommendation to the Government is that

> hereafter instead of hiring old buildings for General Hospitals they should order the erection of a sufficient number of wooden shanties or pavilions of appropriate construction, and fully provided with water for bathing, washing, and water-closets, and ample arrangements for ventilation

and for securing warmth in winter, to accommodate from thirty to sixty each, and to be sufficiently distant not to poison each other. This suggestion embodies the latest and best views as to the construction of hospitals, and its adoption would save both lives and money (p. 8).

Government yielded. The report was submitted in July, and in September of the same year (1861) construction began in Washington on two cheap and temporary model hospitals. They were an adaptation of Brunel's one-story barracks. For 50 patients, it will be remembered, Brunel designed a partitioned ward 100 by 40 feet, 12 to 25 feet in height. The partition was now omitted and for a group of 25 to 50 patients the dimensions adopted were closer to those recommended by Florence Nightingale, to whom the commission wrote at the outset for guidance: for 32 patients, a barracks 111 by 30 feet and 17 feet high. The Brunel hut had been ventilated under the eaves and at the peak of the gable. Civil War barracks, at least in the North, were ventilated all along the ridgepole, a possible derivation from the fire hole of Tilton's Indian hut. The first barracks were arranged, like those at Renkioi, at opposite sides of the corridor with water closets at the free extremity and the nurse's room and dining room next to the corridor. The original Civil War hospitals were for only 250 beds, but later ones were much larger; the West Philadelphia Hospital contained 3,124 beds in wards of 48 beds each.[2]

The same system and plan of hospitals were adopted by the Confederate army during the Civil War. Chimborazo Hospital in Richmond, Virginia (1862–65; fig. 175) accommodated 7,000 patients in 150 whitewashed wooden barracks 100 by 30 feet. Each held 50–60 men, and there were in addition 100 tents for 8–10 soldiers or convalescents each. A large private house north of the hospital was used as medical headquarters, where were also the guardhouse and 5 deadhouses, en route to the cemetery. The hospital owned several hundred cows and up to 500 goats; soup was made in idle tobacco factories and soap manufactured from the leftover grease, the bakery turned out 10,000 loaves a day, beer was brewed and stored in caves at the foot of the plateau and in 5 icehouses.[3]

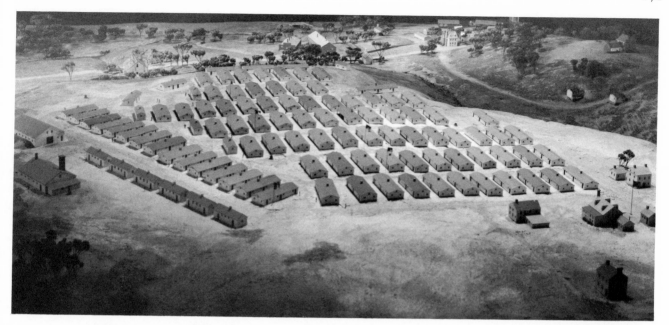

Fig. 175. Model of Chimborazo Hospital by Edward Plumstead, at the Medical College of Virginia Commonwealth University, Richmond.

Chimborazo Hospital, built along Nightingale lines, was an effective, self-sufficient army town in a farming area. Her influence is likewise felt in the highly symmetrical and rational design of Mower General Hospital in Philadelphia (fig. 176). With half the number of patients—3,600—Mower is laid out so logically that one can follow a patient from arrival to discharge. The patient would arrive by train at the passenger section of the depot—freight was taken in at the other —and be admitted at the reception room in the only two-story barrack, opposite the station (which contained, on the ground floor, the hospital laundry as well, and on the second floor rooms for the clerical and nursing staff). Following his admission, our patient would be assigned to one of the 49 single-storied barracks radiating from a covered racetrack corridor half a mile long (as the plan proudly states). He would be fed from a central kitchen, a one-story continuation of the laundry–reception building with a special annex for the "Manufactory for Ice Cream & apparatus for roasting and grinding Coffee by Steam." If he required surgery, he was conveyed to a separate small building for the operating room, on the right side of the huge interior court. The surgeon lived on the top floor of the large building lying crosswise in that court, and on the ground floor were his mess and the general offices. The commanding officer's quarters stood at right angles to the surgeon's; other officers lived in L-shaped buildings at the far corners of the site. If our patient wanted to attend religious services, he had access to a church in the inner court with a Bible classroom attached. In the court dwelt the carpenter; the blacksmith and wheelwright shops as well as

stables could be found in the outlying fields. As our patient improved he would be moved to a lodging, half-hidden in a sizable grove, for convalescents who no longer needed treatment; there he would find a ten-pin alley and gymnastic grounds.

This plan is clearly no mere offshoot.of the *Notes on Hospitals*. Its author, John McArthur, Jr., was one of the outstanding architects of his time, who designed the Philadelphia City Hall and during the Civil War served as architect under the quartermaster general's department in Philadelphia. Between 1862 and 1867 he designed twenty-four temporary United States hospitals. It has been suggested that he wrote the specifications for the timber barracks.[4] His plan for Mower Hospital was adapted in Germany during the Franco-Prussian War as a barracks hospital and after the war as an epidemic hospital in Moabit, Berlin (1872; fig. 177). The German racetrack is long and narrow, the number of patient pavilions is reduced to 30 and of beds to 811, and the pavilions do not surround the track, for to clear the court, the administration, kitchen, and laundry buildings are relegated to the entrance in one of the narrow ends. Workshops, sheds, boiler house, disinfection house, and morgue are ranged in a row across the service road from the free ends of the pavilions, whose interior floor plan is a very familiar one (fig. 178).

One characteristic of Civil War hospitals, present at Chimborazo, is lacking in our bird's eye view of Mower: tents. They appear in a print of Lincoln Hospital in Washington D.C. (fig. 179). As often as not, tents for infectious cases made up half the hospital. Burdett reported (*Hospitals and Asylums*, 3: 753) that

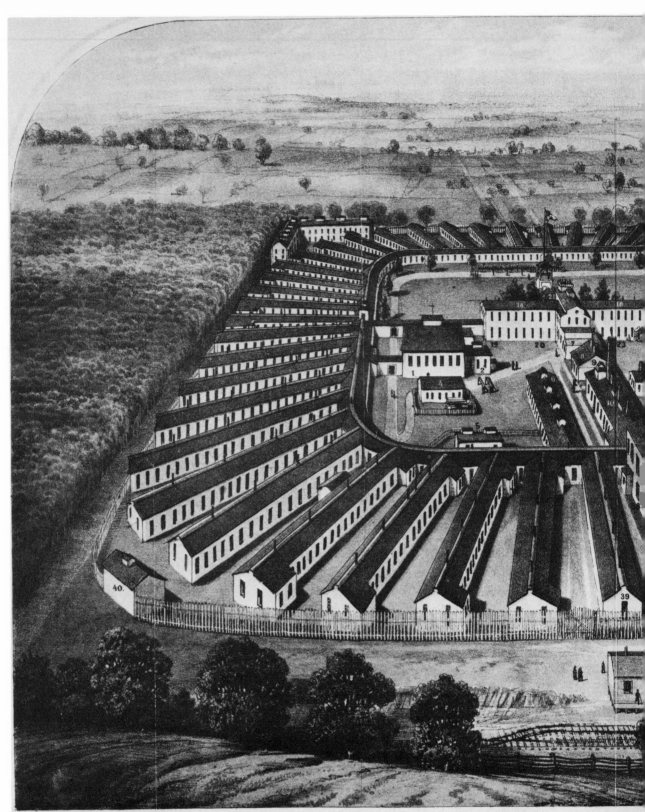

J. McArthur, Arch't.

P.S.

1 Chapel
2 Bible Class Room
3 Post Office
4 Carpenter Shop
5 Band Quarters
6 Dining Room for Attendants
7 Conservatory

8 Engine Room
9 Manufactory for Ice Cream & apparatus for roasting and grinding Coffee by Steam
10 General Kitchen
11 Butcher Shop
12 Milk House
13 Fat & Bone House

14 Extra Diet Kitchen
15 Operating Room
16 Guard House
17 Sutlers Store
18 Surgeon's Quarters
19 Dispensary
20 General Office
21 Comdg Officers Qurs

MOWER U.S.A.

Chestnu

Entered according to Act of Congress in the year 1865 by W. Kiple

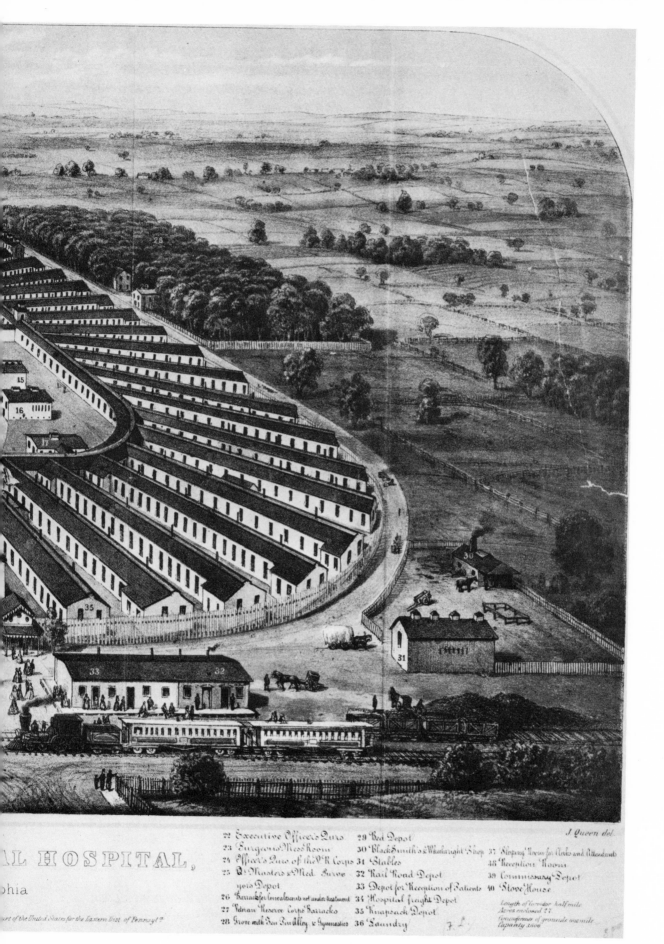

AL HOSPITAL,

phia

rt of the United States for the Eastern West of Pennsylt?

22 Executive Officer's Qurs   29 Bed Depot
23 Surgeons Mess Room   30 Black Smith's & Wheelwright Shop   37 Sleeping Room for Clerks and Attendants
24 Officer's Qurs of the VR Corps   31 Stables   48 Reception Room
25 Q. Masters & Med. Purve   32 Rail Road Depot   39 Commissary Depot
   yors Depot   33 Depot for Reception of Patients   40 Stove House
26 Barracks for Convalescents not under treatment   34 Hospital Freight Depot
27 Veteran Reserve Corps Barracks 35 Knapsack Depot   Length of corridor half mile
28 Grove with Ten Pin Alley & Gymnastics   36 Laundry   Acres enclosed 27
                                                                        Circumference of grounds one mile
                                                                        Capacity 3600

Fig. 176. Mower General Hospital, Philadelphia, Pa., 1865.

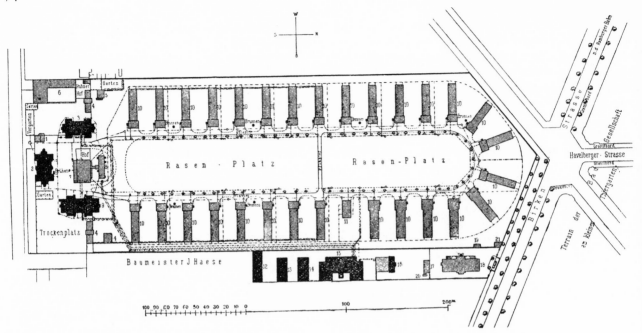

Fig. 177. Plan of the City Hospital, Moabit, Berlin, 1872.

the 60 wards of Lincoln Hospital could hold 1,240 beds, but by the use of tents and a branch barracks nearby, the wartime population rose to 2,575 beds. Tents were favored for wounds or acute fevers by Dr. John S. Billings (army doctor and librarian of the surgeon general's office) because they could be abandoned even more easily than wooden barracks when the ground became infected. Warming them in zero weather presented no problem: "The secret of properly heating such structures, or tents, consists in placing the heating apparatus not in the room to be warmed, but below it."[5] Indeed, the interior view looks cozy enough (fig. 180). A difficulty arose in warm, still weather, when tents are difficult to ventilate.

Burdett visited Lincoln Hospital twenty-five years after the war ended and wrote it up. The site was surrounded by a picket fence 5 feet high, and a road for ambulances ran between it and the free ends of the wards. Two-story houses across the base of the V were for the medical officers. The kitchen, dining rooms, and nurses' dormitories were in buildings in the enclosed triangle. The long, raised covered corridor was made navigable with a railway track two feet wide (this Crimean invention was put to good use) for boxcars conveying food to the wards from the kitchen, one of which can be seen in fig. 179 at the end of the right-hand corridor.

Burdett described the pavilions in great detail (3: 752-53). They were of rough whitewashed boards, the roof boards covered with tarred paper. They were 187 by 24 feet, 16 to 20 feet high, with ridge ventilation (usually closed in winter) that ran the full length of the ward. The walls were plastered inside to about

8 feet above the floor. "Four ventilating gratings, at regular distances in the floor of the ward, communicate by wooden flues under the floor with the air outside, thus giving a full supply of fresh air whenever the weather requires the doors and windows to be closed." There were 62 patients to a ward, 31 on a side, with chair and bedside table between each pair of beds and a free passageway of 11 feet down the center. Night lighting was by kerosene lamps, heating by stoves in winter. At the west end of each pavilion were 4 rooms 15 feet long used for clothing, baths, nurses, and so forth.

Immediately afterward Burdett described a very similar Southern hospital, Sedgwick Hospital in Greenville, New Orleans (a typical barracks plan): 15 one-storied pavilions 145 by 24 feet, plus an administrative building as long and a little wider, radiated from a circular covered way 12 feet wide. In the center were such buildings as housed the kitchens and a distance detached buildings for staff quarters and services. The wards were raised on brick piers 3 feet

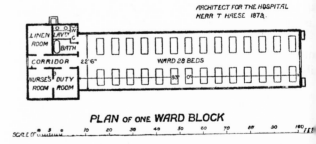

Fig. 178. Floor plan of one pavilion, City Hospital, Moabit, Berlin.

above ground and had ridgepole ventilation. There were 2 beds between each pair of windows and 40 beds to a ward. Perhaps Southern and Northern hospital personnel wrote separately for identical instructions from Miss Nightingale; perhaps both simply read the 1861 Report of the English Sanitary Commission, which advocated a barracks hospital plan. Southerners seem quietly and sensibly to have subscribed to the Northern governmental instructions of July 1864 for the building of hospitals, which stipulated detached pavilions for 60 patients each and detached buildings for administration, to be connected by covered corridors with open sides; ridgepole ventilation in the pavilions, and at either end of them small rooms partitioned off for nurses, a closet, and medical stores; water closets attached where the water supply was adequate, otherwise privies to be built at a convenient distance and emptied every night (Burdett, 2: 751).

Five Plans for Johns Hopkins Hospital, Baltimore

American postwar hospital designers found themselves in a quandary. Barracks saved lives. Tents prevented the spread of infection. The military solution for hospital building seemed the most daring, advanced, and workable one of all. Then why build permanent structures? Block hospitals on the European corridor plan were out of the question, but even pavilions were liable to become infected and therefore dangerous. Perhaps all buildings really intended to make patients well should be planned cheaply for a life span of ten to fifteen years and demolished as soon as they became saturated with morbific particles.

At this juncture the city of Baltimore was offered a university and a hospital, equally and munificently endowed by a local businessman, Johns Hopkins. Seven million dollars were to be divided between the two. University and hospital were to form two separate corporations with separate boards of trustees, but the hospital was to be used as a teaching instrument for the university's medical school, and it was to be no ordinary hospital. It must "compare favorably with any other institution of like character in the country or in Europe," and its staff should be made up of surgeons and physicians of the highest character and greatest skill.[6]

"'To compare favorably with'—what does that mean?" asked John S. Billings, the man more responsible than any other for the design of the new hospital.

It is a peculiar phrase, which, coming from a shrewd business man and a member of the Society of Friends, signifies, I think, to excel, if possible; at all events, that is the safest interpretation. And it was not this or that hospital which

was to be surpassed or equalled, but all other hospitals in this country or in Europe—Africa, Asia and Australasia being put out of the question. It was a large contract.[7]

Johns Hopkins himself purchased the 13-acre site for the hospital and pledged toward the construction of buildings $100,000 a year while he lived. He died within the year and the hospital found itself in a still more favorable financial position: properties worth $2 million had been willed to it and though the specifications were that building was to be financed only from income, that income amounted to $120,000 a year —more or less, as the properties fluctuated in value. After building was completed, the income was to be used for maintenance. A Colored Orphan Asylum was to be founded on a separate site and maintained from the same funds.

In a direct, brief, and eloquent letter of instructions —it runs to three pages, no more—Johns Hopkins indicated to his trustees how he wanted this hospital built and run. There were to be 400 patients. The indigent sick of the city and state, without regard to sex, age, or color, who required surgical or medical treatment or were stricken by any casualty, were to be received free of charge. A limited number of patients who were able to pay were also to be provided for, and the income thus raised was to be applied to the relief of the poor.[8] There was to be a training school for female nurses—so strong was Miss Nightingale's influence by 1873. A religious spirit should be strongly felt but administration was to be nonsectarian.

As to the form the buildings should assume, the knowledgeable, hard-headed businessman made only one concrete suggestion: any site plan chosen should permit symmetrical additions to the buildings that were first constructed. He knew that the shape of hospital buildings made a difference in patient care but he also knew there was widespread uncertainty about what shape was best. One must consult the experts before making a move. "It will, therefore, be your duty," he instructed his trustees, "to obtain the advice and assistance of those, at home and abroad, who have achieved the greatest success in the construction and management of Hospitals. I cannot press this injunction too strongly upon you, because the usefulness of this charity will greatly depend upon the plan which you may adopt for the construction and arrangement of the buildings."[9]

The trustees assumed in full seriousness their task of building the best hospital in the world. Should it be a monument? A tent? The compromise already embodied in the first pavilion hospitals? "It is still maintained," they averred, "by a weight of opinion

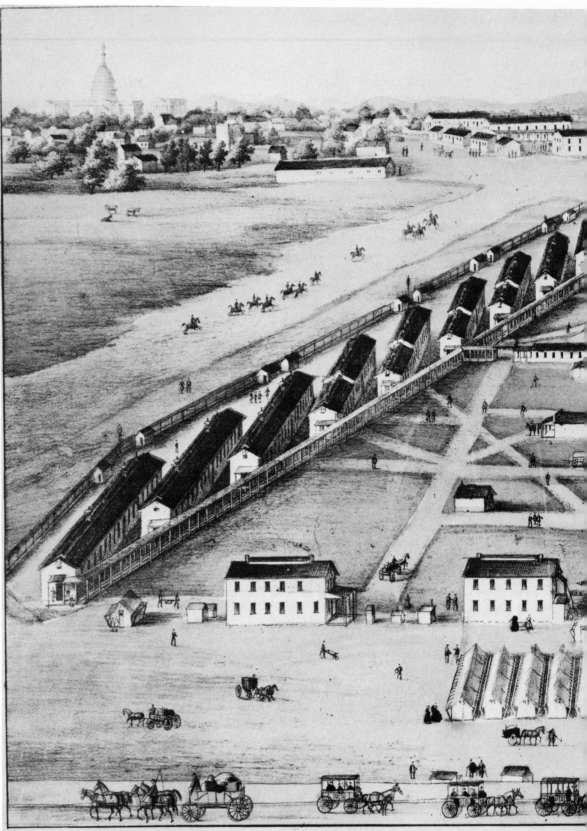

LINCOLN HOSPI

Published by Chas. Magnus,

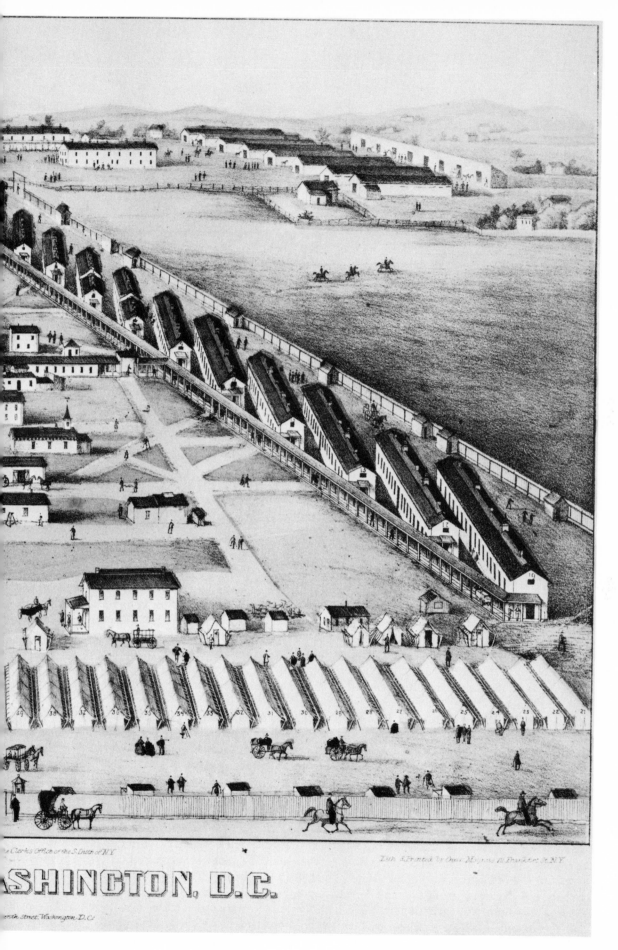

SHINGTON, D.C.

Fig. 179. Lincoln Hospital, Washington, D.C.

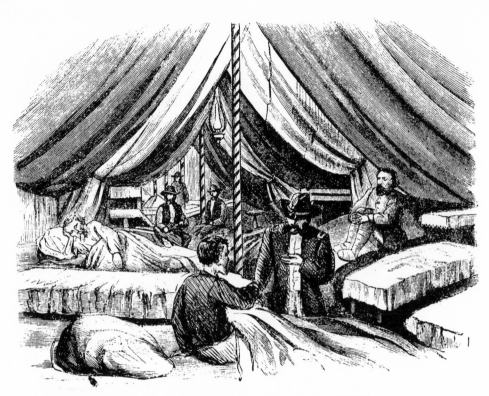

Fig. 180. Interior of a hospital tent during the Civil War.

too eminent and too learned to be disregarded that the reform has not gone far enough, and that it yet remains for some institution, having adequate means at command, to carry the improvement to its highest capability."[10] They wrote for guidance, for suggestions, and for specific plans embodying those suggestions to five distinguished physicians who had made the subject of hospitals their special study.

"We presume there must be some general principles of hospital hygiene and of hospital treatment fixed and immutable in their character, the discovery and proof of which are the result of close, careful recorded observation and judgment," they wrote; today we read the words wistfully. "If these principles can be best applied through the agency of the pavilion system, we wish to adopt that; if by the barrack system, then we will avail ourselves of that form of construction, and if the true rule for our guidance shall be found in the selection of the good features of each, and the combining of them all into a harmonious middle course, then we desire to make that selection and combination." A block hospital was thus out of the question and the five physicians were not given a truly free rein, for the trustees further presumed that "there will be no departure from the now very general method of a central administration building, with wards for the treatment of the sick as carefully separated therefrom and from each other as practicable."[11]

The five replies were to be published, and everyone concerned worked very fast. The letter went out to the doctors March 6, 1875, a deadline was suggested of May 1 of the same year, and the resulting volume of *Hospital Plans* still bears the date of 1875. A thousand copies, privately printed, were sent to concerned individuals and institutions for comment and criticism, and thus the Johns Hopkins Hospital, already an object of excited interest for the magnitude of its endowment, influenced the building of other hospitals in the United States and Europe even before the final form for its own buildings had been decided upon.

The superintendent of the Massachusetts General Hospital of Boston, Dr. Norton Folsom, expressed himself as opposed to tents on principle. His wards were designed to open fully and ventilate as well as any tent (*Hospital Plans,* p. 82). He also had no use for barracks in a civil hospital, however well they had functioned for the military. A ward need not be destructible. He believed that a well-built pavilion, with double brick walls and an air space between (p. 66), could be renewed or refreshed on its inner surfaces (p. 60) as often as necessary and remain as healthy as any barracks and a good deal more comfortable. "I should consider the moral effect of barracks in a civil hospital . . . positively prejudicial" (p. 59). However, the pavilions must absolutely be limited to one story because he proposed ventilating them through the ceiling, and they should be detached from one another as far as circumstances would admit (p. 58). He recommended staggering them on the site plan to facilitate the free circulation of air around them (p. 65). They would be connected by corridors lower than the ward windows, and all thresholds would be eliminated to facilitate delivery of goods and patients in simple trucks with rubber tires on the wheels (p. 59).

For individual wards he proposed a square rather than rectangular format (fig. 181), such as that of the new wards of the Massachusetts General Hospital. "I do not think that the attractive, home-like character of such rooms, in comparison with long, narrow wards, can be appreciated without seeing both in occupation" (p. 76). Heat is more evenly distributed from central fireplaces or stoves facing in the four directions, beds can be more evenly distributed, ventilation works better through ceiling outlets grouped around the chimney stack, and a sense of privacy for each bed is increased because the chimney stack breaks the view across the room. It also breaks up drafts that would go whistling down a long narrow hall. Note the southerly veranda and glassed-in sunroom that faces due south. The three water closets were encased in a wall of brick from the foundation up, forming practically a separate building about 9 feet square (p. 78).

Folsom's isolating ward with single rooms was adopted with a few changes for Johns Hopkins Hospital.[12] For the occasional case so contagious or unpleasantly smelly that it cannot remain under the same roof with others, he proposes "sectional buildings"—what we would call prefabs—"made of pine wood, the different parts of which fasten together by hooks and bolts, so that one can be erected in an hour without the aid of a carpenter." The dimensions of each would be 8 by 7 feet by 7 feet high at the eaves, but this was no tent. Folsom did not approve of tents; however, he recommended a "canvas tent fly" to protect the little building from the heat of the sun. After use the sections could be broken down, aired, revarnished, and stored away again in the cellar of the isolating ward (p. 88).

Dr. Joseph Jones of New Orleans, professor of chemistry and clinical medicine at the University of Louisiana, brought his experience as surgeon in the Confederate army to bear upon the problem. He emphatically favored permanent hospitals of the most durable materials, preferably granite, for fireproofing. The walls should be impermeable cement or tile, the floors made of some fireproof material covered with glazed tiles and a "good oil cloth" that could frequently be removed and washed (p. 112). The only way to keep a permanent hospital healthy is by rotating wards: one-twelfth of the ward space

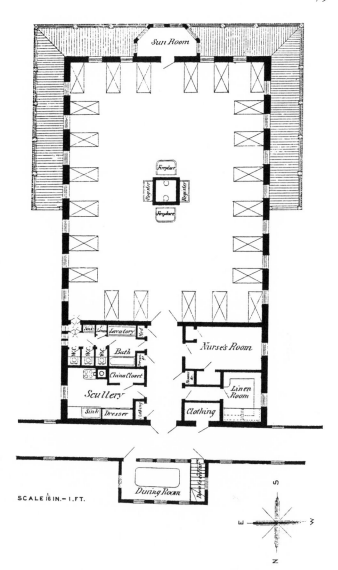

Fig. 181. Dr. Norton Folsom's ward design for Johns Hopkins Hospital, 1875.

should be left vacant at any one time and each ward should be "annually evacuated, cleansed, ventilated and disinfected with chlorine, carbolic acid and burning charcoal and sulphur . . . so that all inconvenience and confusion would be avoided" (p. 113). Thus one would avoid the chief disadvantages of a barracks hospital: danger from fire, and constant repairs to the perishable fabric.

He then proceeded to safeguard these fireproof buildings in accordance with the newest sanitary principles, and, being scared, leaned over backward. The sick should be distributed over as large an area as possible and each sick person should be as far removed from his neighbor as possible (p. 116). The wards were to be erected upon arches; the space of the lower floor, completely ventilatable, might then be used "as a general highway, with a central tramway or railroad, for the conveyance of the food, medicines, patients, clothing, and dead" (p. 117). The distances involved in meticulous separation make Folsom's arrangement look like a cross between the site plan of the new St. Thomas's Hospital and the layout of a model railroad (p. 162). The wards were given many opposite windows, and water closets were situated in nearly detached lobbies at one end of the ward and separated from it by thorough cross-ventilation. "Air is one of the greatest disinfectants" (p. 127). But the principle postulates air in motion since only "a very small portion of the oxygen of the atmosphere is in that active state which favors the destruction of the organic matters adhering to the walls and furniture" (p. 127).

The sanitary theories of Dr. Stephen Smith of New York, physician and expert on health and welfare, were complicated by his rather fuzzy understanding of the new germ theory whereby "a particle of an infective nature may be emitted from the sick, and give rise in another person who receives it to a disease, if not altogether like that in the former, quite as dangerous" (p. 286). If this be the case, separation of patients must be carried much further than ever before. While the pavilion form (now so well established that few details are necessary) would serve as underlying module, the number of patients to a ward, their disposition, and whether the ward would be temporary or permanent would depend on the infectiousness of the disease.

Smith divided patients into four categories: (1) the acutely contagious cases (gangrene, erysipelas, pyaemia, septicaemia); (2) uncomplicated supperations and fevers; (3) acute medical and surgical cases, very slightly infectious if at all; and (4) completely noninfectious chronic diseases and convalescents (p. 288). A pavilion, barracks, or tent could be used as a module, 80 by 30 by 16 feet high (p. 297). Twenty patients of the third category might be accommodated in this much space, or considerably more than that number of patients might be accommodated if they were from the fourth category—chronic and convalescent cases, the only ones Smith would consider placing in two-story wards (p. 296). In the same amount of space, however, only three or four infective patients might be contained in a single row of beds rather than the usual two. Furthermore, the infective patients would likely be assigned to a barracks rather than a pavilion of the same dimensions (p. 298). Smith particularly recommends the tent for such patients because it admitted most thorough ventilation summer and winter.

Whenever the temperature of the air within a tent is raised to a degree above that of the air with-

out, the air within the tent begins to escape, or rather is forced into the surrounding atmosphere, from which, in turn, it is necessarily renewed; and the rapidity of the outgoing and incoming currents of air will increase with the difference existing between the temperature within the tent and the temperature of the atmosphere at large. . . . It is certain that at our ambulance, where we maintained a constant temperature of about 60° Fah. night and day—when we had fuel—the atmosphere within the tents seemed to grow purer as the weather became severe (*Hospital Plans,* n., pp. 293–94).

No planning consideration is of more importance than the proper separation and ventilation of patients. The two rows of pavilions are staggered, the windows of the individual pavilions are staggered as well, since "beds are not very thoroughly flushed by the air which passes directly across the ward from window to window" (p. 301). *All* service rooms are separated from the patient space by a corridor, while the water closet is removed and located where "the air within it cannot penetrate the ward," that is, in the basement. Smith calculates that half the patients in the hospitals at any given time will be capable of climbing stairs; to others he allows a "small room on the ward floor, with dry earth-closets, a urinal, and a lavatory" (p. 300). The free end of the ward, normally used for water closets, is given large windows or doors into the grounds in order that "the ward walls shall be constantly flushed with air and sunlight" (p. 302).

If half the patients are supposed to walk, certainly the staff can. And 20 one-story pavilions—exclusive of service buildings—laid out on either side of a corridor around the circumference of the entire site would involve a great deal of walking. Dr. Smith proposed an ingenious three-layered corridor that was used in the actual building: a basement story for gas, hot air, and water pipes to facilitate inspection (p. 305), a covered walkway with many windows a little below ground level for the tram passage and the staff in stormy weather, and an open walk above that for staff and convalescents. The corridor divided the patient area from the service area of each ward in a manner also adapted for actual use (fig. 182). To conserve staff energy by building two-story wards and so shortening the corridor was unthinkable. "Even if they were less expensive in every respect than one-story pavilions, but in any degree less healthful for the sick, the latter should be preferred" (p. 295). The only plausible excuse for multiple-storied wards is inadequate ground space, for instance in cities, but hospitals should not be built in cities anyway: "All modern scientific in-

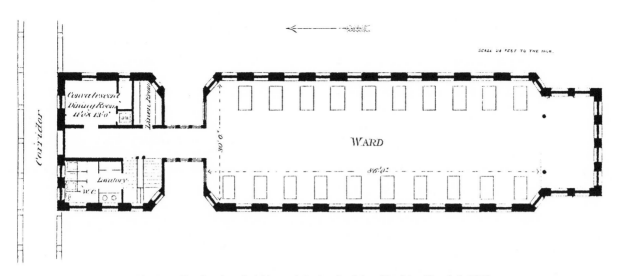

Fig. 182. Dr. Stephen Smith's ward design for Johns Hopkins Hospital, 1875.

quiries into the conditions under which the sick re-over, tends to prove that hospital sites should be selected where there is ample area, and hence in suburban rather than in urban districts" (p. 296).

This plan expresses an infinite division of patients: by age ("one or more wards in each group must be set aside for children," p. 288); color ("separate wards can be assigned to persons of color in each group, if it is found necessary"); ability to pay ("pay patients . . require isolation, and many of the comforts and conveniences of home"); degree of contagion; and sex. "The two sexes of patients cannot safely be allowed to intermingle even on the grounds. They should not only be as widely separated as possible, but there should be an effectual bar against their approach to each other" (p. 305). This can be implemented only by assigning the pavilions along one long side of the lot to males and duplicating them with pavilions for females on the other long side. Four hundred patients in one-story wards, separated by sex, calls for 20 pavilions for each sex. Smith's accompanying plan, which shows only ten to a side, fills the site. He does not face up to this dilemma but suggests a gradual beginning: a couple of wards built on either side, "and the remainder can be added as patients increase, or as circumstances require" (p. 306).

Of the five hospital experts, Dr. John S. Billings, assistant surgeon of the United States Army, had the clearest notion how germs actually reproduce. He realized that they are living particles and that dilution of the air does not altogether solve the problem.

> The probabilities of coming in contact with one are correspondingly diminished; but if it chances that one particle falls on the wound, the results will be nearly the same as if no dilution had been made.
>
> If you are standing on a plain across which a

file of men are firing, your chances of escape are of course better if there are but ten men shooting instead of one hundred; but if one of the ten does chance to hit you, the practical difference will probably not be appreciated (p. 13).

Ventilation alone cannot afford perfect security against hospital diseases, not even if the usual cubic space is doubled and the air supply tripled (p. 14). Does this then mean the use of destructible barracks throughout any type of hospital? Billings once thought so; he toyed with the notion of dividing any hospital endowment in half, using one half to build temporary barracks with a life expectancy of fifteen years and investing the other half at 6 percent interest, on which basis a complete new hospital could be furnished every twelve years for an indefinite period to come (p. 16). But although barracks work well in military installations, they are not the universal solution. Military hospitals differ from civilian in several ways. They have ample site room and need not be located in cities. The patient population is homogeneous, adult, male, and of a better class than the charity patients of a civilian hospital. No medical school or other institution need be consulted in building or running a military hospital, and it is under the direct charge of one medical man whose power is very great (p. 17). And factors such as number of attendants and cost of fuel need not be taken into account.

Billings carefully differentiated between the two raging issues of his time: permanent versus destructible buildings, and one-story versus two-story wards—a totally different issue to which he could give no authoritative answer "for the reason that there are no trustworthy observations as to their relative healthfulness" (p. 27). It is Billings's opinion that for 75 percent of the patients a two-story pavilion would be as healthful as a one-story pavilion, and a hospital of

two-story pavilions would certainly be more economical (p. 28). Two-story pavilions have other advantages: they keep visitors from entering without
authorization and patients from escaping. "Much
of the disease which will be treated in this Hospital
will be due directly or indirectly to Alcohol and Ven-
ery, and it is desirable to prevent patients with de-
praved appetites from perpetuating or renewing their
maladies by recourse to the original cause."

A methodical system of isolation will accomplish the
job ventilation alone cannot effect. The first step is
to separate acute from chronic and convalescent
cases (p. 39). Then one must decide on ward size,
"bearing in mind that the larger the ward the more
difficult it is to secure the isolation and classification
of patients, and the smaller the ward the greater is the
labor and cost of supervision and attendance. . . .
Twenty-four bed wards should be the very largest
ones in this hospital, and numerous smaller ones
will be desirable" (p. 40). Billings estimates the number of acute cases requiring more or less isolation
at about 25 percent of the total population. For the
contagious he recommends hospital tents of the United
States Army pattern, fifteen of them, to be kept on
hand and to be used methodically as isolation wards
(p. 43).

Probably Billings was chosen as consultant because he carefully and sensibly tried to balance all
the elements that went into building a hospital at a
time when germs as well as filth were first recognized
as a cause of hospital fevers. He also had the good
sense to understand that one cannot include one advantage without giving up another. "An attempt is
almost always made," he wrote, "to combine three
things which are incompatible, namely: satisfactory
heating, ventilation, and economy. We can obtain
without much difficulty any two of them, but I have
not yet seen any plan which combines the three, if
the word economy be used in its usual sense" (p. 21).

The fifth planner of this hospital symposium, Dr.
Caspar Morris of Philadelphia, considered economy
the key issue. Though he claimed no originality and
presented a plan essentially that of the hospital of
the Protestant Episcopal Church of Philadelphia,
whose new pavilion had recently engaged his attention, his was the voice of the future: in the interests
of economy, he recommended multiple stories. It
must be understood that Morris was not reverting
to block plans of the early nineteenth century but
actually looking ahead to skyscraper plans of the
early twentieth century, which came into being where
space was at a premium and economy of operation
once again assumed real importance. It is not irrelevant to add here the dates of the first safe elevator
at the Crystal Palace Exposition in New York, 1853;

the first passenger elevator at a department store in
New York, 1857; the first European elevator at the
Paris exhibition, 1867; and the first elevator in a struc-
ture of modern skyscraper proportions in the Eiffel
Tower, 1889.[13]

Johns Hopkins had asked for a city hospital, and
Dr. Morris took him up on that.

> A *city* hospital must be adapted to the require-
> ments of city life, and must be constructed on
> the same principles as the city itself.
>
> Light, air and space are essential to life; and a
> *certain amount* of each is absolutely necessary
> to existence. . . . But the necessity of concentrat-
> ing action, and combining in concerted effort
> for business purposes, compels a majority of [the
> healthy residents of a city] to sacrifice the com-
> fort, and elegance, and superior advantages in
> relation to health, of villa and suburban dwellings
> and to mass their houses on the smallest area
> which furnishes the requisite amount of light
> and air, in order to economize time and strength
> in the co-operative pursuit of common purposes.
> So must the sick and wounded of such a popu-
> lation submit to similar concentration in order
> to secure advantages which cannot be had with-
> out such sacrifice. . . . The supply of medical
> and surgical attendance and nursing is limited,
> and cannot be spread out indefinitely (*Hospital
> Plans,* pp. 178–79).

Morris likened contemporary plans for one-story
barracks hospitals in cities to a utopian dream of
substituting for city apartments a village of cottages.
Certainly cottages would be healthier; and equally
so a nurse for every half-dozen cases; also, a pro-
portional supply of medical and surgical skill would
reduce hospital mortality. On the other hand, the
modern hospital, made up of properly proportioned
wards even though one may be piled on top of another,
was so much better than the living quarters of its
pauper patients that it must seem like a veritable
village to them (pp. 179–80).

Every ward of 24–30 patients is a hospital in itself.
A general hospital is but the aggregation of such
wards, and now the question is: "Shall the number
of wards necessary be spread out upon the one level,
each ward separated from the other by a space at
least double its height? or shall the same amount
of floor and air space be furnished by superimposing
one ward upon another?" He calculates that the cost
of a building's foundations and heating and lighting
installations, and all the various forms of service, is the
same for one story as for two and argues that "the cost
of nursing and support might almost be said to increase
with the square of the distance, and the difficulty of

supervision and administration in the same proportion" (p. 181).

The important thing is not spreading out over a vast area for its own sake but *isolation,* however achieved; "and if this be secured, economy, in construction and convenience of service, may be perfectly justifiable" (p. 182). Isolation is achieved when miasmal infection is not transferred from one ward to another. But infection travels sideways as well as upward, "by currents of air, or on the persons and clothing of those exposed to it, and in sponges, and dressings, and instruments; and if these pass laterally from the source of contamination, the effect will be transmitted by lateral passages as surely as by vertical." A solution might rather be long, wide, high, open corridors and a system of ventilation whereby air currents blow *from* these corridors *into* the wards. "And thus there will be no communication from one ward to another, whether they be placed above or beside each other." There is nothing wrong with upper rooms per se. Upper rooms in private houses are known to be lighter, more cheerful, airier (p. 184).

What a hospital needs most is not physical extension but human vigilance. "Vigilance essential to success" should be the motto of hospital management (p. 185). Billings had said he knew of only one way to detect infection, and that was by the smell of it (p. 22); Morris affirms this to be no test at all. "A lethal influence may lurk in the atmosphere and no sensible odor betray its presence, while a foul and offensive smell may give rise to nothing more serious than nausea or disgust" (p. 185).[14] Fastidious universal cleanliness, never-ceasing vigilance will do more for patients than any building principle or even the skill of professional attendants, "for the establishment which has to be kept in such exquisite perfection of cleanliness, is an establishment which never rests from fouling itself" (p. 186).

The logical outcome of Dr. Morris's arguments would be a plan for a multistoried ward, but the trustees had stipulated pavilions and pavilions were what he drew for them, very like anybody else's pavilions and pretty much like St. Thomas's. His principles, however, persisted and were expressed in new plans twenty years later for city hospitals, where space and economy were of utmost concern.

The Actual Plans of Johns Hopkins Hospital

The five plans were published, criticized, and reviewed. John S. Billings, chosen as consultant to the hospital, had excellent ideas but his plans were undistinguished. By his own account, he was asked if he was still satisfied with them and he replied very promptly that he was not.[15] He drew up new plans with the aid of an architect, took them abroad for criticism, and while there examined the model hospitals of Europe. He returned home even less satisfied, and he, the architect, and the building committee drew up a new set of plans that were finally adopted (fig. 183).

They were nothing if not symmetrical: an administration building in the center of the facade with an apothecary building behind it; the two pay wards, one for women and one for men, to either side of the facade; a square kitchen behind them to the left balancing the square nurses' home behind them to the right; and running back into the lot on either side an octagon ward, three common wards, and an isolating ward. At the rear of the lot is the central church, just where one would expect to find it. In the rear left corner is the building for the pathological institute, in the rear right corner that for the laundry. Only the operating building and polyclinic along Monument Street were not exactly balanced by a conservatory for plants along Jefferson Street.

Building commenced in 1877 with the foundations for the administration building and the two pay wards and went as rapidly as possible. The possibilities, however, were limited. It will be remembered that this hospital was to be constructed with income from its endowment, and after it was built the income was to be applied to running expenses. As income accumulated, the trustees would order another ward; when the money was used up, construction ceased. This went on for twelve years. One of the best-endowed hospitals in the world could not hold to its building schedule for lack of funds. Construction costs were higher than anticipated; the annual income progressively shrank.[16] The trustees were under considerable pressure to open the finished sections, but to do so would mean diverting building moneys to administration and fatally interrupting the completion of the plan. They held out, went on slowly adding unit to unit and finally in 1885 dedicated and opened to patients an unfinished hospital. Only the service buildings and wards on the northern side of the lot were completed. The symmetrical plan as originally conceived was carried no further; the empty southern lawn, assigned for a while to tents, was finally built up in an altogether different style. Johns Hopkins Hospital could have been built symmetrically *or* from income alone, but not both.

The section achieved (fig. 184) was remarkable enough. Every detail was of the very best (fig. 185). There were two types of common ward for charity patients, one rectangular and one octagonal, and two types of ventilation were deliberately tried out in them to see which one worked better. In the rectangular ward, intake of air was through vents opening in the sidewall between every two beds. The air

184

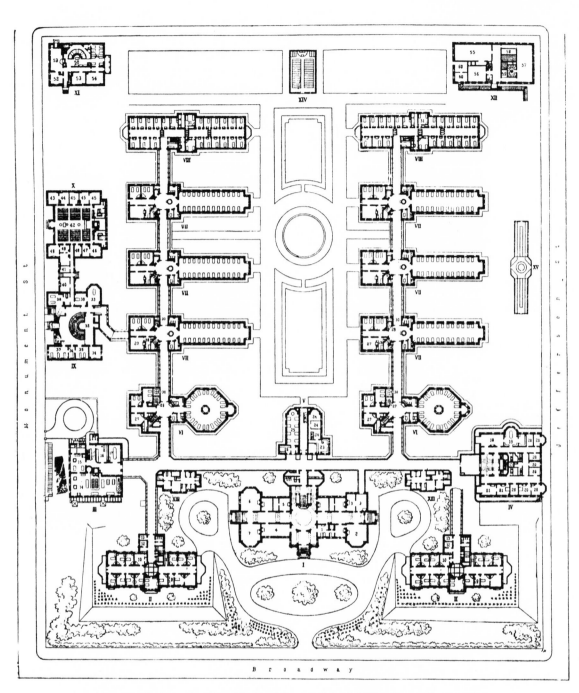

Fig. 183. Final plan for Johns Hopkins Hospital (John S. Billings's second plan) 1876.

was drawn from the basement and the basement was above ground (fig. 186); indeed, we might mistake the common ward for a two-story building but we think on too small a scale. The Victorian planners conceived it as a one-story ward with a full basement serving only as a vast air reservoir, the air being drawn from across the green lawns (i.e., it was the very freshest air available) through as many windows as those in the ward itself. The outer walls of the basement were lined with many coils of three-inch cast-iron pipe for water that could be brought up to a

temperature of 150°.[17] Since the water in each coil could be regulated by a separate valve, the temperature of the air drawn over a coil before it entered the ward could be tempered to suit the individual requirements of the two beds on either side of this particular air intake. Yankee ingenuity was enthusiastically applied to this hospital.

To remove foul air from the ward two series of outlets were used. Both are clearly visible in the view of the ward interior (fig. 187) and that of the longitudinal section (fig. 188). Under each bed was a rounded

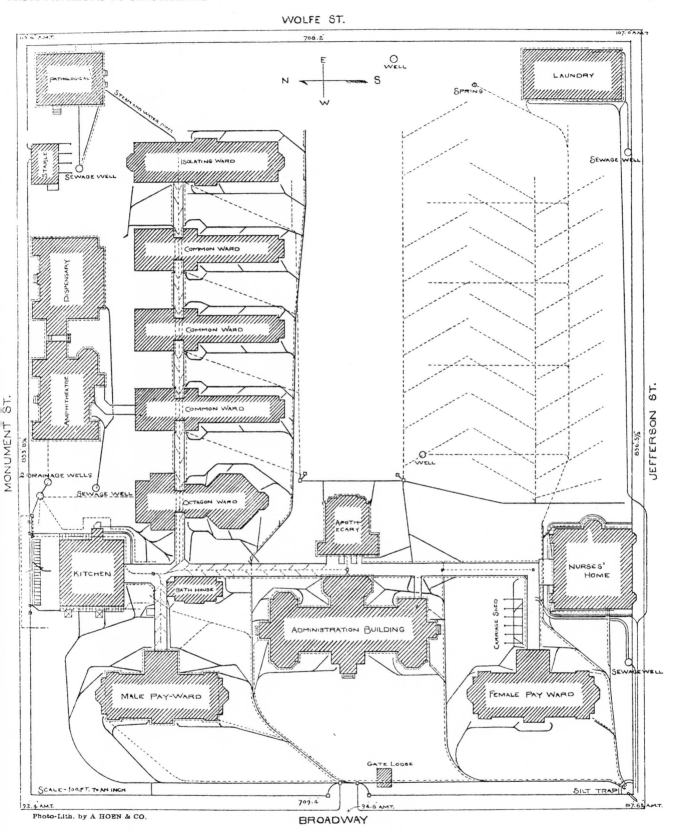

Fig. 184. Site plan of Johns Hopkins Hospital as actually built, 1885.

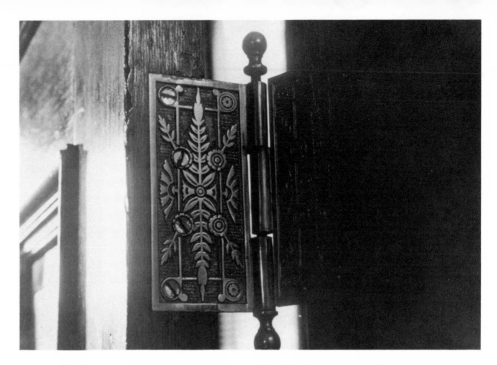

Fig. 185. Brass door hinge in the administration building, Johns Hopkins Hospital.

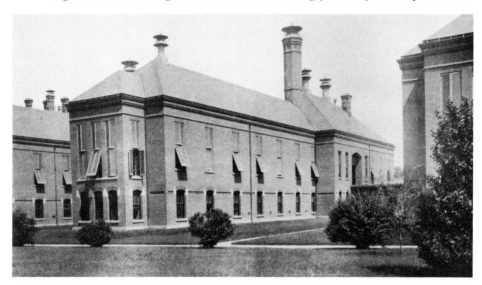

Fig. 186. Elevation, common ward, Johns Hopkins Hospital.

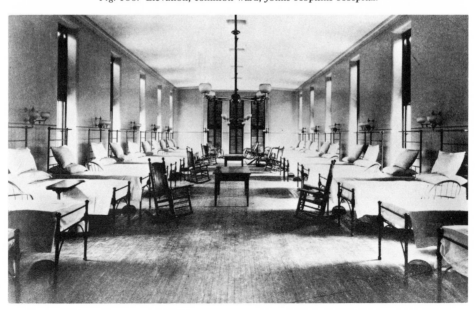

Fig. 187. Interior, common ward.

iron cage leading to a 12-inch galvanized iron tube that ran along the ceiling of the basement to a lower entrance to the main ventilating chimney. And in the center of the ceiling of the ward itself were 6 spaced openings 2 by 2 feet into the upper foul air duct, which ran across the floor of the attic and into the ventilating chimney at a higher point. A coil of steam just above this point accelerated the air velocity through the ventilating shaft. Billings reports that in cold weather only the downward ventilation was used, to save heat, but in hot weather or to flush the ward with air the ceiling registers were also opened.[18]

The one octagon ward that was built, which became quite famous, was in a way a mistake (fig. 189a–c). The architect, J. R. Niernsee, had designed an octagon for the other row of wards (the one that never materialized) because (as one can see on the plan) the rectangular model would have collided with the nursing home. It was an adaptation of the nearly square wards of the Massachusetts General Hospital,[19] and the variation in shape, as well as the fact that this ward was built in two stories with a full basement, called for a different ventilation technique. The direction of air intake is from the circumference to the central shaft, an octagonal chimney 13 feet in external diameter that ran through both stories. The intake air was heated by basement coils in the usual way and entered between every two beds. Foul air was removed from the first-floor ward by a lower and an upper opening on all 8 facets of the chimney, and these openings led directly into its central shaft. But this chimney was very complicated. A boiler-iron tube 5 feet 8 inches in diameter ran up it too, and the openings of the second story entered the space between the boiler–iron flue and the outer chimney, while a ring just above the flue acted as an accelerating coil. The chimney also contained a 12-inch cast-iron pipe to carry off smoke from open fireplaces in the wards, should the addition of fireplaces be found desirable. Over and above these complicated technological innovations for promoting ventilation, one still allowed for the possibility that an open fireplace is the best solution after all.

The three-layered corridor connected the pavilions; its open sun deck was at the level of the wards. The absence of elevators was a deliberate choice. Patients were carried upstairs from the covered corridor at ground level on stretchers, and (see figure 190, an enlarged detail of the middle section of the common ward) the stairs from below (A) did not emerge in the ward itself but at a covered section of the open corridor. Another door, B, led to the anteroom of the ward. Thus no air from one ward could possibly be conveyed to another, and patients in the stretchers were never drenched and only momentarily chilled."[20]

The red brick facade of Johns Hopkins Hospital (fig. 191) is preserved today relatively unchanged, alongside much modern building. It is noble, individual, neo-Gothic. The central hall of the administration building opens to the roof four stories above it; when built it was open to and lit from the lantern of the dome. In this hall the dedicatory exercises were held and one speaker expressed the wish that some friend of the hospital might place under the dome a copy of the statue of Christus Consolator by the Danish sculptor Thorwaldsen[21] to remind physicians, nurses, students, and patients "that over this institution rests the perpetual benediction of Christian charity, the constant spirit of 'good will to man.' "[22] Within two years the copy had been donated and, in the absence of a central chapel that was never realized, in a rather odd manner it does impress the "influences of religion . . . upon the whole management of the Hospital," in accordance with Johns Hopkins's special request.[23] In this busy reception lobby, the cleaning women sometimes pause to pray on their way to work (fig. 192). A Baltimore resident told us, "When I was first brought to this hospital as a very little girl I was scared of the doctors, of what they would do to me. But then I thought, 'He's on *my* side, and he's bigger'n *they* are!' "

The First Skyscrapers

Of the five authors Billings was the only one who took into consideration that the hospital might develop in the future as a result of continuing scientific discoveries beyond any present ability to project or imagine the form it might take. In his own words:

So far as I can judge from my own experience and that which is recorded of others, no matter what plan is adopted, when the Hospital is completed and put into practical operation, it will appear that it can be improved in some particulars, and a certain amount of funds should be reserved for this purpose.

The general principles which I have tried to state in this paper are in accordance with the present condition of our knowledge of the subject, but that knowledge is imperfect, and too much of the teaching of books on the subject of hospital construction is theoretical only.[24]

Nineteenth-century scientific advances, real breakthroughs to understanding the causes of disease, were not fully understood in their time and only in the twentieth century were they translated into changes in hospital design. But very much was accomplished. In 1835 Pierre Louis first used control groups to test the effectiveness of cures—a last blow

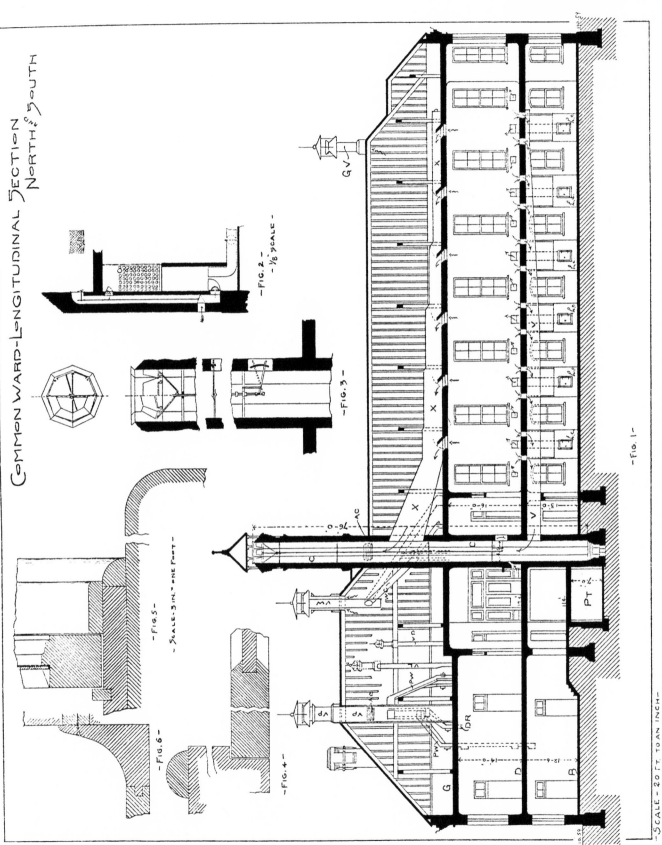

Fig. 188. Longitudinal section north and south, common ward, Johns Hopkins Hospital.

FIG. 1: Longitudinal section of ward.

B	basement floor	DR	vent pipe from dining room, $17'' \times 24''$	
D	main floor	PW	vent pipe from private wards, $18'' \times 22''$	
G	attic floor	GV	attic ventilation, $24''$ diameter	
PT	pipe tunnel, $7'0'' \times 10'0''$	VD	lift vent, $10''$ diameter	
C	central ventilating chimney, $4'8'' \times 4'8''$	VL	linen and patients' clothes room vent, $10''$ diameter	
AC	accelerating steam coils			
X	foul air duct in attic, $48'' \times 51''$	VP	vent shaft (private wards), $36''$ diameter	
V	foul air duct in basement, area 12 square feet	hc	heat coils	
VW	ventilating shaft for water closets, $24''$ diameter			
WC	vent pipe from water closets, $20''$ and $16''$ diameter			

FIG. 2: Section of heating coil chamber. FIG. 3: Section and plans of ventilating chimney showing damper. FIG. 4: Plan of doors showing finish. FIG. 5: Plan of windows showing finish. FIG. 6: Section of washboard.

to untested empirical medicine. Louis's contribution to medicine was that he propagandized for numerical analysis as a valid approach, for example, in proving or disproving the effectiveness of bleeding as a form of therapy.[25] As Richard H. Shryock, paraphrasing Louis, put it, "In the difference here between exactitude and vagueness . . . lay all the difference between truth and error."[26] Once it became possible to measure the results of the heroic remedies—bleeding, purging, overdosing—and they were proved useless, even harmful, they fell into gradual disrepute and were replaced by what were considered more effective methods. The common folk missed them. They had made it seem that something big was happening.

Morphine was introduced into general practice in 1844 and the efficacy of ether was demonstrated at Massachusetts General Hospital in 1846.[27] Then followed a horrible interregnum when operations were performed on the inner cavities of patients who felt no pain at the time but died of consequent infection. Then in 1865 Lister operated under a continuous spray of carbolic acid and halted infection. A later refinement was the aseptic method, in which not the patient himself but everything that came into contact with him was scrupulously disinfected, with results still more fortunate. Steam sterilization was introduced in 1886.[28] Meanwhile, Pasteur was making epochal discoveries: in 1866 that specific bacteria cause the fermentation of wine, in 1875 that fermentation generally is due to the activity of living microbes and each kind of fermentation is the work of a specific microbe, in 1877 that the anthrax bacilli may be cultivated and new cases of anthrax be produced from these bacilli and that vaccination produces immunity; in 1885 that people can be vaccinated against rabies.

In 1882 Robert Koch discovered the bacillus of tuberculosis, a mystery killer up to the very moment Koch delivered his historic lecture identifying and reproducing it. In the 1880s and 1890s he and many other bacteriologists identified causative agents of erysipelas, diphtheria, tetanus, pneumonia, meningitis, plague, and bacillary dysentery—to mention only a partial list of diseases.[29] Until causes are identified no cures can be found. Now cures were indeed found. The first real hospital laboratory was introduced in Paris in 1893,[30] and it was clear that hospitals could never be the same again.

Nevertheless, it took a long time for the new principles to be understood, and people continued to plan in terms of practically infinite separation and segregation. The General Hospital of Hamburg Eppendorf (1885–89; fig. 193) had 1,474 beds distributed in 82 distinct buildings, most of them one story in height, some of them two. Yet Ochsner and Sturm (pp. 479–80) tell us that this was the first great hospital constructed after the introduction of antiseptic methods! The establishment covered 23 acres of land, and still the space around buildings was not considered sufficient to prevent shadows (of buildings and shrubbery) from keeping the ground too damp for satisfactory hygienic conditions. The distances involved in visiting patients were so great that department chiefs rarely found time to make ward rounds, a duty that was relegated to assistants.

A retreat from this extreme seems obvious to us, but in 1905 the Chicago surgeon Dr. Albert Ochsner startled a meeting of the Association of Hospital Superintendents by proposing it.[31] If stories are piled on top of one another, economies can be effected in the areas of space, heating, supervision, cleaning, and the energies of the staff. On a city lot (as Morris had indicated in 1875) hospital space *must* be consolidated. "Were it possible to place hospitals in the middle of our public parks," wrote Ochsner in 1907, "it would be an easy matter. . . . It is, however, rarely possible to obtain more than a city block, containing five acres of land, even for a large hospital."[32]

He illustrates the point by simple diagrams. Assuming, under the most favorable circumstances, a city block of 5 acres for a hospital of 500 beds, he shows it occupied by a 10-story building (fig. 194) with an additional small separate structure for the boiler house and laundry in the rear. This would readily house the wards plus an administration department on the first floor, operating department, recovery rooms, and kitchen on the top floor, and the usual service rooms on each floor for the wards (diet kitchen, bathrooms, toilet rooms, linen rooms, and so on).

Figure 195 shows the same 5-acre lot occupied by 10 single-storied pavilions, also for 500 patients, with the necessary operating rooms, kitchen, boiler rooms, and other facilities. The boiler building is identical. Presumably the ward buildings contained two 31-bed wards that shared a set of service rooms, and gave each patient the same amount of air space as allotted in the previous figure. This would leave two extra pavilions for operating rooms, kitchen, and administration.

But city blocks are not always this large. The next two diagrams are projected on what one might more reasonably expect, a square lot 520 feet on each side. The 10-story building still fits (fig. 196), but when it is translated into 10-story pavilions in two straight lines (fig. 197), what is left of the lot? In which arrangement might patients be presumed to receive more sun and air? In a 10-story structure extending north· and south, each room would receive unobstructed sunlight during some portion of the day: one half of them the morning sun, the other half the afternoon sun, and the hallway the noonday sun. Broad verandas are assumed across the northern and southern ends.

Such thinking was made possible by architectural advances as relevant to hospital planning as new theories of germs as living organisms had been in the medical area. Metal was increasingly being used for the framework of buildings. The weight of a stone structure makes it necessary to thicken foundation walls to bear it, and beyond 12 stories this proves impractical. But when the frame is made of metal— rolled-iron floor beams came gradually into use from the middle of the nineteenth century—the metal will support the weight and walls become mere screens to keep out the weather. Steel skeleton buildings came in about 1900. "The new type of construction which engineering had ushered in," says Talbot Hamlin,

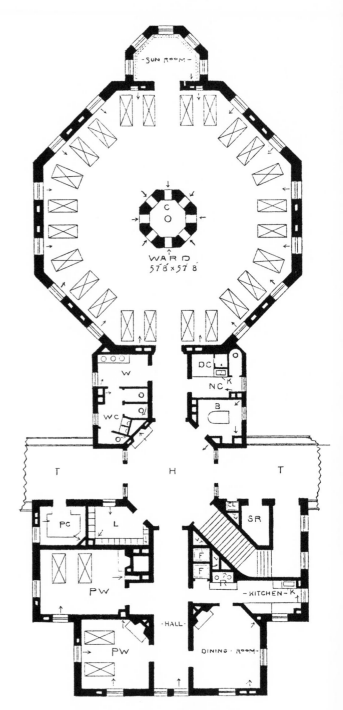

Fig. 189 (a) Floor plan of the first floor (longitudinal section north and south), octagon ward, Johns Hopkins Hospital.

C	central ventilating chimney, 8'0" × 8'0"	VL	ventilator for linen closet and clothes room, 14" diameter
BC	boiler iron cylinder, 6'0" diameter	Co	corridor
AC	accelerating steam coils	PT	pipe tunnel
VWC	vent pipe from water closet, 24" diameter	B	basement floor
		D	main floor
V	ventilator for water closet bath room and lavatory, 32" diameter	E	second floor
		G	attic floor
		DC	chimney damper
VS	ventilator for special wards, 42" diameter	S	smoke pipe

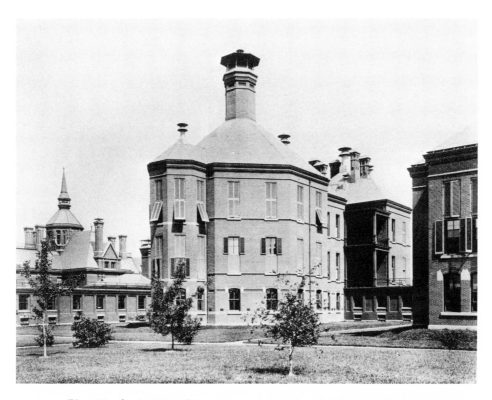

Fig. 189. (b) elevation of the octagon ward; (c) interior of the octagon ward.

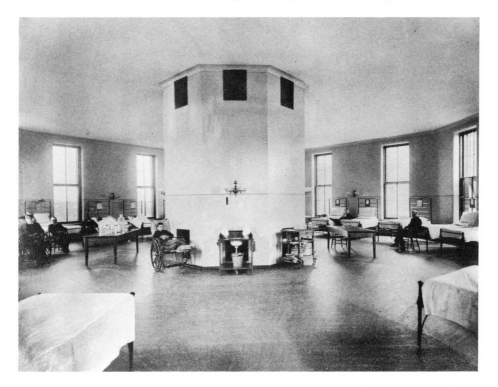

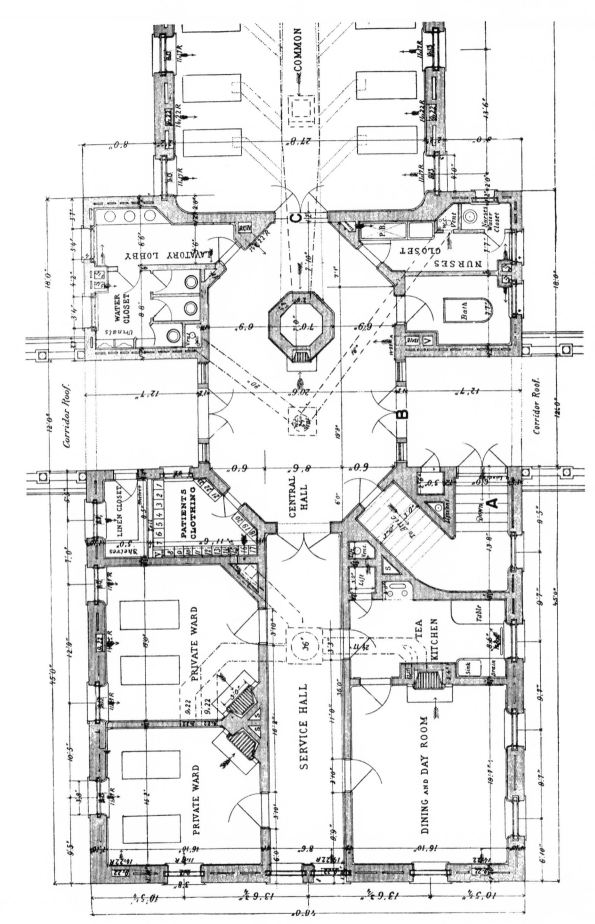

Fig. 190. Detail of the architect's plan of the common ward, showing that stairs from below (A) did not open directly into the ward but into a covered corridor; another door (B) opened into a central hall, where still another door (C) led into the ward.

"was so fundamentally different from anything that had gone before that it made eventual architectural design of an entirely new type inevitable."[33] So in early twentieth-century cities, hospital buildings stretched skyward in company with many other functional constructions: factories, business offices, apartment houses. The trend was toward skyscrapers.

The quest for a sanitary environment had now to be reconciled with a new emphasis on functionalism and efficiency. The discipline of architecture was reduced to the theory of functionalism: "the idea that forms must be designed for specific purposes first and foremost, and that the best answer to a practical necessity of purpose or structure would automatically create successful design."[34] The life of Frederick Winslow Taylor (who died in 1915) was spent in devising ways to economize on motion, getting things done with the fewest waste movements possible, speeding up the production line. "Inventor of efficiency," John Dos Passos calls him, "who had doubled the production of the stamping-mill by speeding up the main lines of shafting from ninetysix to twohundred and twentyfive revolutions a minute."[35] In 1913 Dr. W. Gilman Thompson applied the principles of efficiency to nursing techniques.[36] He made nurses wear pedometers to see how far they walked a day (7½ miles). He weighed the very heavy wooden trays on which patient meals were carried (8 pounds unloaded, 15 pounds loaded) and suggested the substitution of wheeled trucks. He noted that the three screens used to surround and isolate the bed of one patient in an open ward weighed 31 pounds apiece. They were stored in the hall 240 feet away, which meant that every time a patient wanted a bedpan, someone had to haul not only the bedpan but 93 pounds of screens 480 feet.

"An acceptable plan for the construction of ward buildings of many stories in crowded American cities has long been needed." With these words Dr. S. S. Goldwater, superintendent of Mount Sinai Hospital in New York City, introduced in 1910 a detailed plan for a hospital of multiple stories that would fit into the average New York City block, measuring, then as now, 200 by 60 feet. "Better sites . . . are often to be had in other cities, worse ones for the erection of a large general hospital cannot well be imagined."[37] The wards of this hospital must be well lighted and surrounded by a suitable zone of aeration. It should be possible to add further stories to the original four or five when needed without detriment to the latter. The surrounding buildings for supportive services should also be capable of expansion without damaging the wards hygienically. And the whole complex should not be too near the street.

He suggests a T-shaped plan (fig. 198). The open

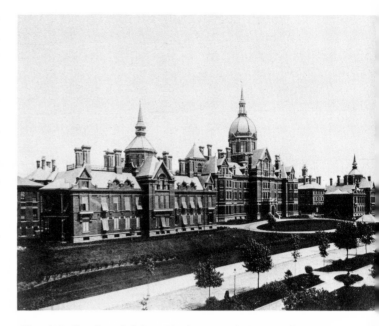

Fig. 191. Facade of Johns Hopkins Hospital, seen from the northeast. The rounded dome is that of the administration building. The red brick architecture is very rich and beautiful.

ward is placed at right angles to its services, permitting visitors to proceed directly from elevator to ward without passing through a long line of auxiliary rooms as in the orthodox Nightingale plan. These 26 beds are supplemented by 5 others in quiet rooms located among the service rooms—3 of them have 1 bed and one is a 2-bed room. One sunny balcony next to the dayroom is reserved for noisy convalescents, the other is for acutely ill cases needing quiet; both can be well supervised by staff from the nurses' utility room or pantry. The corridor of the service rooms at the top of the T is intended as a true cross-ventilating corridor.[38] The section for service and single rooms can be lengthened and/or the open ward shortened, depending on the degree of separation required by the patients.

Skyscraper Possibilities

Skyscrapers used as hospitals present a number of problems, the most serious of which is their inflexibility. Goldwater assumed that his T-shaped hospital would be used only for wards and their annexes, that auxiliary services would be placed in separate structures elsewhere on the lot. As hospitals rose 20 or more stories the temptation was naturally great to fit everything within one shaft or pattern—square, rectangular, X-shaped, or irregular. As a result of new, dramatic medical discoveries in the twentieth century, it was not the services that had to conform to the shape of the wards but the wards that were constrained by the requirements of the services. When

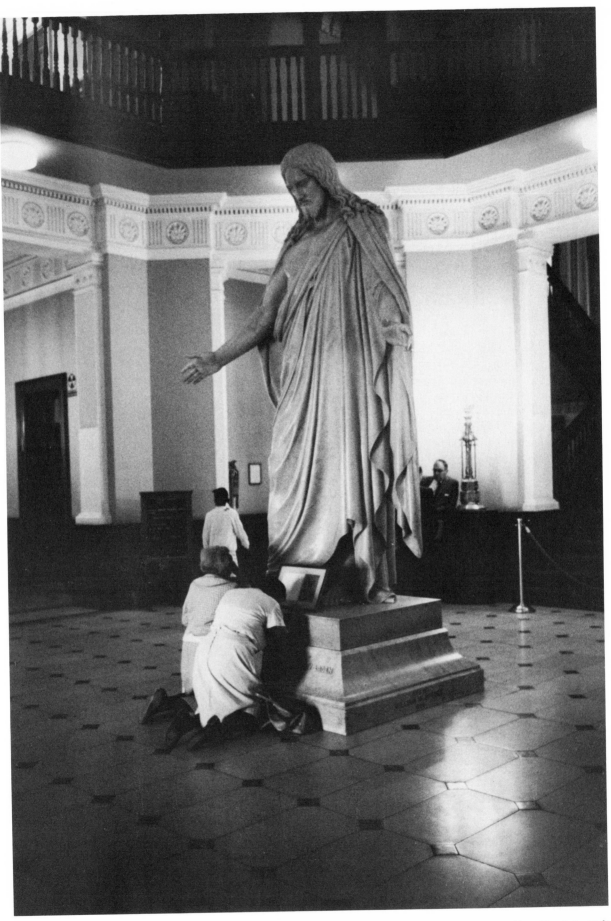

Fig. 192. Cleaning women on their way to work, reception hall, administration building, Johns Hopkins Hospital, 1969.

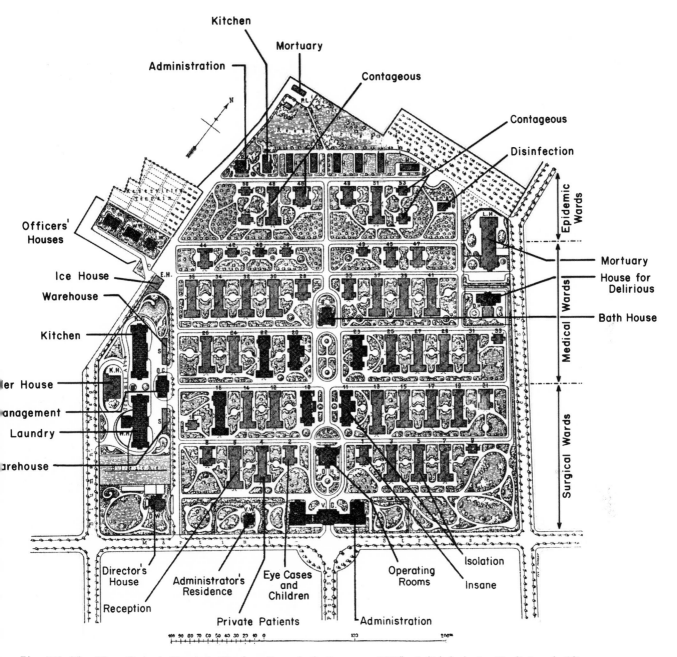

Fig. 193. The New General Hospital, Hamburg-Eppendorf, Germany (1884); 1,474 beds in 82 distinct buildings, most of them one story in height, some two stories.

an operating room on the bottom or top floor (depending on current theories as to whether foul air rises or sinks) must assume a certain shape and size for maximum usefulness, all the wards over or under it took on that shape and size, whether or not it was favorable for nursing. Or they were made to conform to the outline of an ever more important laboratory, or an expanded X-ray department.

Furthermore, once the shape of the hospital had been determined, that was it. The expensive multistoried investment was as frozen in steel and cement

as the monumental philanthropies of the eighteenth century had been frozen in stone. By 1924 Goldwater was pleading for hospital flexibility to allow for expansion, new discoveries, new windfalls, and pressures from within and without. "No hospital," he declared, "can escape its future." "When concentration and simplicity are carried too far," he added in the same essay, "the hospital is forced either to live in a strait jacket or to cast off its original garment and acquire a new and more appropriate one."[39]

Vertical arrangement may turn out to be not much

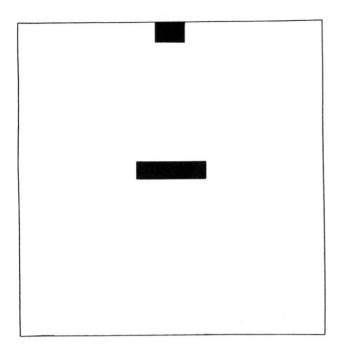

Fig. 194. Albert Ochsner's diagram of a 500-bed hospital in one 10-story building on a 5-acre lot, 1907.

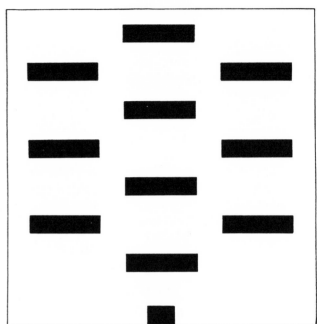

Fig. 195. Albert Ochsner's diagram of a 500-bed hospital in 10 single-storied pavilions on a 5-acre lot.

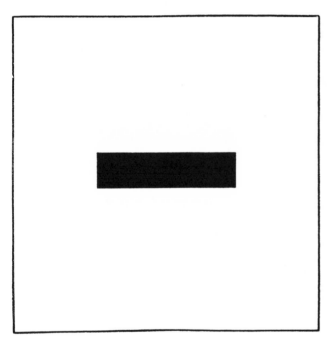

Fig. 196. Albert Ochsner's diagram of a 500-bed hospital in one 10-story building on a city lot 520 feet square.

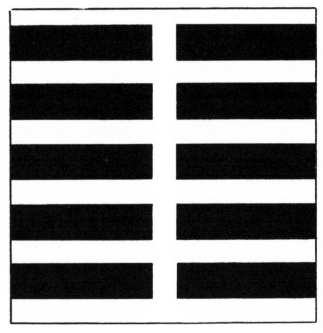

Fig. 197. Albert Ochsner's diagram of a 500-bed hospital in 10 one-story pavilions on a city lot 520 feet square.

simpler than horizontal. Staff personnel were no longer walking their legs off from pavilion to pavilion, but when the same building included, one on top of another, kitchen, outpatient department, public wards, operating rooms, and private wards, there was bound to be a wild jumble of patients, staff, and visitors in the elevators. "For the thoughtful hospital planner," Goldwater wrote in 1929, "the most sig-

nificant contrast is not one between hospitals with vertical and horizontal lines of communication, respectively, but between hospitals in which interdependent departments are conveniently and those in which they are inconveniently grouped."[40]

The skyscraper hospital came to France with the Hôpital Beaujon, opened in Clichy near Paris in 1935. Frankly inspired by American forms, it was hailed as "strictly French in its scale and dimensions . . . characterized by remarkable practical sense . . . ornament of the Assistance Publique . . . one of those human achievements whose importance goes beyond the boundaries of the township, of the province, nay of France itself. . . ."[41] This might be regarded as a realization at long last of the hospital on the outskirts of Paris for 1,200 patients (actually 1,100), ordained by royal decree at the end of the eighteenth century and delayed by uncontrollable events but now achieved in full radiance and at considerably augmented expense—the original estimate had been 10 million francs; the cost in the 1930s was 106 million. The hospital plan is interesting as an attempt to separate yet coordinate wards and services.

The entrance facade faced north. Outpatients were directed for examination and treatment to a series of identical pavilions on either side of the entrance but completely separated from the main block. Medicine and its specialties occupied the pavilions to the left and surgery with its specialties the pavilions to the right. From the southern facade jutted out four rounded stacks containing the inpatient wards (fig. 199). Each ward had 16 beds and a solarium at the rounded end, and because of the southern exposure every window received sunlight at some hour of the day (fig. 200). This was also true for the single rooms for gravely ill patients, which were located between the jutting bays in a proportion of 5 single rooms to 16 beds in the ward. The area we would call a nurses' station, between the single rooms and opposite the elevators, commanded a view of all corridors. Facing north across the corridor from the wards, were supporting services for each ward: the chief medical or surgical doctor's office and examination room, and a small X-ray room and laboratory supplementing the elaborate central radioscopic department, and central laboratory for the entire hospital. Figure 201, a cross section, shows each floor as a self-contained service. Every inpatient service was included, from two wards on the ground floor for venereal diseases (one male, one female) all the way up to short wards for TB cases near the roof, whose cut-back ledges might be used as porches for the sunshine cure.

At the new Westminster Hospital in London (1939) each story was similarly given over to a service (fig. 202), but outpatients as well as inpatients are cared for on each floor. The elevator shaft goes up through the middle of the building and, depending on whether one were an inpatient or outpatient, one turned right or left upon reaching the proper floor. Thus in this hospital, pavilions for outpatients, instead of standing horizontally parallel to one another in front of the ward block, are placed *vertically* parallel: the hospital was described as having been "set on end."

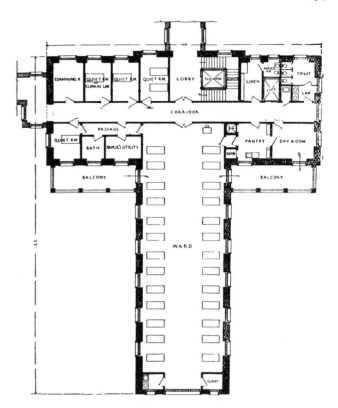

Fig. 198. S. S. Goldwater's proposed T-shaped hospital for a city lot, 1911.

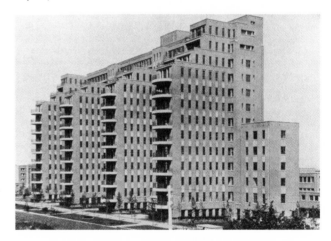

Fig. 199. Beaujon Hospital at Clichy near Paris, 1935.

The vertical planning was inspired by "magnificent hospitals" in Scandinavia. On the roof is the chapel, instead of a reservoir as at Beaujon. Exemplary continuity of personal contacts and written records is claimed for this plan because the same staff is responsible for the patient whether it treats him in the clinic or in bed.[42] Certainly the plan facilitated and perpetuated the English system of assigning certain beds to one group of doctors, called a "firm," but at the expense of occupancy. At Westminster Hospital, occupancy of a ward strictly depends on the specialty it serves. The plan is rigid. In addition, the central

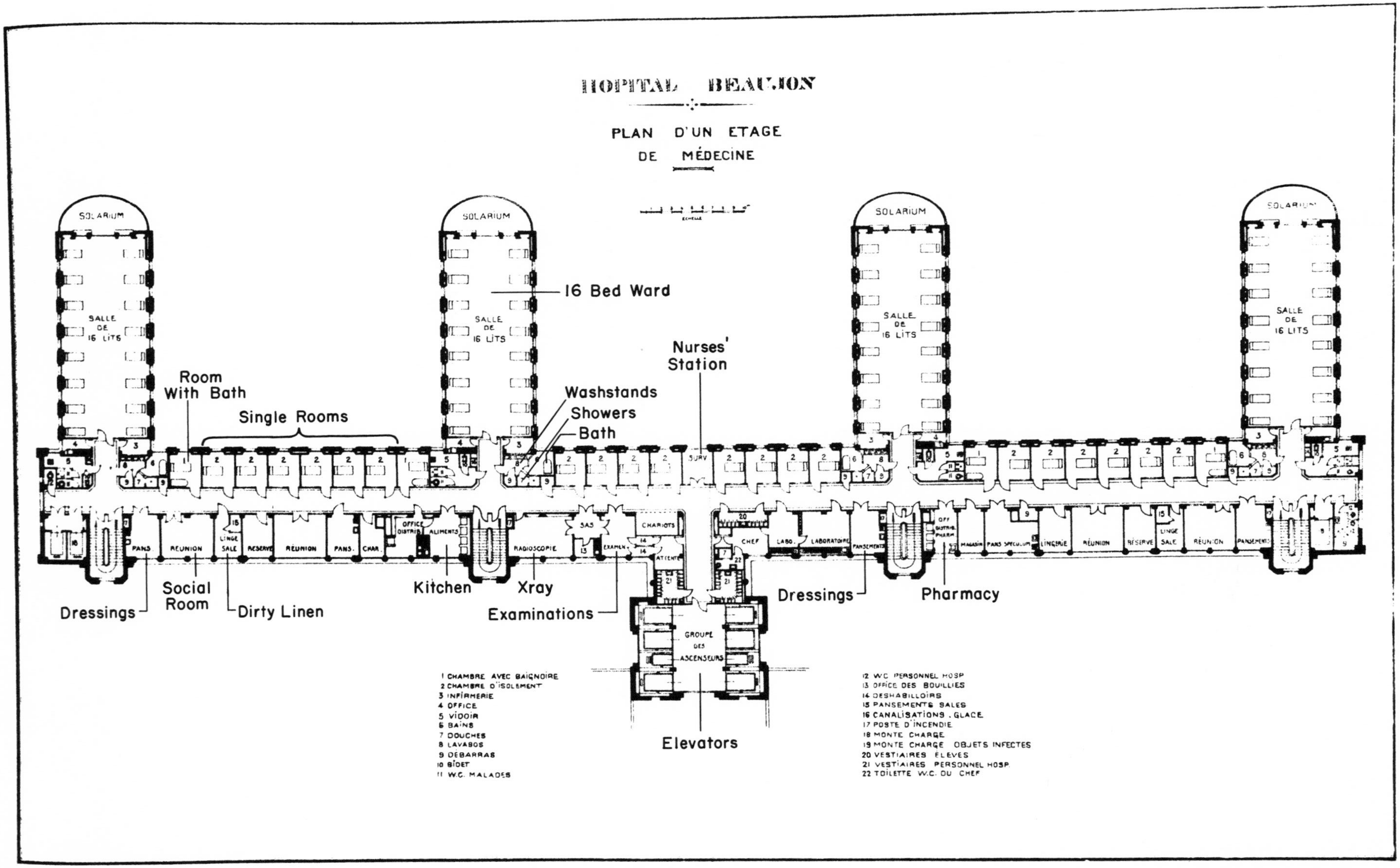
HOPITAL BEAUJON
PLAN D'UN ETAGE
DE MÉDECINE
ECHELLE
SOLARIUM
SALLE DE 16 LITS
16 Bed Ward
Nurses' Station
Room With Bath
Single Rooms
Washstands
Showers
Bath
SURV
CHARIOTS
SAS
EXAMEN
ATTENTE
RADIOSCOPIE
ALIMENTS
OFFICE DISTRIB
CHAR.
PANS.
REUNION
RESERVE
LINGE SALE
CHEF
LABO.
LABORATOIRE
PANSEMENTS
OFF DISTRIB PHARM
MAGASIN
PANS SPECULUM
LINGERIE
GROUPE DES ASCENSEURS
Dressings
Social Room
Dirty Linen
Kitchen
Xray
Examinations
Dressings
Pharmacy
Elevators
1 CHAMBRE AVEC BAIGNOIRE
2 CHAMBRE D'ISOLEMENT
3 INFIRMERIE
4 OFFICE
5 VIDOIR
6 BAINS
7 DOUCHES
8 LAVABOS
9 DEBARRAS
10 BIDET
11 W.C. MALADES
12 W.C. PERSONNEL HOSP
13 OFFICE DES BOUILLIES
14 DESHABILLOIRS
15 PANSEMENTS SALES
16 CANALISATIONS . GLACE
17 POSTE D'INCENDIE
18 MONTE CHARGE
19 MONTE CHARGE OBJETS INFECTES
20 VESTIAIRES ELEVES
21 VESTIAIRES PERSONNEL HOSP
22 TOILETTE W.C. DU CHEF

Fig. 200. Plan of a medical floor, Beaujon Hospital.

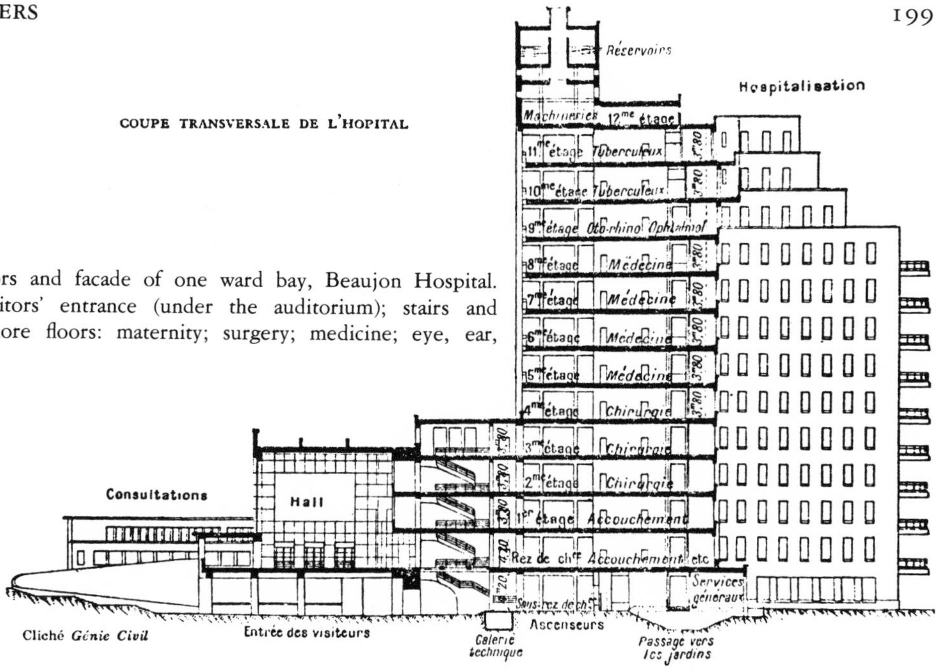

COUPE TRANSVERSALE DE L'HOPITAL

01. Longitudinal section of service floors and facade of one ward bay, Beaujon Hospital.
left to right: consultation rooms; visitors' entrance (under the auditorium); stairs and
ors; the services, taking up one or more floors: maternity; surgery; medicine; eye, ear,
and throat; tuberculosis.

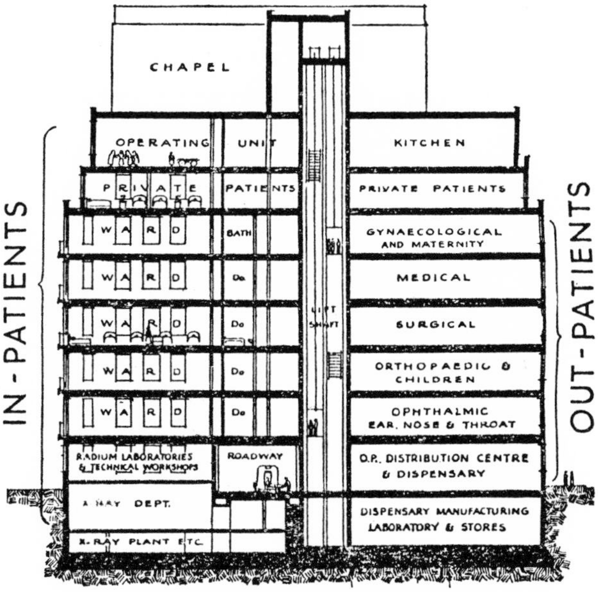

Fig. 202. Longitudinal section of the new Westminster Hospital, London (1939), showing the relation of wards to services.

Fig. 203. Bridgeport (Connecticut) Hospital before expansion.

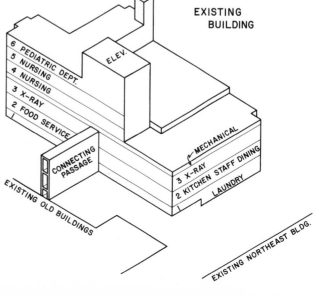

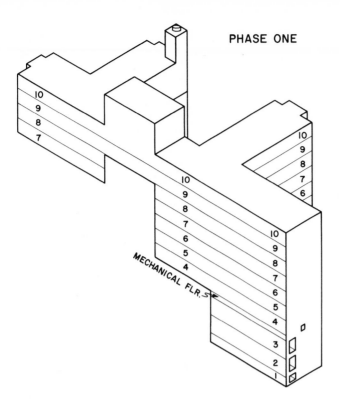

PHASE ONE

10
9
8
7

10
9
8
7
6

10
9
8
7
6
5
4

MECHANICAL FLR.S

10
9
8
7
6
5
4
3
2
1

Fig. 204. Expansion of Bridgeport Hospital, 1970–71; John Thompson, consultant. Phase One: expansion of serv (floors 1–3) and multiple-bed wards (floors 4–10).

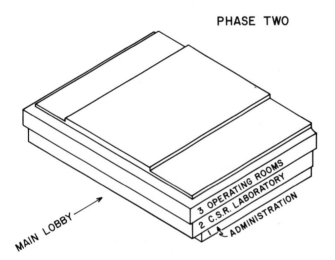

PHASE TWO

3 OPERATING ROOMS
2 C.S.R. LABORATORY
1 ADMINISTRATION

MAIN LOBBY

Fig. 205. Expansion of Bridgeport Hospital, Phase Two: podium.

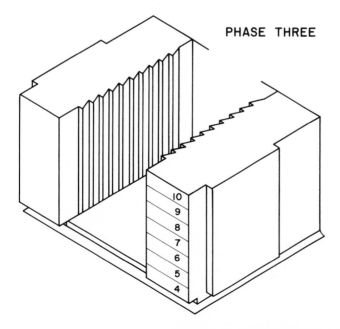

PHASE THREE

10
9
8
7
6
5
4

Fig. 206. Expansion of Bridgeport Hospital, Phase Th the towers, mainly composed of private patient rooms.

COMPLETED BUILDING

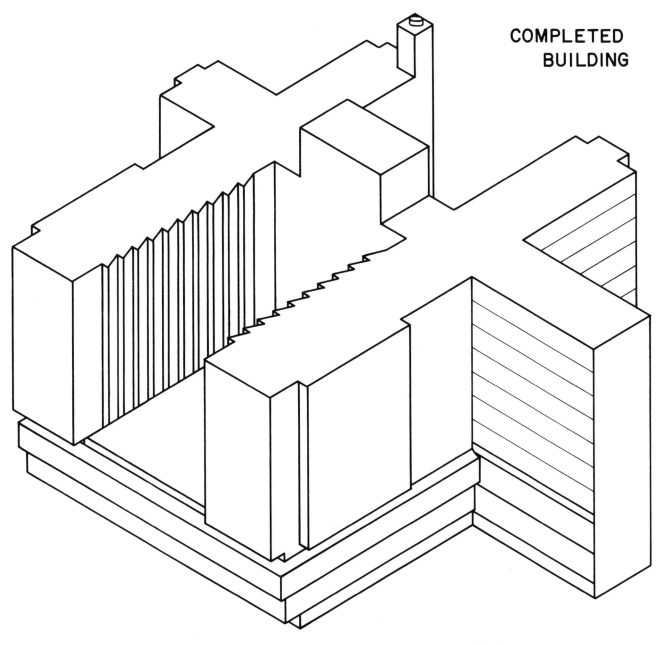

Fig. 207. Bridgeport Hospital: all phases assembled in the completed building.

x-ray department—there are no others—has been found to be too remote from the departments it serves.

Recently, auxiliary services have been altogether removed from nursing areas to a differently shaped but not separate building. The wards are usually on top of the services: round wards over a low, broad podium for services, or a round broad podium with square wards over it (the form referred to as a "matchbox on a muffin.") When stacked wards no longer had to conform to the shape of a laboratory, kitchen, X-ray department, outpatient department, or any other nonnursing facility, they were freed to take on any shape deemed best by those who thought they

knew—and many thought they knew, as will be seen from contemporary American and English arrangements discussed in the following two chapters. Square, round, rectangular, and hexagonal wards have been proposed, built, debated, and defended in recent years and we are still in the throes of the argument.

In the modernization of the Bridgeport (Conn.) Hospital (1970–71), an older multistoried building, with wards and services set in the same mold, was transformed into a tower, wholly made up of wards, set upon a podium wholly given over to services. None of the original building (fig. 203) was sacrificed. Patients were relocated in a series of hopscotch moves

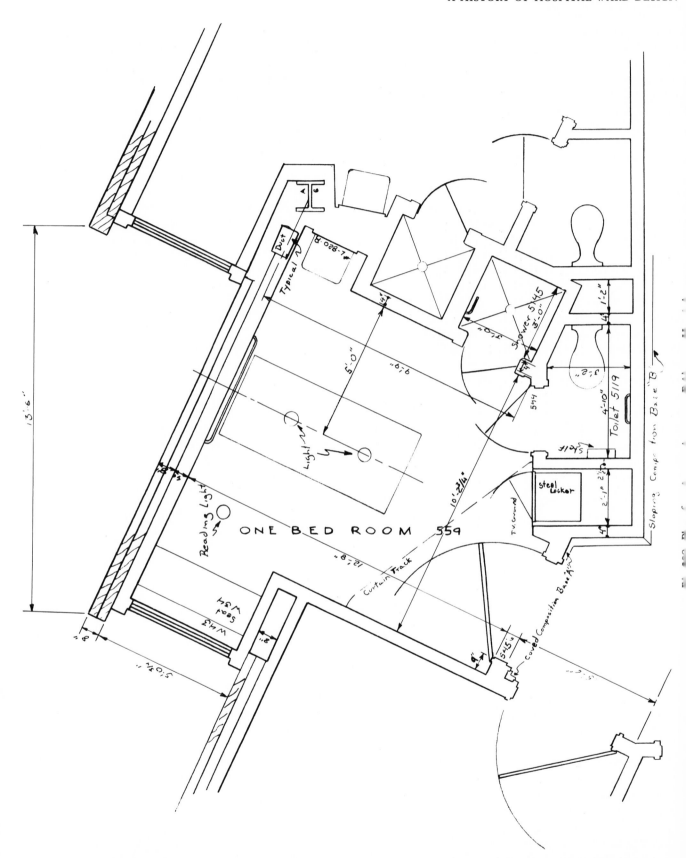

ONE BED ROOM 559

as the superstructure of Phase One (fig. 204) was fitted over the existing plant. The first, second, and third stories extended the service facilities of the original; floors four through ten were made up of wards for two to four patients apiece. Phase Two (fig. 205) extended the podium still farther by joining to the original service areas and the added space on the first three floors of Phase One a large, three-story, square frontal section for admission, administration, laboratory, and operating room. Above this platform rose Phase Three (fig. 206), two ward towers from the fourth to tenth floor—this time mainly of private rooms. Because additional space existed at the rear of each tower, one 4-bed and one 2-bed ward was added on each floor. In the completed building all elements are grouped around a central elevator stack made taller by three stories (fig. 207).

Figure 208 shows in detail one of the private rooms in the saw-toothed towers. Into a space only 12 feet 8 inches by 10 feet 2¾ inches an island bed has been introduced—that is, a free-standing bed whose head alone is against the wall. This gives nurses space on both sides of the bed to handle the patient, and fairly heavy equipment can be installed on either or both sides of the bed when needed. For extremely sick cases requiring more equipment, a few larger private rooms are provided in another part of the hospital. These private floors are intended for wealthier pa-

tients not desperately ill, and many amenities of privacy are included: a standard locker, a private shower, and a separate and private toilet room. The sink is not in with the toilet but in the room itself, closer to the patient, more convenient for staff.

The room is completely air-conditioned, another technological development that changed the shape of hospital wards in recent years. This means the window cannot be opened for the patient but can be opened to be cleaned. It need not often be cleaned, for there are double panes of glass and the venetian blind lets down between them; it and the inner surfaces of the glass will require attention only once every three or four years. The window is directed toward a fine view of Long Island Sound, yet patients in the parallel towers cannot see into other rooms or be seen from them. A patient can see into the hall and be seen from it if he desires; if not, a curtain may be drawn diagonally across the doorway (not around the bed).

This meticulously designed private room, assembled like a watch from its necessary elements, is an end product of a long process of development in the twentieth century. It could not spring full-grown from the "amenity rooms," "quiet rooms," "rooms for the dangerously ill," and "rooms for the exorbitantly rich" with which we have so far had to deal. The story of its evolution is a chapter in itself.

PART 2

Twentieth-Century Ward Planning in the United States and Great Britain

A Loud, Loud Noise about Privacy: A Review of Contemporary American Literature on the Hospital Room

No hospital problem has generated more heat in modern times than the issue of privacy, particularly in the United States. Our history of nursing ward design revealed that for hundreds of years two forms of privacy in the well-run hospital were regarded as axiomatic: the single room for medical reasons (plague, leprosy, violent insanity) and the single room for social reasons (for the high-born or wealthy patient). Those who advocate single rooms in our time include far more than the customary categories of patients. They want a single room for everybody. To judge from much recent American hospital literature, this one design component now overshadows in some planners' minds both economy and adequate nursing supervision.

Many assume without question that privacy is an undiluted boon and that one should arrange for as much of it in the hospital as one can pay for. A private room for every patient is the ideal. The attitude is reflected in captions of some recent American articles chosen at random: "Lack of privacy in semiprivate room may affect medical care." "Consultant recommends all private rooms." "Community hospital provides privacy for all." "All rooms are private in new children's hospital." In 1962 a leading American hospital planner issued a manifesto (the capital letters are his): "I WOULD LIKE TO MAKE A PREDICTION! THE SEMI-PRIVATE PATIENT ROOM WILL BE AS ANTIQUATED IN FIVE TO TEN YEARS AS THE FOUR BED WARD IS TODAY!"

On the other hand, a title of 1963 inquiring, "Do patients prefer single rooms?" reports on the tentative results of a questionnaire in which 19 of 85 patients said they preferred single rooms, 51 chose two-bed rooms, and 15 liked four-bed rooms.[1] The factor of class is found to affect the desire for privacy. In general, the poorer classes, who were never alone in their lives, resent being left alone in a hospital.

After reading widely in the American literature of the past century about privacy we conclude that (1) it is still an open question; (2) arguments for either side come close to canceling each other out; and (3) therefore, no strong preference for or against privacy should be stated as an axiom. A patient pays

more for privacy; no way has yet been found to controvert this fact. Not all patients, even of the upper classes, want privacy. In the very nature of the case, privacy means and will always mean a sacrifice of continuous supervision. As for ensuring a sanitary environment, no experiment yet undertaken has proved that a patient's recovery or relapse was determined by his degree of privacy in hospital.

A steady trend toward more privacy in every aspect of twentieth-century life accounts in part for an overemphasis on the single room in hospitals. The Victorian attitude toward privacy in general was vastly more indifferent, and the major Victorian hospital planner, Florence Nightingale, carried it further than that when discussing private rooms in hospitals. She was against them. Privacy, even relative privacy, was equated in her mind with the "holes and corners" of ill-built English military hospitals such as Netley, "eight or ten little bed-rooms, miscalled wards, a little kitchen, everything, in fact, on a little scale, like a collapsed French hospital."[2]

Because a hospital ward must primarily allow for ease of supervision, privacy's very opposite, Miss Nightingale said she would rather place even 40 patients together in one large ward that could be efficiently overlooked by one head nurse than the same number in four 10-bed wards that could *not* efficiently be overlooked by one head nurse. As for privacy, neither type of ward provided that. Privacy is not relative but absolute. "Much has been said about the benefits of small wards for from six to ten sick," she wrote, "about the greater comfort and privacy of such wards, and the greater facility for ventilation which they afford. It is simply an error to assume that small wards afford any such advantages. Privacy, in an hospital, does not extent beyond any two adjacent beds."[3] She hoped that the virtues of efficiency would make up to the patient for his loss of privacy. "The extreme punctuality in well-ordered hospitals, the rule that nothing shall be done in the ward while the patients are having their meals, goes far to counterbalance what unavoidable evil there is in having patients together."[4]

Miss Nightingale could not conceive of an exceptional case that would fare better in a small room. The very sick and the dying she would place in the large ward right next to the nursing station, where they would receive most attention. Noisy or offensive cases, who must be removed so as not to disturb the other patients, she would not relegate to a small room attached to the general ward but would group them in a large "casualty ward" quite apart, with its own staff. However, such a ward must not be used for convalescents, who would be "comparatively removed from inspection, and often play tricks there."[5]

The first hospital where Florence Nightingale was able to dictate the design of the wards, Herbert Hospital, was built between 1859 and 1864 without a single isolation room. The design was acceptable only to one who did not believe in contagion—and Miss Nightingale did not, save as a consequence of imperfect sanitation.

> In the ordinary sense of the word, there is no proof, such as would be admitted in any scientific inquiry, that there is any such thing as "contagion." There are two or three diseases in which there is a specific virus . . . such as small-pox, cow-pox, etc. But these are not "contagious" in the sense supposed. . . . Infection acts through the air. Poison the air breathed by individuals and there is infection."[6]

As it happened, the facts of contagion did not bear Miss Nightingale out. The separation room crept back into St. Thomas's Hospital which was opened in 1871. Each ward still has 30 beds, but two of them are in a small room opposite the nurse's. Later hospitals, adapting the Nightingale ward, provided isolation rooms in varying proportions to the number of patients in the open ward. Presumably all patients were isolated for medical reasons. The English writer Burdett published in 1893 what he considered medical indications for allotting a private room to a ward patient. He divided candidates into two types: first, those that because of their nature are better off apart: eye cases, hysteria, cases needing special quiet, to whom Burdett would assign a small room near the general ward. We may imagine single rooms in the many Nightingale wards all over Europe peopled by just such patients. In the second category were cases that would endanger other patients: infectious fevers, erysipelas, dirty and offensive cases, and so forth. He recommended that they be housed in isolation wards cut off from the hospital and entered only from the open air.[7]

Along with these single rooms for medical reasons, private rooms for social reasons were furnished in increasing numbers, usually in a separate hospital.

At the beginning of the century privacy had been the privilege of the well-born or those who could pay well. Now it was granted to those who were merely genteel and could not pay very much. Some patients of the middle class without family or friends (upon whom the burden of caring for the sick usually fell) shrank from receiving charity yet needed hospitalization. It would not be right to place them in the paupers' ward, so pay rooms were made available that were to be private, or nearly so. Brian Abel-Smith describes a pay hospital opened in London in 1842 for the nursing and medical and surgical care of persons belonging to the middle classes. It had eight single-bedded rooms. This "first pay hospital in Britain" had to be abandoned after three years of successful operation because of an insufficient initial endowment.[8] In 1877 the first Home Hospital was proposed for persons "comparatively friendless and alone, such as clerks and young men living in town away from their relations, governesses and others. . . . Patients of the class of which we are speaking . . . would require a greater amount of privacy, with separate rooms, or, at all events, wards containing only two or three beds in each." A four-bedded ward had to be abandoned because "when a visitor comes to a patient in a ward with more than one bed, those who have no friends quietly overhear all the visitor has to say."[9]

In 1881 the administrators of St. Thomas's Hospital, which was overbuilt and without funds, with only 13 of its 21 ward blocks in use, decided after vigorous controversy to devote one of its empty blocks to paying patients. The single rooms were rented out at 12 shillings a day. Then, because a Nightingale ward has plenty of windows, thick, striped linen curtains were used to divide the ward into compartments, and each was furnished as a bedroom with its own window and "containing every needful requirement." But the *British Medical Journal* doubted that the cubicles would prove popular "as it is evident that there can be little real privacy under such an arrangement."[10]

Henry Burdett found a different system in operation when he visited the United States in 1893. He was much impressed by American pay wards—the dominant accommodation rather than a noteworthy exception. Americans never had a nobility or gentry; social class was determined by ability to pay. Also, in that Calvinist society, there was a horror of pauperism. Pay and indigent patients lay side by side in adjoining beds in the public hospital wards, the one difference between them being that the indigent were expected to help out in the work of the wards when they were well enough to do so. Rich patients were cared for in very many private pay hospitals. Burdett

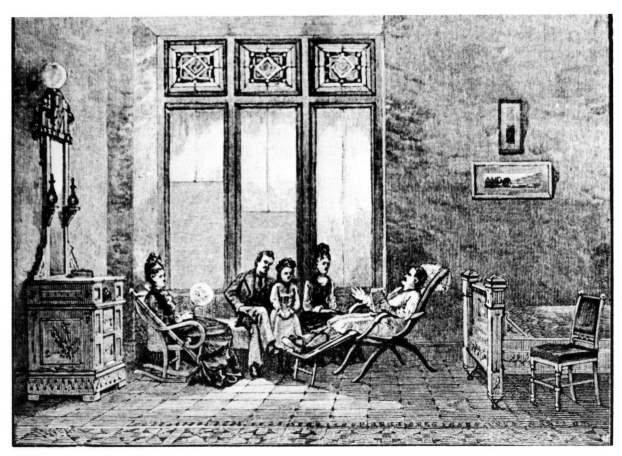

Fig. 209. Private patient's room, New York Hospital, New York City, 1878.

described one such institution of 150 beds with ward as well as single rooms. The single rooms were "fitted up with Eastlake furniture, Turkey rugs, and plate-glass mirrors." The wards had "tesselated flooring, brass fixtures, small Axminster rugs by each of the beds, and electric signals to all parts of the building. . . . A feature of this modern pay hospital is the recreation room, in which the attractions of a conservatory are combined with those of an aquarium. A platform for a band has been placed at one end of this room."[11] In 1878, *Harper's* printed a view of a private patient's room in New York Hospital that seems to belong in the same price bracket (fig. 209).

By comparison with this languorous scene and Burdett's upholstered description, the private room of the pay ward of Johns Hopkins Hospital is a rather barren affair (fig. 210). However, we are told that it was finished in ash and handsomely furnished, with an electric bell for each room.[12] Also, at Johns Hopkins, when you paid you bought privacy. Thirteen rooms on each of the two pay floors are singles, and one is a two-bed room. The pay wards were in a building of their own, as were the single rooms of the isolating ward, a very different form bristling with ventilation (figs. 211 and 212). The isolating ward was

based on Folsom's plan (cf. fig. 181). Each isolating room, assigned for medical reasons, had its own fireplace and chimney, and the bed stood on a floor with 5,000 quarter-inch holes in it, the object being to have a large amount of air pass constantly upwards, "so that no portion of this air shall be rebreathed or come a second time in contact with the patient, thus placing him in the condition of being out-of-doors in a very gentle current of air."[13]

Johns Hopkins's forward-looking plans were imitated in other hospitals even before its buildings were finished. In this one institution were combined the plush housing of private pay hospitals with the stripped, utilitarian common wards of the voluntary charity hospital—but not in the same building. The next step was to plan for expensive rooms in a private wing within the general hospital. A quarter of a century after publication of the Johns Hopkins plans the synthesis was not yet taken for granted. In 1914 S. S. Goldwater felt it necessary to defend the advantages of running the two services under one roof as follows.

Charity patients would greatly benefit. Rich potential donors were frequently first interested and involved in the hospital's charitable work during their hos-

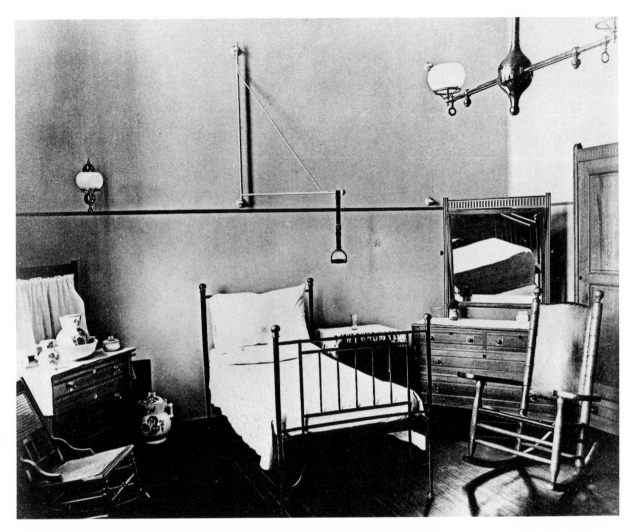

Fig. 210. Private patient's room, pay ward, Johns Hopkins Hospital, Baltimore, Maryland (1885).

pitalization in the private wing. A doctor could donate more time to charity patients if he did not have to spend a good part of the day visiting his private patients in their homes all over town. A hospital scaled to the exacting standards of private patients is bound to be better built than one intended only for charitable work. For private patients, also, efforts are made to find the best way of doing things regardless of cost, and since in the hospital there is a tendency toward the creation of a single standard of surgical technique, therapy, and even nursing care, charity cases would benefit from the presence of a private wing. Nurses who plan to take up private nursing require contact with patients of the class by which they will be chiefly employed after graduation. Finally, the private patients themselves will be better off. By 1914, scientific paraphernalia had already become so elaborate and expensive that private hospitals could no longer keep up with the latest discoveries, and only large institutions could afford to offer the

best in medical care. To be fair to the rich, a community must not place itself in the attitude of offering to the poor opportunities for the restoration of health which are denied to the well-to-do.[14]

The argument takes into account only two social classes—the two extremes. A rich man who wanted privacy could buy it, a poor man who needed privacy was given it at community expense. What about the hospital patient with only moderate means? In 1910 C. Irving Fisher discussed before the American Hospital Association "The Need of an Intermediate Single Room Service in Hospitals." He affirmed that now a really poor ward patient, paying nothing at all or a nominal sum, was provided for in a hospital "so perfected as to be nearly beyond criticism."[15] Admittedly, ward treatment presented a few drawbacks: lack of privacy, a chance of agreeable or disagreeable neighbors, diet that did not cater to individual tastes, and the inevitable movements in an open ward at night. "To such things as these, however, the average patient in the ward is already well-accustomed." Rich patients were also adequately cared for in the costly private rooms. But the middle class, "the great bulk, the most important part of the community," was still not provided for.

> They do not live when well on the same scale with wealth, and they cannot afford to be sick on that scale either. . . . But they want in sickness that to which they have been accustomed in health, a degree of privacy and personal choice of companionship which the open ward does not admit, and the satisfaction which the genuine soul finds in paying its own way with the product of its own industry and thrift.

For these patients "plain single rooms, or very small wards, with service a little better, or even identical with the ward service, would give privacy and make possible larger privileges in visits from friends, and a fee could be charged in proper proportion." Aside from present financial gains, it was important that middle-class patients receive a good impression of their hospital stay. The philanthropy Goldwater anticipated from the wealthy, Fisher hoped for from the upwardly mobile middle class.[16]

To some it seemed that for such patients only a private room would fill the bill. And the proponents of privacy for patients of moderate means began to express themselves with increased urgency, for often enough they were no longer thinking of patients in the abstract; they themselves were the patients of moderate means or, as hospital personnel, they sought the most favorable conditions for their patients of moderate means. "When I return, put me in a closet rather than in the ward!" exclaimed a discharged patient to the superintendent of Chicago's Presbyterian Hospital, Asa S. Bacon. And Bacon responded (1920) with a finely wrought plan for a hospital made up of private rooms.[17]

A hospital is often called a hotel for sick people, says Bacon. This hotel argument is still invoked today, but Bacon had the good sense to realize that from the patient's standpoint there is a distinct difference. A man is prepared for a hotel; hospitalization always catches him unprepared. He is given no choice of accommodations, he must take what he can get. For the patient in moderate circumstance, unable to pay for an expensive room, this means a ward bed. Ward beds, however, are for charity patients, and labor conditions had so changed by then that the average workingman did not want charity. But the sick man's earning capapcity is often cut off by his illness. Very well, the job of an efficient hospital must be to make him well and productive in the least possible time.

The efficient hospital, Bacon believes, is one of all private rooms. Let us review in detail Bacon's arguments in favor of private rooms, for we will be hearing them over and over and over. A ward does not permit maximum capacity. "The proportion of cells for men's or women's beds does not remain the same, and certain diseases seem to come in epidemics. This makes imperative some scheme for flexibility in the use of beds." The private room absolutely solves problems of flexibility because it allows the occupancy of all the beds all of the time. (This economic argument for privacy was only finally refuted in 1969 in a study that demonstrated by computer simulation that a hospital of all private rooms does not necessarily experience a higher rate of occupancy.[18]) One need not worry about contagion. Patients need never be moved. Better examinations can be made, better case histories taken. Room temperature can be kept at the patient's liking and visiting rules can be relaxed.

With a practical sense amounting to genius, Bacon thinks through the implications of a hospital of all-private rooms. He foresees a private toilet and lavatory in each patient's room instead of special duty rooms and general lavatories;[19] a central kitchen and serving station instead of floor diet kitchens; a central linen supply instead of floor linen rooms; elimination of long corridors (the diagram shows an X-shaped hospital floor with four short wings); dumbwaiters direct from the central supply rooms to each floor section; pneumatic tubes to carry written requisitions from each floor to the central supply station and also to carry any supplies that can enter the tube. We have come to take these conveniences for granted. In a single revolutionary paragraph in 1920, Asa S. Bacon proposed them all (see "Efficient Hospitals," p. 124).

Like many another innovator, he found out soon enough that he was not the first. The all-private-room hospital was not only feasible but had actually been in operation for 12 years. The 75 beds of the King's Daughters Hospital in Temple, Texas (1908) were all in private rooms, for charity and pay patients alike. "It is seldom that the nurse in attendance knows whether the patient is a pay or a charity patient," wrote one of its doctors. "It goes without saying that we do not put the charity patients in the most expensive rooms."[20] A thoroughly efficient administration made and enforced a rule that the hospital's bill must be paid before the doctor's. It had long since adopted the plan suggested by Bacon of central cooking and central linen distribution, which it found exceedingly satisfactory. Indeed, the hospital personnel were generally pleased with their decision. "We . . . would by far prefer to furnish the charity patients with one

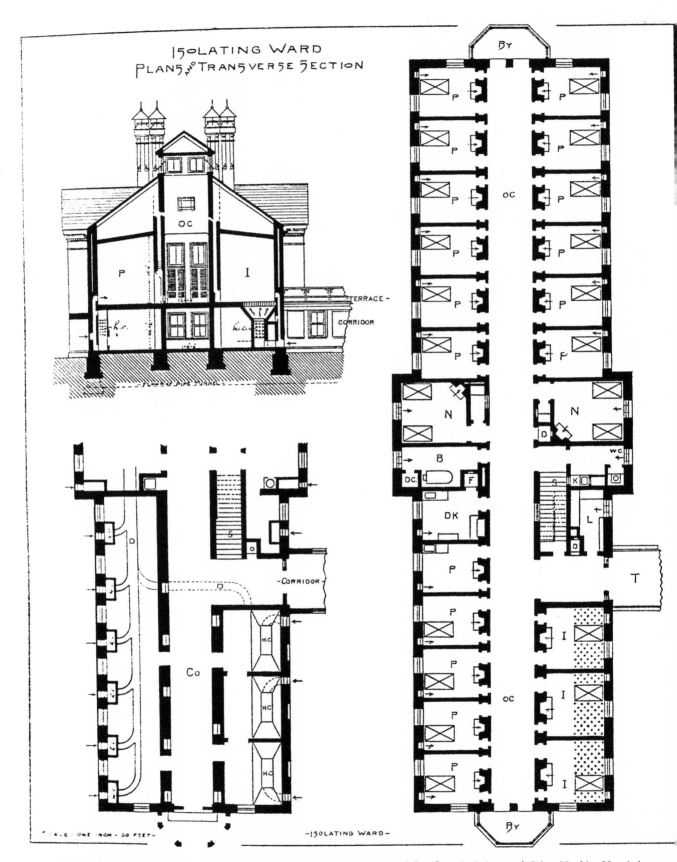

Fig. 211. Transverse section and plans of the north end of the basement and first floor, isolating ward, Johns Hopkins Hospital.

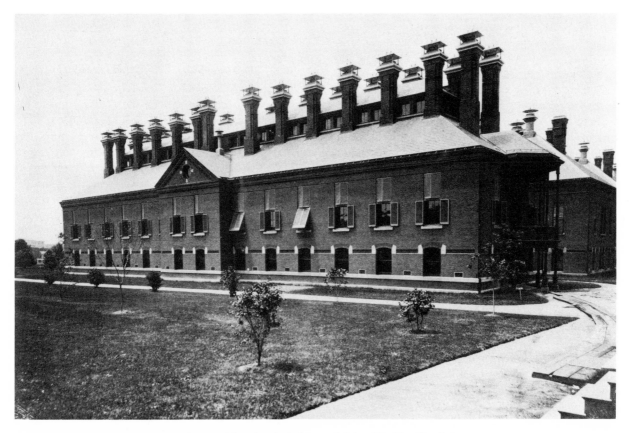

Fig. 212. Elevation, isolating ward, Johns Hopkins Hospital.

of our less expensive rooms rather than return to a ward plan, which is unsatisfactory both to the patient and to his attending physician."

Far less practical than Bacon, L. J. Frank, superintendent of New York City's Beth Israel Hospital, categorically stated his preference for privacy (1921).[21] "If an individual of ordinary intelligence were asked, when he was ill, whether he would prefer to be in a private room in the hospital or in a bed in the ward, he would invariably choose the private room." A ward patient, to his mind, is no better off than a convict who has lost his identity. He is number so-and-so, no longer "an all-important, suffering, sinning, and sinned against human being." As soon as he can afford it he seeks privacy. He does not want to impose upon his neighbor; he is embarrassed to attend to nature's wants in public. In the ward he must wait for his bedpan because it happens to be visiting hours, meal hours, or round hours. He is assailed by "unaesthetic, disagreeable odors emitted by his neighboring sufferers." He must watch his neighbor go off to the operating room and worry about him when he gets back. Still more harrowing, he is an involuntary spectator "when the doctors begin crowding around one patient, when the nurses hurriedly and ominously surround a bed with the white screens. . . . He

hears the shriek of the patient in agony and then the death rattle." How different is a private room! One can have quiet, drawn shades, peace for tired nerves, and at night "rest, real rest. . . . Nor will the patient at any time of the day be disturbed by the lights, bells, signals, and other hospital noises."

Frank attempted to design an ideal ward. He understood that private rooms involve hospital employees in extra traveling, which he attempted to avoid by proposing individual utility rooms. Without them the private-room system might not be economically feasible. "With the utility room between every two rooms, I think that all such problems are solved." Each utility room would be equipped with "water closet, bed pan disposal, wash basin, sink, stove, cold drinking water, etc. etc., and the room will have all connections to make certain examinations such as x-ray, electrocardiograph, etc., and certain treatments such as Brand baths for typhoid fever, continuous baths for skin and nervous diseases, etc." One wonders what other amenities he envisaged in his four etceteras.

Frank appended the usual arguments for private rooms: isolation of contagious patients, danger in moving patients, planning for maximum occupancy, (etc.) and the advantage of entertaining visitors at will.

The last is "both a therapeutic advantage and an administrative advantage. . . . The fact that visitors are
allowed at any hour will reduce the population at any
one time, and in case of panic will not tax the exit facilities." This type of reasoning caused the administrator of Mt. Sinai Hospital in New York City, S. S.
Goldwater, to protest that whereas one or two quiet
rooms were once considered sufficient for a ward unit
of 25–30 beds, and twice that number somewhat later,
"It has remained for hospital idealists of recent times
to voice a demand for a separate room for every patient, regardless of medical or social classification,
cost of service, or any other consideration."

In 1925 Goldwater and his friend E. M. Bluestone
made a serious attempt to define privacy in the hospital.[22] First they distinguished between the two
types of single rooms: "(a) for all patients who *desire*
and can *afford* to pay for them and for the additional
service which is indispensable for their proper care"
(privacy for social reasons); and "(b) for all patients
who *need* single rooms and individual service, whether
they can afford to pay for them or not" (privacy for
medical reasons). They added, "The real point at
issue is whether or not all patients need single rooms."
Those needing single rooms for medical and social
reasons were divided into eleven categories, and the
two authors together with members of the Mt. Sinai
medical staff undertook to evaluate the patients then
in their hospital in an attempt to discover what percentage of the total number fell into the eleven categories. Five hundred patients, drawn from a cross
section of the several clinical services, were examined
as candidates for segregation over a period of four
months. "A group judgment, formed in circumstances
which favored the reduction to a minimum of the
personal prepossessions of the individual" was that
72 of the 500 patients, or 14.4 percent, should be
placed in separation rooms. This was one of the first
valid and objective pieces of research into the subject of privacy. The final figure, 14.4 percent, was
quoted as gospel for decades and turns up even now in
American hospital literature, although most of the
diseases in the eleven categories are no longer a
menace and in our time nearly all of them are treated
differently.

The deserving poor were to be given private rooms
whether or not they could pay for them. The rich
who were permitted to buy private rooms must pay
a fair share of their maintenance—which Goldwater
calculated as not only extra services required in the
day-to-day upkeep of luxury accommodations but
also as a fair share of the capital investment (*On Hospitals,* p. 65). The private wing was built by money
donated for the poor. Had the money been invested
for the poor, the poor would enjoy interest on it. On

this basis the income from private facilities must be
calculated and applied to the charitable work of the
hospital.

Now, what about the middle class—those who "not
being able to afford the superior comfort of single
rooms, must content themselves with the semiprivacy of intermediate wards" (p. 272)? This may be
the first reference to semiprivacy in hospital literature (1926). But the term is not used to mean the sharing of a room by two persons or by four. It is Goldwater's way of describing that familiar figure, the
patient of moderate means, who "craves particularly
a measure of privacy during his stay in the hospital."
If he could pay the full, real costs of a private room,
"he would present no special problem, and the long
debate which his supposed wrongs have engendered
would never have started." Already, in 1926, it had
been a long debate. Already, physicians and surgeons
acting as spokesmen for this kind of semiprivate
patient were clamoring, "Give us plenty of cheap
private rooms!" Goldwater replied,

> What these spokesmen for the refined patient
> of limited means have in mind is a private room
> which the hospital will be prepared to rent at
> approximately ward rates; but if adequate ser-
> vice is to be given in private rooms, and if the
> service is to be quite self-supporting, there is
> no such thing as a cheap private room. Individual
> private rooms may, of course, be made larger or
> smaller, but whether large or small, the average
> semiprivate patient, by definition a person of
> limited means, cannot pay what it costs to pro-
> duce and maintain such a room, and to render
> adequate nursing service in it (p. 273).

What can you do with these patients? You might make
them part of the ward by assigning to them the separation rooms that the ward patients need on medical
grounds. In that event the ward patients would probably envy the superior privileges of the semiprivate
group, who in turn would probably resent being
classified among charity cases. You might scatter semiprivate among private rooms, forcing the administration to give the semiprivate group an unduly expensive grade of service at public expense. Goldwater
offered no answers, but he defined the disadvantages
of his alternatives.

Without private nursing, absolute privacy and adequate supervision cannot be reconciled. Goldwater
and Bluestone cited recorded instances when the
nurse did not arrive in time to prevent a private patient from falling out of bed or from leaving his bed
in a foggy state and wandering through the halls.
"Privacy with adequate attention is one thing; separation with neglect is another."[23] "A hospital which

places a sick person alone in a room, without immediate and constant supervision, assumes a serious responsibility; the patient who is thus left alone runs a serious risk."[24] The price of a private room must include further additions to the nursing staff as a safety measure. "Besides, the sick are often terrified by loneliness; it is as true as ever it was that misery loves company."[25]

An attempt was made by hospital planners to provide nurse substitutes—to compensate by mechanical devices for the defects of supervision of a single room. By a simple bell on the pillow and light over the door, contact was established between the patient and the nursing station, but this arrangement worked only one way. A two-way communications system, the executone—adapted from the speaker between boss and secretary in business offices—was installed in American hospitals as early as 1947 and has since been refined to transmit the patient's very breathing. Whether this is a satisfactory substitute for constant visual observation is still subject for controversy. One member of a recent conference at The Hospital Centre in London remarked that he had never understood why it was so important that a patient should be *seen* to fall out of bed. A principal matron observed that a nurse could stand at the bottom of a patient's bed and not realize he was dead.[26]

"Are the chances of care invariably improved, is the period of treatment unquestionably shortened, is the patient's comfort necessarily enhanced, is the safety of the patient always promoted, by placing him in a single room rather than a larger ward?" asked Goldwater and Bluestone in the early 1920s.[27] The questions remain unanswered.

However, in the United States the trend was toward increased privacy. Absolute privacy having been discovered to be too expensive for ward patients or even for Goldwater's semiprivate patients, planners since the 1920s have had to ask themselves: Privacy to what degree? As expensive dress creations are mass-produced for the general market in an inferior material, so the expensive commodity of privacy was offered to the many in a relative form. Just before World War I, the American architect Edward F. Stevens visited the Rigshospital of Copenhagen, where the Nightingale ward had been redesigned to provide more privacy (1909; fig. 213). Beds were turned parallel to the windows, two deep on either side of the central aisle, and subdivided by screens in groups of three or four. The screens did not go up very high or reach down to the floor, lest the free circulation of air be fatally impeded, but, socially,

Fig. 213. Plan of a ward unit, Rigshospital, Copenhagen (1910): beds turned sideways to the windows in groupings of four; nurses' room and special care room in center of ward.

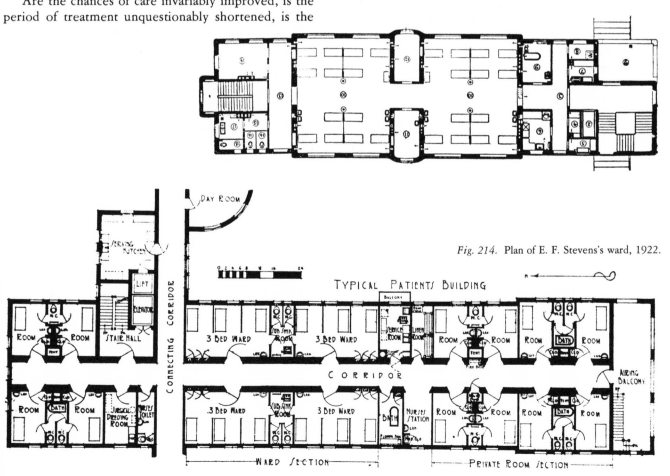

Fig. 214. Plan of E. F. Stevens's ward, 1922.

patients were now citizens of a small group rather than of the entire ward. One really private room for medical reasons was walled off in the center of the ward opposite the nurses' room.

This "Rigs ward," copied in many parts of the world, greatly impressed Stevens. He designed (1922) a pavilion combining private rooms and wards and greatly augmenting the proportion of private rooms (see fig. 214). Whereas in the Rigshospital there were 26 beds in groups of 3 or 4 to one single bed in the separation room, in Stevens's pavilion there are 12 one-bed rooms to 4 rooms of 3 beds each. The degree of privacy is increased even within the multibed rooms. Each bed is partitioned off from the others by a screen reaching to within 1 foot of the floor and up 7 feet or to the ceiling, depending on the classification of patient. For ease of supervision the partitions were left open toward the ward door. Though Stevens willingly fell in with the American trend toward more privacy, he by no means advocated single-room hospitals. People, he said, often try to liken a hospital room to a private hotel room with its private toilet. The two cannot be compared. "The sick patient is generally helpless and needs diligent care and watching, which care cannot be as economically given in single rooms as in open wards." Nor, he adds, have we at present enough nurses and attendants to do so.[28]

With a truly American concern for plumbing, Stevens gave 8 private patients their own toilet and had them share a bathtub with a neighbor. Four of them share a toilet with one other patient and do without a tub. Between two wards of 3 patients each he inserted two toilets, back-to-back, which *must* open to the outer air. The 12 ward patients—and 4 of the private patients—managed with one public tub, but, Stevens admitted, the bathtub is used little by the average patient.

In the United States by the end of the 1920s we find large open wards for the poor, large private rooms with toilet and bath for the wealthy, and a large open question of what to do about the middle classes. Almost overnight, the depression changed all that. Elegant private rooms were the first to empty out for want of patients who could pay for them. Some hospitals closed down whole floors, others remodeled private as semiprivate accommodations, and still others whisked two beds into every private room where there was space for them. Suddenly the country was flooded with semiprivate accommodations. What was first proposed as a compromise for sensitive patients became the dominant arrangement. In certain homogeneous communities whole hospitals were built of two-bed rooms. It is impossible to overestimate the influence of Blue Cross on this development; for years it paid its maximum subsidy for 4-, 3-, or

2-bed rooms. Nationwide insurance enabled patients who would have had no choice but to enter the 30-bed ward to select a 4-, 3-, or 2-bed setup fully covered by their policies and to pay out their small savings for the services of a private doctor. It must be remembered that at this time the type of accommodation determined the type of medical supervision. Ward patients were given no choice but to be treated by the house doctor. Semiprivate patients were permitted to choose their own private physicians and were taken care of at a certain fee, whereas private patients treated by private physicians were charged about twice as much.

The 25- and 30-bed wards shut down, less quickly than the luxury singles, but inexorably. One by one they were remodeled as smaller units or demolished. A great argument against private rooms had been the additional cost of partitions and plumbing. When nothing larger than a 4-bed room was being built, the difference in building costs was minimized. Then came World War II and early ambulation. Suddenly there was a real use for a private toilet. It was discovered that getting out of bed right after an operation actually helped patients to recover faster. The case for private rooms was strengthened by an urgent drive to give each patient his own, or an exceedingly convenient, toilet facility.

In addition to the real forces favoring single rooms, two-bed rooms had proved disappointing. Russell T. Sanford, a patient, described what could go wrong with them in an article called "Bedpandemonium" (1951).[29] A sudden attack of some sort had sent him in acute pain to the hospital, where he was paired with a teenager laid up in a cast for eight weeks and acutely bored. The teenager needed TV and his large clan of noisy relatives as much as Sanford needed rest and quiet. To switch to private accommodations would have cost Sanford an extra $127.50 because Blue Cross would only pay half the subsidy toward the more expensive private room. The doctor warned him that the cost of his services would exactly double if the patient took a private room. "Such an arrangement," Sanford complained, "can only be justified on the assumption that privacy is a luxury, and that incompatibility, indignity, noise and turmoil are good enough for the average citizen no matter how sick he may be. Naturally, as long as this situation holds, hospitals are going on building a minimum of private rooms and a maximum of two-bed rooms."

The problem, still urgent, is yet unsolved. In the late 1950s and 1960s Americans came to feel that a two-bed compromise between the private room and the four-bed ward was too much of a compromise because it simultaneously attempted to satisfy administrative need for flexibility, the patient's need or desire for privacy, the physician's preference for privacy, the nurses' need to save steps by working a shorter corridor, and the hospital's urgent necessity to keep costs down. One room could not do all that. The semiprivate room—thought of as a two-bed room when the four-bed room became the "ward"—really satisfied nobody. If one had to have roommates, three instead of one gave a patient three times the chance to find someone congenial. In a semiprivate room there is no escape from an unpleasing companion but to be transferred. Slogans were coined that found wide circulation: "You wouldn't ask a person to share a hotel room with a well stranger, why should he share a room in a hospital with a sick stranger?" "There is no such thing as a condition of semiprivacy, any more than there is a condition of semipregnancy."

From an economic point of view, two- or four-bed rooms had one undeniable advantage over the single room: twice as many patients could be lodged along the same length of corridor. With help scarce and expensive after World War II, it was important that the nurse not have to walk far to tend patients (her every step became a precious commodity). A room for two or three patients with beds parallel to the window takes up no more corridor space than a single room with an island bed, that is, a bed parallel to the window, jutting out into the room, and with space on both sides of the patient's head. Thus six-bed wards, three on a side, are the most economical of all, but whereas this bed conformation is popular on the Continent and in England, it never caught on in the United States, probably because of a stronger predilection for privacy. Two patients in a six-bed ward have no privacy at all. The patient near the window can turn toward the window and find a space of his own; the patient near the corridor has his own corner too; but the patient in the middle finds no retreat—whichever way he turns he is in company.

The problem in designing an inexpensive private room is to give each patient his own space without increasing the length of the corridor. This involves a contradiction. The controversy over the "nonexistent cheap private room" is probably endless because the planners are battling two contradictions, this one and the impossibility of simultaneously achieving perfect privacy and perfect nursing supervision. This quandary explains why planners who are carried away by one alternative or the other often talk perfect nonsense.

Attempts to solve the insoluble impasse proceed along two lines. The designer may think in terms of rearranging the unit as a whole, in which case invention focuses on the corridor. If this is wrapped around itself, if it is conceived of as a double or racetrack corridor having an inner service core, artificially lit

and ventilated, with several shortcuts through that core from one corridor to the other, fewer nursing steps will be needed no matter what the shape of the rooms. With the advent of really effective air conditioning this plan has become popular, and not only in the United States. Another ward plan with *three* corridors was experimented with in the Kellogg Foundation Medical Center, Walnut Creek, California (1954).[30] The central corridor is reserved for staff and nursing activities, and the public is excluded from it. Alcoves along both sides of this working corridor are fitted up, alternately, as nursing stations and utility rooms on one side, kitchen and drug units on the other in such a way that each set of four services takes up just the corridor space of the eight it serves. The two side corridors are for visitors, who enter each room from an outside door. For the rooms to be well lit, the side corridors must be open; therefore the plan would not do for a colder climate. Another California institution, Community Hospital of the Monterey Peninsula (1963), grouped four rooms on two floors around a patio (on the ground floor) or semiprivate balcony (on the floor above it) opening to the outside—also a plan calling for a suitable climate.[31] In the St. Paul Tower of Mercy Hospital, Baltimore (1968),[32] the idea was ingeniously adapted to an *inside* corridor, where four 1-bed rooms opening off a common vestibule take up the corridor space of three (fig. 215).

This is one possible approach. The other concentrates on the individual patient room. Planners (1) try to reduce the nurse's travel distance by bringing within the room the chief utilities she would be travel-

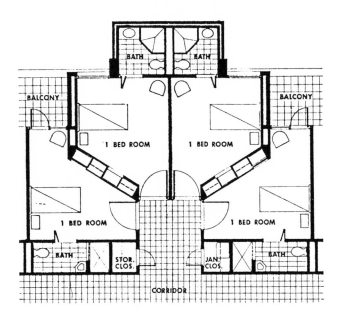

Fig. 215. Plan of private-room cluster, St. Paul Tower, Mercy Hospital, Baltimore, Maryland, 1968.

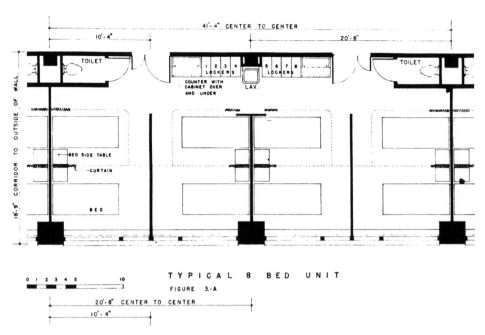

Fig. 216. Plan of I. Rosenfield's cubicled ward, 1952.

ing to, (2) subdivide the space of a multiple-bed room into cubicles narrower than the specifications for a single bed room, (3) decrease the width of the room along the corridor by relocating the bed, or (4) redesign a smaller room from scratch. The new expedients of room or corridor are not necessarily mutually exclusive, although a champion of one or another often writes as though his alone were the universal solution. Much heat has been generated in the controversy, and very little light. Let us try to bring some order into it by examining sample room plans from each of the four categories, in the above order.

Expedient number 1. In 1947 Isadore Rosenfield, architect and hospital consultant, wrote as follows: "The proverbially long hospital corridor is long only if it is necessary to traverse its length countless times a day. When the nurse can perform most of her duties without leaving the patient's room, the corridor length ceases to be a problem."[33] He proposed a cubicled ward for eight patients with two entrance doors and two toilets (fig. 216). The beds are partitioned two by two and each bed may be curtained off. The cubicles, like Stevens's, are left open to a common hall within the room. The beds, unlike Stevens's, are arranged parallel to the window. The plan is made to work by placing cabinets within the room, not for the patients' use but for the nurse's. The principle was developed further by Gordon A. Friesen, hospital consultant, who in 1960 crossbred Rosenfield's cabinet for the nurse with the old hotel "servador" and produced a "nurserver" installed in a space beside the door, which opened both into the room and into the corridor.[34] Vertically, half of it is given over to

clean supplies, half to dirty. Dirty supplies are taken away regularly, but not by nurses. Clean supplies are brought by vertical conveyor from a central supply room and delivered to the nurserver as far as possible without the aid of human hand or footsteps—without, particularly, the nurse's. She is to be saved for nursing. Friesen estimates that 50 percent of a nurse's time in the average hospital is spent gathering supplies (an estimate that has never been verified).

Expedient number 2. The need to subdivide a semiprivate room is self-evident and was the one Sanford fell back upon to escape from bedpandemonium. In trying to find an economic justification for his privations, he noted that "seemingly the only argument for nursing economy is mileage" (although in his semiprivate room, nursing services were seldom rendered to both patients simultaneously). How might as many private as semi-private beds be installed without lengthening the hospital corridor and alienating Blue Cross? He suggested a folding fabric divider in a semiprivate room that would muffle noises and draw back to allow easy maneuvering of large beds and heavy equipment.[35]

The architect Carl A. Erikson designed Sanford's room for him. Erikson too was galled by Blue Cross regulations in favor of the two-bed room, a concept that more or less ignores the fact that many people prefer to be in either a private room or a four-bed unit.[36] Until thus hampered, Erikson had planned to design a hospital of all-private rooms because the doctors with whom he was working were opposed to the two-bed room. He got around Blue Cross favoritism with what he called the "private

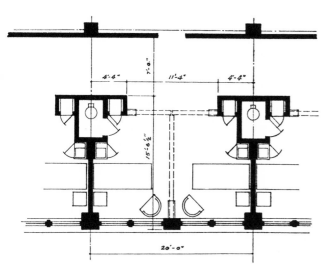

Fig. 217. Plan of C. A. Erikson's "private two-bed room" 1951. The dashed lines indicate folding fabric walls.

two-bed room" (fig. 217): a common corridor, two beds facing each other, and fabric folding walls that could be kept closed until the Blue Cross inspector arrived. The curtains would deaden sound, though they were not soundproof. Each patient shared his toilet not with the other occupant behind the curtain but with the patient next door. The design could be sold as a two-bed room to patients with insurance, as two small private rooms at less than the usual private room cost, or in emergencies even to patients of opposite sexes.

Fourteen years later in 1965 a similar facility, dubbed a "duo room," was hailed as a "new approach to the double–single room."[37] In the later design, beds were placed with their heads to the window and each bed had not only its own window but also its own door to the hospital corridor. A toilet used in common was placed between the two doors. "A soundproof folding partition between the beds permits either double or effectively single occupancy at a low rate." But alas, in a report on a double room with sliding partition at Paradise Valley Hospital, California (1968), the whole argument in favor of the duo room recoils upon itself. The sliding partition was seldom opened, and there was difficulty in attaining acoustical separation. In addition, the disadvantages of mixing patients, which is characteristic of multibed rooms, recurred in these rooms.[38]

Expedient number 3. It was suggested that in order to fit as many private as semiprivate patients into the same length of corridor, beds in separate private rooms should be turned with their heads to the outside wall. Then the corridor, instead of allowing for the length of a 6-foot bed with a 3-foot clearance at the foot of it, need only allow for bed width plus window width. This solution presupposes a corner bed placed

directly against a sidewall because if space were allowed on both sides of the bed head, one would be no better off than with an island bed parallel to the corridor. So the private room with corner bed was introduced into the hospital at about the same time that large, bulky, but extremely effective machines for treatment and the very maintenance of life were coming into use for exceptionally ill patients.

Even without mammoth machinery to be installed, somehow, about the patient's head, the corner bed constituted a nursing problem that was recognized as early as 1929 by Charles Neergaard.[39] As a patient in an island bed, he had had the opportunity to count the number of times nurses had to get at him from either side. He wondered what was going to happen in the cubicles, open at the foot, proposed for an about-to-be-built hospital of which he was a trustee. He pictured the inconvenience of working from one side only or of having to pull the bed crosswise in the cubicle or out into the public space of the ward. He too took refuge in a curtain between cubicles instead of the solid partition that had been planned. Let the nurse encroach on the space allotted to the next patient. The cubicles, at least, might be given flexible walls. But the corner-bed rooms of which they were forerunners had real walls that would not bulge or bend and that inherited the problems Neergaard foresaw for the cubicle.

In 1930 S. S. Goldwater flung all his authority into a passionate warning against the flock of corner beds he could see were about to descend upon the hospital. "Nothing but the free-standing bed, in my opinion, is admissible in hospital practise," he stormed. "If a reason can be adduced to the contrary, I should like to hear it."[40] He cannot imagine a patient being freely and thoroughly inspected from only one side; he cannot imagine a nurse moving the bed or the patient deriving any comfort from being moved. But really, how often does a corner bed have to be moved to enable a nurse to treat the patient from both sides? In how many instances is there insufficient space for heavy equipment around the patient's head? John F. O'Connor conducted a study at the Genesee Hospital, Rochester, New York (1959), to try to determine the acceptability of the corner bed. Despite its favorable reception at the Genesee, very few hospitals were installing corner beds; most followed Goldwater. O'Connor affixed a form to the foot of each bed in the 32-bed unit with spaces to evaluate any activity performed on the patient in bed. Ward nurses, aides, and patients cooperated splendidly. Participation of the physicians could not be enforced, and from the start private duty nurses strongly disliked the tiny rooms; they had charge of very sick patients requiring bulky equipment for which the bed had to be moved at an angle, creating cramped quarters. This study came to the conclusion that if patients are acutely ill and a lot of equipment is involved, they are better off in an island bed with a 3-foot clearance on each side. But for patients not acutely ill, there was an average of only 2.4 movements of the bed in 24 hours.[41]

At the Genesee Hospital one of the few controlled tests to date on the question of privacy was conducted by its assistant director, Charles Lotreck (1952).[42] Rochester was a good town for an experiment in privacy. It had a liberal Blue Cross willing to credit the highest semiprivate room allowance toward the private room; also, the doctors there did not increase their fees for private patients. The town had a tradition of private rooms. In 1941 Dr. Basil MacLean quietly and without fanfare installed at Strong Memorial Hospital a 6-story wing of all private rooms, mainly for medically indigent patients. The rooms had in effect a corner bed standing maybe 6 inches from the wall, and staff and patients unanimously agreed that these rooms (8′ × 15′) were adequate in size even when an oxygen tent or fracture frame was used. Corner-bed rooms at the Genesee were 8 by 17 feet. A few larger private rooms (17′ × 17′) had to be converted into permanent two-bed units because of a continuous high census. ("Those opposed to this [corner bed] arrangement say that the room is inflexible and may never be doubled in any emergency," comments Anthony J. J. Rourke. "The proponents feel this to be a major virtue.")

A previous test run by another hospital had indicated that fewer than 25 percent of its medical and surgical patients would ask for private rooms even if the price were identical to that of semiprivate rooms. Genesee Hospital was understandably eager to get at the truth of the matter. Studies seemed to show that building private rather than semiprivate rooms would increase the area of a 250-bed hospital by only 5 percent and, presumably, construction costs proportionately. A comparison of routine service costs at the Genesee found that the multibed floors cost $10.99 per patient day and the private floors $11.35. Difference in nursing costs was negligible: $5.79 per patient per day on the multibed floors, $5.72 on the private floors. (All sorts of questions arise in considering nursing services. Do semiprivate patients feel better cared for if they see the nurse in the room more often, though she is attending to someone else? Do they make demands on the nurse that would otherwise not have occurred to them simply because they see her in the room?) Nurses liked the private toilets, which could convert any room into an isolation room at need. They liked the privacy; they felt it gave them a closer rapport with the patient, who would be neither reluctant nor embarrassed to ask for help and advice. They did not object to the corner bed according to this study, and they thought even the luxury private room might prove to be too small for large equipment. Among the doctors, 73 percent favored a private room for a patient of moderate means; when questioned about future construction, 81 percent preferred compact, low-priced private rooms to semiprivate rooms.

Now what about the patients? Upon entering, a little more than a third of them asked for private rooms; the remainder were equally divided between a preference for semiprivate rooms and an inability to make up their minds. By the time they left, almost two-thirds would have preferred a private room, while again the remainder were equally divided. Had there been no difference in price, 84.4 percent would have chosen a private room, 14.8 percent a semiprivate room. These patients were then asked what factors would be most important to them in the future in choosing a hospital room. They rated the private toilet highest, companionship lowest. The third-most-important item on the list was privacy, which meant even more to patients over fifty years of age than to younger people. This is significant: our population gets older every year, and more old people fall sick. Patients in semiprivate rooms rated companionship higher than did those in private rooms, but only 8 of 122 patients stated that they did not get enough companionship during their hospital stay. "Either the needs are not as great as they seem or they are filled in other ways," Lotreck speculates.

If the economic factor were removed, would patients still choose semiprivate rooms? The hospital ran another test. Each day, until the quota of 75 was reached, two or three average (not emergency) patients were offered the compact private room at the same price as a semiprivate room. (The usual price was $2.50 more.) Of those who had intended to take a semiprivate room, 68.4 percent changed their minds when they heard that the price was the same for a private room. In all, 69 percent asked for the private room under those circumstances. The remainder who held out for semiprivate accommodations were put by the hospital into the compact private rooms anyway, so that in the end 93.3 percent of all these patients were in private rooms. Only one was dissatisfied enough to demand to be switched to a semiprivate room. When these patients left, they were asked which room they would choose if they had it to do over again, and 81.6 percent said they would take a private room. Thus it is found in many areas of patient preference that patients ask for what they are familiar with and that they tend to preserve the status quo.

Then the patients were asked which room they would choose if the private room cost a dollar a day more than the semiprivate instead of being the same price. At that rate, only 73.7 percent came out in favor of the private room. The extra dollar changed the minds of 8 percent of them and again Lotreck speculates, "It may be that to 8% of the patients, privacy is not that important."

Indeed, the further one inquires into the importance of privacy to the patient, the more questions arise. For instance: the narrower a room is, the less protected the patient is from being seen from the corridor when his door is open. A patient in a corner bed has to face the door—yet most corner-bed patients at the Genesee, who could not see out their windows, kept their doors open a good part of the time. How important was privacy to them? Privacy from what? Privacy in relationship to whom? To visitors in the hall, to the medical staff, to a sick roommate?

And one last question: what relationship, if any, exists between the provision of privacy and the outcome of illness?

In hospital literature to this day one can watch planners, administrators, and architects writhing this way and that to escape the mathematical limits of the compact private room. They play fantastically with expedient number 4 by designing in unusual shapes: for instance, in circles, for which great hopes were entertained in hospital planning in the 1950s. But that was not the first time; it will be recalled that there was quite a run on circular wards during the last decade of the nineteenth century (fig. 173). In a circular unit with rooms shaped like a piece of pie, if the bed projects from the curved crust there is extra room just where it is needed—to either side of the patient's head. But the point of the pie will be too narrow to accommodate a private toilet, and if the toilet is placed against the outer wall all that was gained is lost again. Thus in one pioneering circular unit of private rooms (Rochester Methodist, N.Y., 1958),[43] an island bed projected from a sidewall and the toilet was tucked against the crust. A circle is self-limiting: there is no way to build onto it, and if it is enlarged beyond a certain point there is bound to be waste space in the center. This is exactly what would happen with a circular unit of all-private rooms accommodating as many patients as the semiprivate. The private unit would have to be much bigger with a core so vast as to undo the intended economy. It is no accident that a successful functioning circular unit such as that of the Valley Presbyterian Hospital in Van Nuys, California (also 1958),[44] has two-bed rooms with island beds projecting from the back walls. The experimental 12-bed unit at Rochester was assigned to intensive care.

Well then, how about a different approach—a square room built on the tiniest scale possible? Dr. N. A. Wilhelm, director of the Peter Bent Brigham Hospital in Boston, observing with admiration Pullman car roomettes designed in terms of inches rather than of feet, wondered (1951) whether a far smaller room than had been thought practicable could not be designed for hospitals: a workable, economical room offering "that precious ingredient everyone desires—privacy—and at a reasonable price!"[45] The "minimal room" Wilhelm envisaged (fig. 218) tried to get everything into 20 square feet—all the necessary facilities, washbasin with running water, drinking water, mirror, toilet. The patient could be bathed from the basin, wash his own teeth and hands, get his own drink of water (but only if he were lying down; this became impossible when the bed was rolled up to a sitting position). And although "this hospital, like all others, doesn't want its patients to service themselves when they need a urinal or bedpan," in a pinch the patient could help himself to those too. The windowsill served as end table, storage space, and stand for flowers, leaving no room for the window to be opened. Forced-air ventilation in the form of a wedge-shaped insert near the corridor wall was installed in the room and toilet. (No longer do toilets have to be located on an outside wall.) Wilhelm admitted that "one would not care to be quartered too long in such a small area, but for a few days it was most acceptable."

Hexagonal single rooms planned in 1959 for the Davis Medical Foundation of Marion, Indiana, were another attempt to design a novel receptacle for modern nursing paraphernalia (fig. 219).[46] It is a shame that this excellent plan was never built but foundered on a technicality that never passed the local building code. The rooms had the advantage that from his bed the patient could see both out over the countryside and through double doors into the hospital corridor. He was certainly approachable from either side, thanks to the hexagonal design, but there is some question whether there would have been enough room at his head for heavy equipment. Each of the 6 walls was to be 6 feet 8 inches wide. A bed alone takes up nearly 4 feet, including adjustable sidebars. Bed and table occupy nearly 6 feet—6 very full feet if you add an overbed table. What about oxygen equipment ($1\frac{1}{2}'$ in width) and a nurse to operate the oxygen equipment, whose controls are on the side of the machine away from the bed? What about stretcher and nurse (3' wide collectively, given a thin nurse)? For a very sick patient, the bed would always have to be pulled out into the middle of the room. But the plan did not founder on a question of size. There was to be a toilet next to the bed that could be folded up out of the way when not in use,

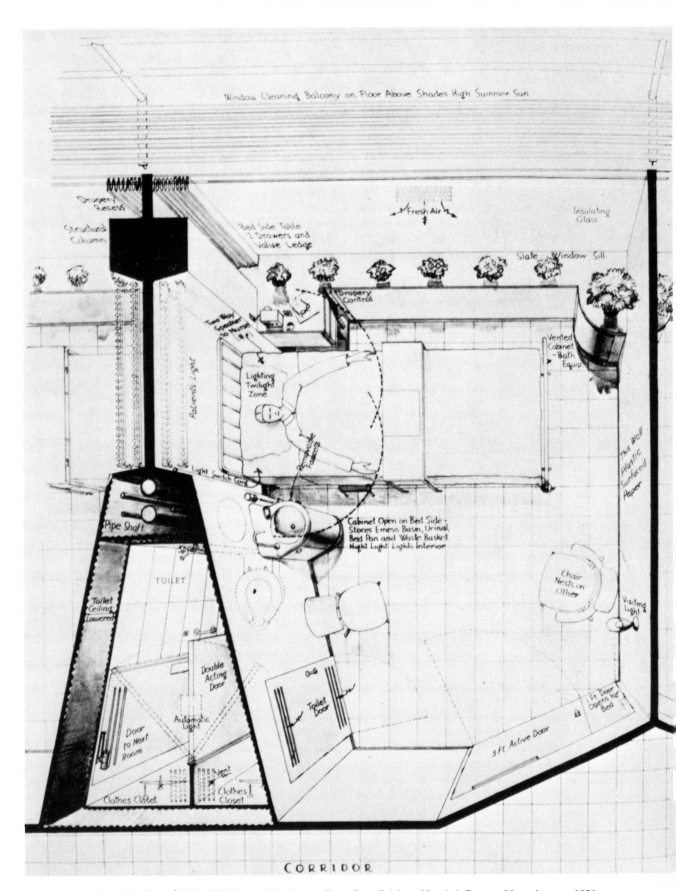

Fig. 218. Plan of N. A. Wilhelm's minimal room, Peter Bent Brigham Hospital, Boston, Massachusetts, 1951.

like the toilet of a Pullman compartment. This involved a flexible drain, and the drain was what never passed certain building codes, so the plan fell through. It was extraordinarily compact—40 rooms dovetailed in an approximate square around a central corridor —and should have been built to permit evaluation of its design.

Gordon A. Friesen (1968) suggested equipping the individual patient room as a special care unit by installing a lightweight extension boom in the middle of the room to carry all services: power, communication, and medical gases.[47] This would free the bed to be moved out from the wall altogether, and the staff could circulate around it in every direction. A design halfway between corner and island bed was proposed by James S. Moore (1962).[48] The bed is turned at an angle, its head against the slanted wall of the toilet (fig. 220). The toilet has flitted back to the outside wall. Corridor length can thus be reduced to 8 feet 6 inches, only about two-thirds of the 12 feet required for an island bed. The patient is brought nearer the corridor, and a jutting toilet room no longer hides his face from the nurse standing in the doorway. Of course, with the washstand in the toilet room at the far side, the temptation in such a room is to add a second washstand near the door for the convenience of doctors and nurses.

This plan does not permit a 3-foot clearance at the patient's head. However, Moore filled his room with machinery and people and called in photographers to prove it could contain the lot. He very strongly advocates all-single-room hospitals and has influenced the construction of many of them: among others, Providence Hospital of Seattle and Paradise Valley Hospital of National City, California. "Highly respected and experienced nurses," he reports, "have said that caring for patients in private rooms takes no more nursing time than caring for those in semiprivate rooms or four-bed wards." In private rooms moving costs are avoided (he estimated the cost of moving a patient at $20–$25 a move; others put it as low as $5–$8), as well as the errors in identification and medication that moving patients can bring about. "Also, would a person want to share a hotel room with a sick stranger? Yet, when he comes to a hospital and is not well, he is asked to do this." He admits that some studies done at Yale "actually did find that some patients who were interviewed were willing and preferred to share a room. We believe that the person desiring to share the room was assuming that his roommate would be the right sex and race, would like the same TV shows, wouldn't smell, snore, or smoke cigars, and would have only attractive, quiet visitors." He darkly prophesies that hospitals being built now with semiprivate and four-bed wards "may

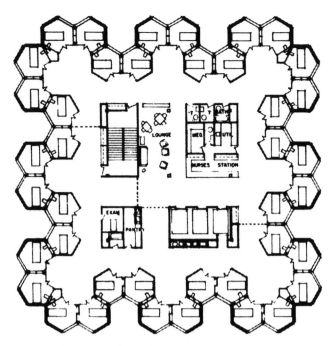

Fig. 219. Plan (never built) for a floor of hexagonal single rooms, Davis Medical Foundation, Marion, Indiana, 1959.

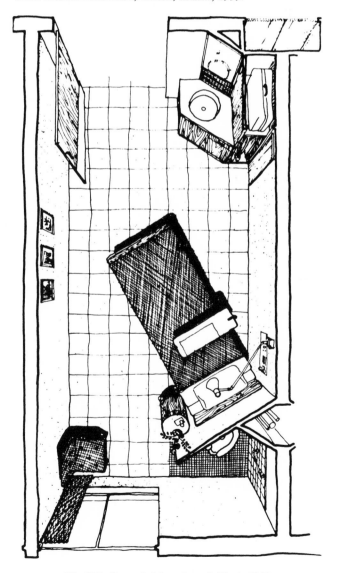

Fig. 220. James S. Moore's angled bed, 1963.

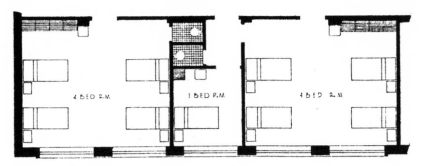

Fig. 221. Plan of John D. Thompson's four-and-one combination, Montefiore Hospital, New York City, 1955.

in the next 5 to 10 years be forced by competition as well as by patients to operate these as single-bed rooms."

The studies we did at Yale in 1957, to which Moore alludes,[49] definitely linked a preference for privacy to the social class of the patient (thus independently confirming hospital practice of half a millenium). We classified according to income the 505 patients answering our questionnaire by employing the five categories of the Hollingshead–Redlich Index of Social Class. It was demonstrated that among patients from Classes I and II, the upper 12.4 percent of the population in terms of income, almost 60 percent wanted private rooms. So did almost 50 percent of Class III, the next 21.4 percent of the population as far as income was concerned. But among patients belonging to Classes IV and V, the lowest 66.2 percent of the population in income, only 20 percent preferred a private room. This means that 80 percent of the members of the largest social class, who were patients at the time we ran our study, actively preferred to share a hospital room with others. "Being alone often frightens Classes IV and V," we reported at the time. "At no point in their lives have they experienced privacy, and they do not wish to be deprived of company in their time of trouble."

This was not our first encounter with an expressed preference for multibed rooms. In 1955, one of the authors introduced into Montefiore Hospital, New York City, a module of two 4-bed rooms with a small single "administrative" room tucked between them (fig. 221).[50] The 1-bed room was assigned for medical reasons and shared the toilet facilities of one of the 4-bed wards. It cost no more than a 2-bed room and consequently the full amount was covered by Blue Cross. A floor for 38 patients made up of these 4- and 1-bed rooms occupied the same square footage as one for 30 patients with the standard mix of 1- and 2-bed rooms, and such a floor was found easier for the nurses to work in, cheaper to build, and adaptable to the needs of semiprivate patients. Noisy or ex-

tremely ill patients were cleared out of the wards and assigned to the single rooms, a move that went far to reconcile the ward patients (who had expected their semiprivate accommodations to mean a 2-bed room) to remaining in the 4-bed ward. But their expressed satisfaction was not as startling as the expressed dissatisfaction of patients assigned to the single rooms. They resisted being moved into them. It was not because these rooms had the connotation of "death rooms" but rather that the patients claimed they would be lonesome or bored in a single room. Most of them welcomed the time when they might move back into the 4-bed accommodation. The same conclusion was reached at an eye hospital in Philadelphia in a questionnaire given to 510 patients (1968). It indicated that these inpatients, regardless of sex, age, degree of vision, or cost, preferred multibed units.[51] In an eye hospital, it may be surmised, boredom would be particularly acute.

"Patients like to have their own needs determine the degree of privacy they wish," Dr. Carl Walters affirmed in 1959.[52] This seems to be borne out by Dr. Ernest Dichter, who is a psychiatrist, when he discussed the hospital–patient relationship in 1961:

Everything that gave the patient a sense of belonging, sharing and participation helped him in his emotional integration to the hospital situation. This raises, of course, the question of the emotional value at times of the private room. But it also indicates the profound possibilities in interpatient activities. The patient as he convalesces becomes increasingly a social being. It is part of his emotional recovery from helplessness and childlike dependence. . . . Even the relatively free access to visitors allowed the private patient in one hospital did not make up for the sense of isolation from the hospital family. . . . The patient, it was found, longs for someone to talk to, other than visitors who are quite often merely formal. He wishes to share his hospital experience. . . . The other patient becomes in a sense either an older brother or sister, teaching and helping, or . . . the younger sibling. . . . The sharing in either form is therapeutic.[53]

But the proponents of the all-single-room hospital, free of doubts and filled with a religious ardor, are intent on converting the world. No one is more active in the cause than Gordon A. Friesen, and there has been a perceptible response even in England to his American dream. It was recently decided to rebuild St. Anthony's at Cheam, Surrey, and to incorporate in it every advanced method of hospital design and medical care.[54] This end in mind, the sister administrator toured Britain, Germany, Sweden, Italy, and Ireland and then flew to America to consult Mr. Friesen in Washington. She returned with a "revolutionary plan" for a 300-bed hospital of all single rooms, complete with nurseservers, central supply system, and a closed-circuit television network for patient–nurse communication. In a published statement the hope was expressed that this hospital, then scheduled for completion in 1971, would permit almost 100 percent bed occupancy, that automation would effect a 30 percent saving in domestic and other ancillary labor, while enabling nurses to give 100 percent patient care. Said Sister Mary Perpetua, "Why should patients today have to lose themselves in a hospital 'dormitory' when we don't do this—or want to—in any other aspect of our public lives? When we go to a hotel we don't expect to have to sleep in a room with several other people. . . ."

CHAPTER 8

The All-Private-Room Hospital:
An Eighteenth-Century Reprise

In 1788, four years after the opening of the Allgemeines Krankenhaus in Vienna, two hospital planners of Mainz engaged in a debate on the desirability of hospital privacy for its own sake. Dr. Strack, the university authority on hospital science, opposed private rooms in a hospital. Dr. Hoffmann, who championed them, was the Elector's private physician, a very successful practitioner but not a university man. Each was put in charge of remodeling a convent as a hospital. (It will be recalled that the ultra-modern Allgemeines Krankenhaus of Vienna was a converted poorhouse.) Strack tore out the partitions between cells of the St. Clara Convent and created 9- or 10-bed wards. When the work was two-thirds completed, the Elector asked Hoffmann to inspect it. Hoffmann objected to the 10-bed wards, whereupon the Elector gave him permission to set up 10 one-bed rooms at the Altenmünster Convent, which were then to be compared with one 10-bed ward at St. Clara. A controversy in pamphlet form developed between the two hospital planners,[1] Hoffmann demanding that work at St. Clara be abandoned and that the Altenmünster Convent, still in its original single-cell form, be cheaply and readily adapted as an all-single-bed hospital.

Hoffmann had visited Paris, as had all good European hospital planners of his time, in search of the perfect hospital form. He thought he found it in the Charité —spacious wards, one patient per bed, the beds placed at a proper distance from one another. Due regard was paid there to cleanliness, and doctors, surgeons, and nurses were attentive. He visited this "unimprovable" hospital several times until one evening he found a patient in the throes of death.

> His breast was boiling. This horrible noise could be heard throughout the entire ward and struck me as a truly terrible sound, and must have struck the poor patients as an even worse one. The greater part of the patients attempted to hide their ears in their pillows but all wished the patient a speedy end to his misery. Because of the horrible noise I left the saddened place, but the patients had to stay, like it or not.

After this experience Hoffmann noticed how often one patient disturbs another "by heavy snoring, coughing, clearing the throat, gargling, vomiting, moaning, sighing, groaning." Patients' sleep was disturbed by this and their recovery retarded. "I now thought I knew that the Charité also was imperfect, and that these imperfections could not be removed unless each patient was given his own bed and room."

The late eighteenth-century controversy between Hoffmann and Strack on the subject of the private hospital room was carried on in a spirit of acrimony equaling our most virulent modern debates. Strack admitted that the chief objection to his 10-bed wards and thus "the most probable reason" for having private rooms would be danger of infection. He defines an infectious disease as occurring "when a totally unknown substance emitted from a sick body enters into a healthy body and there causes the same disease."

Totally unknown? Hoffmann proffers the information that some doctors say infectious material of a certain disease can infect a body and bring forth a similar disease, and that proofs of this are no less certain than Harvey's theory of the circulation of the blood. "If this matter were not totally unknown to Dr. Strack, I might ask him indeed what he had against these proofs."

Strack responds that in some diseases direct contact with the patient is not necessary. There may be a general cause that brings forth a certain disease in many bodies simultaneously. Diseases infectious under some circumstances are not so under others. Typhus for instance is far more infectious among the poor. He realizes that with his best efforts some diseases will remain infectious in his model hospital —smallpox, crabs, scarlet fever, and some kinds of dysentery—and for such patients he will have ready special spacious wards. But most ordinary infection can be driven out by moving air and an open fire. A splendid ventilation system will make his wards much safer than those of Vienna, London, Paris, Strasbourg. This ventilation system will depend on a fireplace and on an air intake through the outside walls (the air being warmed on its way toward a vent in the middle of the room), and along the roof there will be exhaust pipes that turn with the wind, and so on. Infectious patients will have open chimneys, *two* intakes, and *two* exhausts.

Hoffmann begs to differ. "No ventilation system, Dr. Strack's included, suffices to stop infectious diseases." He instances the spread of typhus and dysentery in army hospitals where the air is constantly freshened.

Small rooms are not immune, Strack reminds Hoffmann, quoting from one of Hoffmann's own papers a statement that smallpox may be carried on anything.

Hoffmann replies that a private room won't stop infection but will lessen it. Both reason and experience suggest that there is less danger of infection in private rooms than in wards. After all, it takes only one patient in a ward of twelve to give all twelve a disease directly. Experience shows that infectious diseases are more of a problem the larger the hospital and the more patients in a ward. There was never an epidemic of infectious disease at the Spanish Hospital of Vienna (with all-private rooms for the rich; it cost one gulden a day and closed down because it was too expensive.)

Nor is relative freedom from infection, Hoffmann adds, the only reason for preferring private rooms. Patients require different temperatures according to differences in their physique and in the illnesses they suffer from. "In diseases we find various emissions, the stool, the urine, sweat, vomit, and breath. Each of these emissions must be treated with a particular room temperature. However, this is impossible in a ward."

"The layman might be convinced by this reason . . . but experienced doctors' are not," Strack retorts. "All these methods demand nothing more than a pure and properly warmed air."

Uniform warmth is a very good thing in some diseases, Hoffmann allows. At a certain point in the progress of the disease it may indeed be desirable, but at another point it would be fatal. In brain fever one requires cold compresses. At the onset of smallpox, warmth can cause death. Dr. Strack is too interested in defending 10-bed wards. "To be sure, he is right, if he does not care whether the patient recovers or dies."

Strack envisages ten different rooms with ten different temperatures, and the doctors running around all the time from one room to another checking the temperatures.

Hoffmann exclaims, Nonsense! Can't you trust the nurse to do that? Besides, a good room will maintain a steady heat for a long time.

The perfect hospital, says Strack, must stand free, "surrounded by its streets like an island, so that the free circulation of air will protect it from even the most dangerous vapors."

"Dr. Strack paints his ideal here in such a way that it fits the St. Clara Convent."

Strack: The croaking of frogs in a swampy neighborbood (the Altenmünster Convent happened to be located in a swamp) and a large number of mosquitoes must disturb the peace of the patients.

Hoffmann: "That could be."

Strack: There should be no noisy occupation, no flour mill, locksmith, smithy, plumber, coopersmith, or barrel-maker in the neighborhood; no slaughterhouse; no tannery or dye works because of the smell; no bakery, so the smoke from it may not fall down into the hospital; "nor should any wine be fermented in the hospital cellar."

Hoffmann never heard of anyone being made ill by the vapors of fermenting wine. There are vapors and vapors.

Strack: "The kitchen wastes must be disposed of daily in order that they do not rot. And the necessary cats should be sterilized in order that their howling when they are in heat does not disturb the patients' sleep."

Hoffmann: "Beware, ye cats! But really, is there no more comfortable means of getting rid of mice in a hospital than by using sterilized cats?"

Strack "And create an unbearable smell by their urine."

Hoffmann wants to know whether sterilizing the cats will prevent the smell of urine.

Strack maintains that in his perfect hospital, strict rules would enforce complete silence in all the wards, and the nurses would wear felt slippers. As for coughing, vomiting, and so forth (noises one can't do away with), one must remember that patients in a charity hospital are not of a sensitive class accustomed to all comforts, "but are the kind of people who in their small, narrow dwellings are used to a much greater amount of noise than they will experience in a well-run ward."

"That is to say," Hoffmann objects, "that a patient doesn't need to have a separate room even though the disease has made his brain more sensitive. . . . Even the lightest rustling can immediately induce gout and unconsciousness, though these noises are not harmful to a healthy man. Such conditions can arise in a patient even if only a small amount of light is let into the room."

What about privacy during confession? Strack says the curtains can be pulled around the patient's bed and those of his nearest neighbors, and he can be confessed without anybody noticing.

Hoffmann: They can't see his face, but they can hear him.

Strack: "And should the patient be deaf, the priest can speak to him through an ear horn, so that the neighbors will not hear the least noise."

Hoffmann: "This is certainly a comic notion!"

Strack: Anyway, one of the rules of the hospital is that each patient should receive the sacraments upon admission.

Hoffman: "A proper rule on many counts."

Strack: And if a patient die in the ward, the body can be "noiselessly pushed out" through the swinging door to the corridor that is used to bring in and out the closestools.

Hoffmann: "Noiselessly? I am amazed!"

Strack: "Patients who make a good deal of noise while out of their senses will be carried into another room."

Hoffmann: "But what if moving them in such a way is dangerous for them?"

Strack: "Surgical operations where screaming and moaning cannot be avoided must be performed in the surgical amphitheatre already set up in the St. Clara Convent."

Hoffmann: "Special rooms after all!"

Strack says that when he was in the Altenmünster Convent before it was abandoned, you could hear everything anyway because the cell walls were so thin.

Hoffman retorts: Had you thought to close the doors?

Strack accuses Hoffmann of having chosen the Altenmünster Convent as his hospital because the cells were still intact (requiring a minimum of alteration). But obviously the St. Clara Hospital is almost finished.

Hoffmann: Yes, but you're going to have to tear it down and start over.

Strack: At the Altenmünster, the cells are too small —8 feet 2 inches by 10 feet 10 inches. They haven't enough air.

Hoffmann: I will take care of that by good ventilation. Besides, those are only the smallest ones, there are others much larger.

Strack: "A bedstead for an adult should be 6 feet long and 3½ feet wide. And if you were to add a chair and small tables, how much room is left? In a small cell, a bed must be placed along its length along the wall, which is the worst position for a sickbed, since a sickbed must necessarily be free on two sides so that one can comfortably approach the patient from all sides."

Hoffmann: "Necessarily? Has Dr. Strack ever found such arrangements in private homes? . . . Dr. Strack is basing this argument on the false information that all rooms in the convent are too small." (A nasty thrust. Strack had been convent doctor at the Altenmünster for 27 years; he obviously knew perfectly well that there were larger rooms.)

Strack: "For instance, should a broken bone have to be set in such a narrow cell, there would not be enough space for the surgeon and his assistants."

Hoffmann: "Although the smallest cells have sufficient space for this operation, nevertheless such a patient would receive a larger room."

Strack: "It was ordered by the Elector that young doctors should receive bedside instruction at this hospital. We must note that besides the physician who teaches, barely four interns could fit into such a cell."

Hoffmann: There are rooms in the convent large enough for twenty or more interns.

Strack: "And how many minutes would they be able to remain without danger to their own health?"

Hoffmann: "Just as long and just as easily as in Dr. Strack's wards." In fact more easily, there being not twelve patients but rather one from whom to receive the contagion.

Strack: The narrower the space, the faster the pollution.

Hoffmann: If the windows aren't opened and the ventilator isn't turned on.

Strack: What about a patient with dysentery, gangrene, smallpox—what an intolerable stench in the small room!

Hoffmann: "Isn't it wonderful that Dr. Strack describes doctors and surgeons to the public as so exceptionally stupid that it doesn't once occur to them that they could open the windows when the room stinks? Why do his wards have ventilation and he thinks my rooms will be totally closed in? I have ventilators just as good as his and even better, which will definitely cleanse my rooms from their dangerous air ten times as fast as is possible in his wards with his system."

Hoffmann does not doubt that doctors would approve of single rooms for the peace and quiet they provide and the freedom from infection. But doctors think of the multiplication of staff and the expense, they remember the Spanish Hospital and they ask, Where will we find the money for such an establishment?

Hoffmann presents a system whereby no more nurses will be required for ten individual rooms than for a 10-bed ward. Picture, he says, a 10-bed ward with the nurse walking up and down the aisle between the beds. Let us assume that the one nurse can take care of all ten beds. Next, "let us imagine that the space in front of the beds has been separated off by a wall and that each bed has been enclosed with side walls." Provide each room with a door. Now "the nurse can go along the corridor just as easily as he went along in front of the beds, for the space is the same." Imagine a pane of glass in each door, through which the patient's bed can be seen. And imagine the nurse looking in on him, supervising yet not disturbing each patient, "who loves nothing so much as peace and quiet." The nurse wears fur soles. The glass in the door will be curtained for privacy while the patient is on the closestool.

But if a patient needs a nurse, he can call him.

> Should a string be placed next to each bed, as is the custom, by which a small piece of wood which is fastened to the string, for instance a box top, is pulled up high, and should it be so done that the piece of wood which has been pulled into the air remains there, then the nurse can see either when he is at his post or as he goes along the corridor that a patient wants him, because he notices the piece of wood which has been pulled up. . . . If it is desired that a bell should ring when the string is pulled, nothing more is necessary than to arrange the matter so that the little piece of wood moves a bell when it is pulled up. In the same way, each nurse who needs another nurse to help him when he is with a patient, can call the second nurse in from the corridor by ringing the bell.

Moreover it must be remembered that "at any time," as Hoffmann triumphantly concludes, "only a small number of the patients in the hospital are totally helpless, and the rest can take their chamber pot and their beverages from a chair or table in front of the bed, and can usually serve themselves."

In a private room or in the larger ward, helpless patients have a private nurse. Delirious patients could be bound with cloth bands and be watched and cared for from the corridor just as other patients are, with the advantage that they would not upset other patients in the ward. And with all-private rooms, convalescent patients, wearing felt shoes, could visit one another in their rooms or walk and talk in the heated corridor.

Now Dr. Strack must be given his chance to register objections, which he does emphatically. "This proposal can only be accepted when one is considering the cost all the time, as the author himself admitted he was doing . . . but a doctor need not decide how the patient will be cared for in that case."

Hoffmann admits: "It is true that I have removed all removable expenses wherever possible. The Spanish Hospital in Vienna was closed simply because it

was too expensive. I should not like my hospital to falter for the same reason."

Strack: "Charity commands, however, that the poor patient be provided with nursing care, drink, healthy food and pure medicine, in the hospital, just as well as a prince that is in his palace."

Hoffmann: "This may well be the case in an imaginary world—but in our good one . . . !"

Strack: What if the patient becomes unconscious, falls into convulsions, without the nurse suspecting that this would happen? How can he pull his little string?

Hoffmann: He cannot.

Strack: What happens to him then, until the nurse comes by his room again?

Hoffmann: "He will remain lying unconscious or in convulsions until these conditions cease. The entire difference will consist of the fact that in the one case the nurse looks on while the patient lies unconscious or in convulsions, and in the other case the nurse will not see this, but in neither case can the nurse give any help. Moreover, if the nurse goes up and down the corridor as he should, then the difference in time cannot be greater than a minute. If the doctor must be called, then the cases will be very rare where a minute is important."

There are several fictions, particularly of timing, in Hoffmann's reasoning, but Strack outdoes them with his next question: "What if another patient, while the nurse is absent, hangs himself on the little string as a result of a sudden increase in fever?"

"We will make the little pieces of string too weak for the patient to hang himself on," Hoffmann snaps. "That will do, won't it? All of those who are saved in this manner must owe their lives to Dr. Strack's timely warning. But just between us, Mr. Minister," (Strack was also Minister of Health) "wouldn't (the bell) ring if the patient tried a little bit to hang himself on the little string?"

Strack: Perhaps the patient would jump out the window. How responsible is such a system in that case?

Hoffmann: Then the patient must have a private nurse. Or put up iron bars on the window. "My God," he exclaims, "what kind of imaginings he indulges in in order that private rooms may be cast into disrepute!"

Strack: "Now take the case of a patient in full possession of his senses, but the nurses, because they are taking care of someone else, are not in the nurses' room. How long will the patient have to pull his little string or wait until he gets, say, a closestool?"

Hoffmann: "It is in the corridor, and therefore hardly a second longer than if a nurse is taking care of another patient in a ward."

Strack: "Or should the closestool perhaps actually stay in the hospital room?"

Hoffmann: "To be sure, and it still won't make even the least stench, not even when the refuse is being carried across the corridor. Dr. Strack can be quite unconcerned about this matter."

Dr. Hoffmann does not mention how he would deodorize the closestool. He doesn't explain his toilet accommodations either. Strack describes toilet channels opening into the Rhine, flushed by rainwater from the roof gutters, guarded by valves from a back-up of vapors in the pipes. Hoffmann airily remarks that his system is so much better than Strack's that he's going to write a separate article about it, not waste it on this one.

Strack computes how many nurses it would take for an all-private-room hospital if the nursing were done as he would have it done. He comes up with the figure of 80 nurses for 40 patients—one by day and one by night. He then projects this to a big-city hospital with 600 beds, achieving a total of 1,200 nurses and a mammoth policing problem.

Hoffmann reports that in the Spanish Hospital of Vienna they had five nurses for every ten patients in their private wards. He suggests women nurses: by their nature they only work part time, they have trouble getting any other kind of job anyway, and they're always desperate for work or they wouldn't be working at all. Therefore you can get better women than men for the job and you can dismiss them for the least negligence. He has heard stories about women nurses who would go down on their knees and promise not to do it again in order to keep their positions.

For these nurses, figure a twelve-hour shift. The off shift will be one of pure recuperation. You can't expect a nurse to do other work during those twelve hours and keep up strength for the nursing. Therefore you must hire servants for housework, which makes staffing even more expensive.

In describing the removal from a private room of a patient who died of an infectious disease, Hoffmann approaches fantasy. The corpse should be placed in a sack and pulled through the ventilation hole in the ceiling up to the attic, through a door to the roof, and so out of the house. "The pipe that usually stands above the hole in order to take away the stale air from the room, and lead it out over the roof, must therefore be movable." This is an advantage to private rooms that modern planners have lost sight of. The mattresses and featherbeds were to be levitated by the same route and aired in the attic until all the dangerous vapors are dispersed.

And as literally the final advantage of the private room, Hoffmann cites the patient's ability to "call his wife, his child, and his friend to him and discuss his household circumstances with them, or how he would have things done after his death, and converse in privacy without anyone else hearing it."

Since the little volume we have reference to is Hoffmann's and he quotes Strack at length only to refute him, it is not surprising that the author concludes that Dr. Strack failed to prove it was not a good thing to give every patient his own bed and room, and believes that he has shown every reader how pleased a patient will be to have his own room and bed. This was in 1788.

CHAPTER 9

Supervision/Observability: A Review
of Contemporary British Literature
on Privacy versus Supervision

In modern Britain, emphasis is placed on the design elements of supervision and economy at the expense of the absolute or relative privacy so dear to an American heart. St. Anthony's practically stands alone in its commitment to a private-room pattern. To examine contemporary literature in England on the subject of supervision—or as the British term it, "observability"—is to approximate more or less the thinking of other European countries where an attempt is made to provide on a limited budget a decent standard of hospitalization for all citizens. Under such circumstances, planning must be in terms of 4- or 6-bed wards or units larger still.

The specifically British emphasis on supervision derives from Florence Nightingale. From 1861 to the beginning of World War II, the Nightingale ward was the dominant accommodation in Britain, indeed very nearly the only available design for a nursing unit. Designed by a nurse, the ward was beloved by nurses for its ease of nursing supervision. What matters most to a good nurse is to see her patients, be able to respond instantly in an emergency, and reach the patient having trouble in the shortest time possible. In the Nightingale system of progressive patient care, the sickest patients were grouped around the nursing station at the entrance to the ward, and the ones nearly ready to go home were down at the far end close to the balcony, if there was one, and the sanitary facilities, such as they were.

Because private rooms interfere with supervision, Florence Nightingale put little stock in them, and sure enough, the single rooms inserted among the service rooms of the entrance hall did not work for very sick patients. A nurse tending a difficult case in a single room could not know what was going on in the ward, and vice versa, so the singles came to be used as "amenity beds"[1] for moderately ill patients paying a modest fee or for members of the medical or nursing staff when they fell ill. There were never enough amenity beds to meet the demand. These singles were not suitable for infected patients, because they lacked their own sanitary facilities. They

did come in handy for dying patients by giving them more privacy and getting them out of the ward where a death would only depress the others, but as a medical man who worked in these wards for twenty years recently remarked to his compeers of the House of Lords, "If you have only two single rooms in a ward of 25 or 30 people and you say to one of your patients, 'I think you need more rest and we ought to put you [in] a room to yourself,' he thinks he is going to die. And he is usually right."[2]

It may seem strange that a single design could keep everybody reasonably content for eighty years (1861–1941) but as Hugh and John Gainsborough point out, nursing practice is basically very stable, certainly in comparison with meteoric developments in medicine or surgery, and "a ward that is correctly designed for basic nursing does not become obsolescent in a functional sense."[3] The Nightingale ward was designed at a time when rest in bed was the standard remedy for most ailments, a very long hospital stay was expected, bedpans were taken for granted, nurses were eager, plentiful, and not very highly paid, and meals and enemas alike were given on a military schedule. The beds stood at attention in two immaculate rows, and like marching soldiers all patients were supposed to do the same thing at the same time. A few screens were kept on hand for very ill or dying patients, bedpan rounds, and dressings. Only with the introduction in the 1940s of the mass use of penicillin (first discovered in England in 1928) and of other antibiotics that led to fundamental changes in medical treatment and nursing practices, did the defects of the Nightingale ward become evident.

During World War II, antibiotic treatment helped to turn patients out of hospital beds in record time. It was discovered that early ambulation benefited nearly all of them. This insight finally and decisively cracked the happy harmony between nursing practice and the Nightingale ward. What happened may be likened to the fate of the first classic Nightingale wards of St. Thomas's in London as a result of bombing during the blitz. For a long while it was thought that the original buildings could be saved and the interiors modernized, plans were drawn up for remodeling, and then it was found that the foundations had been too badly damaged. It was decided to demolish the existing structure and rebuild on the site in an entirely new mode. Similarly, the open ward still evokes loud expressions of affection and earnest pleas for its preservation, but with early ambulation more generous provision of day space and sanitary facilities became imperative. There has been a trend toward units with fewer beds. When nurses express nostalgia for the old days of absolute supervision, they may be understood to mean not only having the patient under visual control but also having the whole ward politically under their thumb. During an evaluation of one of the new subdivided units the sisters (that is, head nurses) expressed the feeling that they do not have the independence that was, and still is, enjoyed by the head nurse of a Nightingale ward.[4] Along with the ward inherited from Miss Nightingale each sister must receive some portion of her autocratic spirit.

The Nightingale ward had 2 toilet cubicles to a ward of 25 or 30 beds, and those were at the end of a very long walk. Even if patients were strong enough to cover the ground or could be wheeled in a toilet chair, the mathematical probability was that they would have to queue up. There was likewise a shortage of baths and washbasins (2 of each). The space could not well be subdivided by sex or by diagnosis, though for some years at St. Thomas's certain smaller specialties shared a ward by erecting a dividing wall down its full length—this, of course, did away with cross ventilation. In an ordinary ward, after meals or bedpan rounds when the nurses went around flinging windows open, there was entirely too much ventilation down the back of one's neck. A glare struck one's eyes from the windows opposite. There was no day space except in the middle of the ward. There was entirely too much space in the middle of the ward for extra beds: in times of overcrowding as many as 10 beds could be added without even the privacy of a back wall for those patients. The deficiencies of the open ward were recognized during the war years, but war damage and lack of funds prevented new hospital building. By 1960 the cracks in the foundations became unmistakable, patience wore thin, and exasperated comments were heard similar to those made earlier in the United States: "The truth is that the open ward is an anachronism. It is socially undesirable and medically unsound. In 1960 the public, the doctor, and the nurse should no longer be expected to put up with this scandalous impromptu." "We will try to prove that the open ward is now archaic, and a lie from those who tell

us we live in an affluent society." "After the war, we belatedly gained some appreciation of the frankly indecent conditions of life in the open ward."[5]

By the time real action was taken, the wards were not only anachronistic but obsolescent. The impoverished hospitals of Britain were nationalized in 1948, but for ten years thereafter national priorities were given to the rebuilding of bombed-out housing and of schools. Stopgap measures were resorted to in an effort to make the large wards more livable. To give a better view the nursing station was placed in the center of the room and surrounded by beds of the gravely ill. Or a ward would be subdivided into 4-bed cubicles with beds parallel to the windows, as in the Rigshospital of Copenhagen in 1911; this expedient was adopted at Hertford County Hospital in the 1930s. Progressive patient care being by this time formally operative in the world at large—it had always been a feature of the Nightingale ward—the cubicles were graded on a descending scale of gravity of illness. This could involve a bewildering moving-about of beds, but patients liked it and felt safe in the intensive area before operation and encouraged when moving toward self-care and home.[6] On paper, schemes were worked out for turning the open ward into 18 private rooms opening off a corridor[7] and for building a "gazebo ward" from prefabricated elements with sawtooth walls and a little niche for each bed—a kind of jagged Nightingale ward where the patient was given the privacy of one partial sidewall and could not see his neighbors, although sister could see him well enough and the television at the end of the ward could be viewed by all patients from their beds.[8] In plans for privacy, lack of human companionship is regularly compensated for by a television set. The subdivided single and gazebo wards were never built, because official investigation moved along quite other lines in rethinking the whole matter. In the 1950s funds for basic research in hospital management and planning came not from the National Health Service but mainly from independent voluntary organizations such as the Nuffield Provincial Hospitals Trust and King Edward's Hospital Fund for London.[9] The Nuffield studies in particular provided basic formulas for hospital building in the coming decades, when more government money became available.

The Nuffield researchers followed nurses in three different types of old wards as they performed a full day's tour of duty and laid out their movements on a plan of the ward with cotton yarn. Where the yarn lay thickest the traffic had been heaviest. Immediately they detected the difficulty of supervising auxiliary private rooms. A higher percentage of single rooms could be recommended only if they were so situated that nurses could conveniently divide their attention between the patients in them and the rest of the patients. But how many single rooms should there be, and for what kinds of cases? As Goldwater and Bluestone had done in 1925 in New York City, they asked the doctors, and 24 senior specialists representing every clinical specialty came up with essentially the Goldwater–Bluestone categories: patients who were infectious or susceptible to infection, seriously ill or dying patients, and those likely to disturb others or who required special attention. But the 1925 figure of 14.4 percent of patients in single rooms for medical reasons was nearly doubled in 1955. Even in Britain, the modern trend is toward privacy. The Nuffield provision for privacy is on a scale of 20 to 25 percent, yet it is specifically stated that "in planning the experimental wards the Investigation regarded ease of supervision as a crucial factor in the design." Clearly arrangements for privacy in Britain must provide for the "fundamental need—that the nurse should be able to keep a continually watchful eye on the patients as she goes about other work."

The five types of patients requiring private rooms were boiled down to two, with supervision as the criterion. Class A patients comprising the very ill, the dying, and cardiac cases had to be kept under close observation; Class B patients, the infectious, or those "otherwise socially unacceptable" did not require supervision by the nursing staff. Class A single rooms should be immediately adjacent to the nursing station, but Class B single rooms might be anywhere in the periphery of the ward.

The nursing station should be but a *pied à terre,* "a small unenclosed area of the ward, near the ancillary rooms and near the patients."[10] The English have not blindly accepted the modern American conception of a nursing station, represented on at least one U.S. Public Health Service plan as a mere office.

> There are 7 charting seats for nurses and the ward clerk (apart from the doctors' charting seats), and one must ask how can you accumulate so many staff in one place at one time if the nurses really go into the patients' areas, even in this admittedly intermediate care ward. To make it worse there is a conference room largely for nurses' use. . . . Whenever we meet doctors from the U.S.A. they always complain of their nursing difficulties and it seems that these plans are the overt expression of their troubles.[11]

The first experimental wards built according to Nuffield principles were financed by regional boards in Scotland and Ireland. The unit attached to Larkfield Hospital in Greenock (fig. 222) is an initial attempt to reconcile the claims of privacy and super-

vision, to increase sanitary provisions (assuming that most patients will be able to go to the w.c. and washing cubicles), and to determine independently and rationally the proper size of both a ward and a multiple-bed room (Nuffield *Studies,* p. 25).

The size of both wards was reasoned out as follows: it was first asked how many patients one trained nurse could handle. The answer arrived at was a minimum of 8 at peak periods and twice that in nonpeak periods. Multiples of 8 led to a ward unit of 32 beds with its own ancillary rooms on either side of a central staircase and an elevator, which would thus economically handle traffic related to 64 patients on each floor. (As it turned out, site space was lacking, and the second 32-bed ward was built above the first.) The 32 beds were divided 16 and 16 on either side of the service rooms. Of the 16 beds one-quarter, or 4 beds, were placed in single rooms: two type A rooms across from the nurses' station and two type B at the end of the hall. One room at the end of the hall for an infectious patient had its own toilet. All 4-bed groupings have a toilet *en suite,* as the English (and French) would say, instead of across the hall, and all beds are in alcoves entirely open to the central corridor (pp. 19–20). The Rigshospital influence is strong. The bed complement is very close to that of a Nightingale ward, however it was arrived at. The layout has some features in common with that of the American Public Health Service double-loaded single corridor (that is, a central corridor with wards and private rooms opening off both sides of it). But few American designers would tolerate the open bed bays and nurses' stations.

At the Musgrave Park Hospital Experimental Ward in Belfast (fig. 223) it was decided to increase the number of patients per nurse from 8 to 10 in the interests of economy. Forty instead of 32 patients could thus be served by one set of ancillary rooms, 80 instead of 64 would fit on a single floor, and the basic unit was increased from 16 to 20. If the building had been further extended by groups of fours and singles it would have become more expensive to build and more expensive to operate in terms of nursing steps. A squarish building is more economical than a long thin one. Therefore the beds for 12 patients in each grouping of 20 are in 6-bed wards, that is, they are lined up 3 deep from the window, and the 4 extra patients have been given bed number 3 in each of the 6-bed wards. There are still only 4 single rooms. Privacy has been reduced in two areas, but oddly enough so has visibility: toilets, washbasins, and patients' lockers are lined up as a kind of wall closing off the 6-bed wards from the corridor. However, the nurse is centrally located in a compact rectangle with the 4-bed room behind her, the 6-bed

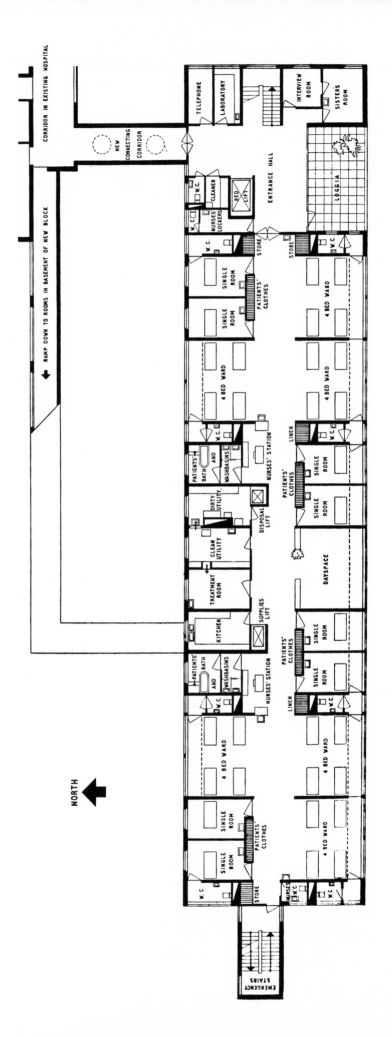

Fig. 222. Plan of experimental ward unit, Larkfield Hospital, Greenock, Scotland, 1956.

rooms on either side, and the singles across from her. With a minimum of moving she can look in on all her charges. This is an improvement on the Larkfield nurses' station midway between patient and service areas, with the patients' washing area behind it and only two private rooms in front. At Musgrave Park the noise of the utility rooms has been removed from the neighborhood of patients requiring privacy. Type A and type B single rooms are here indistinguishable (pp. 21–22).

But 6-bed rooms present a problem in lighting. For a physician it is important to see his patient in daylight since most artificial lighting falsifies colors and may lead to mistaken diagnosis. The Larkfield wards with only 4 beds were generously sized, and planners went to great lengths to solve the problem of lighting. Windows were extended to the ceiling. Wall and floor finishes were kept very light, and a baffle [the "Nuffield eyebrow" (fig. 224)] was designed across the window. The purpose of this baffle was to reduce the area of sky visible by the patient in the bed nearer the window, thus reducing excessive glare. At the same time the baffle had a reflective upper surface that bounced light onto the ceiling of the ward and thence onto the bed farther from the window. The experimenters admit that the baffle considerably reduces the total light, but since it was intended to reduce light contrast inside the room this was not decisive. However, it was also found to be structurally very expensive, and this was fatal (pp. 94–96). Musgrave Park needed a Nuffield eyebrow to light that third bed, but the investigation concluded that a 6-bedded ward could be adequately lit from a window on one side only (p. 99). This meant that permanent artificial lighting for at least a portion of the area became inevitable at Musgrave Park—the price that had to be paid for economy.

Designs for Larkfield and Musgrave Park were published by the Nuffield Trust in 1955, and the experimental units were actually built but were unique in their time. The figures tell the story: from 1948 to 1958, $240 million was spent on new hospital construction in Britain. Then the hospitals' turn for government building funds finally came and from 1958 to 1968, $1,200 billion was spent. Each year new buildings to the value of more than $240 million are being completed.[12] Whereas principles arrived at by the Nuffield studies are being applied right along to new construction, the single-corridor plans of Larkfield or Musgrave Park were soon challenged. The double-corridor, or racetrack, ward, a wartime expedient proposed in the United States in 1942 by Charles Neergaard, was the acknowledged model for the Wycombe General Hospital near Oxford (1958–66). Although British hospitals

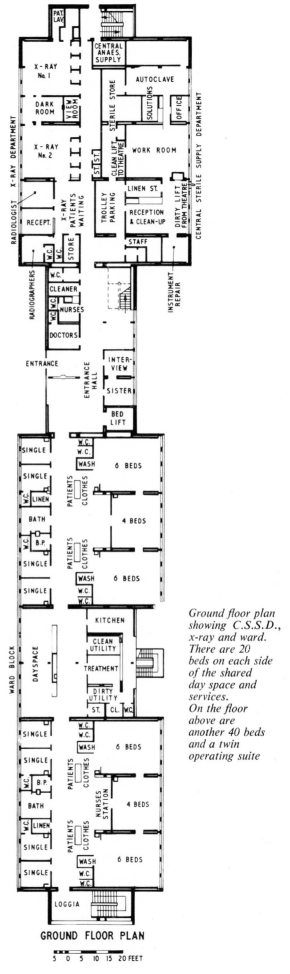

Ground floor plan showing C.S.S.D., x-ray and ward. There are 20 beds on each side of the shared day space and services. On the floor above are another 40 beds and a twin operating suite

Fig. 223. Plan of experimental ward unit, Musgrave Park Hospital, Belfast, Ireland, 1957.

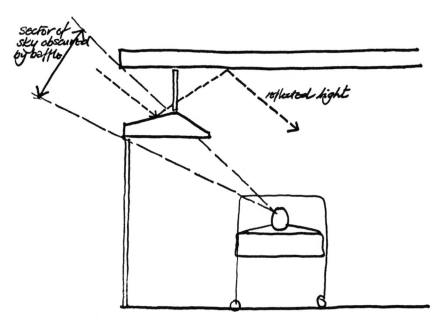

Fig. 224. How the "Nuffield eyebrow" or baffle works to keep light out of the eyes of the patient in the bed nearer the window while bouncing it to the inner bed. Diagram by Brian Brookes, not to scale.

adopted the concept of placing wards around the periphery of a squarish building and services in the central core, the name was resisted; it was said that "neither nurses nor patients are horses to be running round and round a course."[13] The racetrack ward, of which Wycombe was the first example in Britain, came to be known as "deep planning."

The designers of the new Wycombe Hospital (fig. 225) had intended to construct a single-corridor ward on the model of Larkfield. But the site was too short, so a double-corridor plan was resorted to, with considerable misgivings; although the plan had been in operation in the United States for many years, "the architects had little data on which to base their ideas."[14] A Larkfield-type ward was built on an ample site at Swindon at about the same time (fig. 226) and the two were compared. Wycombe won on nearly every count except capital and running costs. "The ward block at Wycombe had not long been commissioned when it became conspicuously apparent that the ward which was the standard unit for the 224-bed block was functioning very successfully in terms of patient care."[15] The question was, Why?

The answer came in terms of supervision, or as it had come to be referred to by then, observability. The corridor at Swindon was long, narrow affair and from their station the nurses had their choice of view into the two single-bed rooms behind them or into the patients' toilet accommodations across the corridor. At Wycombe the wards were wrapped, so to speak, around the nurses' station: the two singles behind it, two 6-bed wards to either side, a 4-bed

ward diagonally across on one hand, and two more singles diagonally across on the other. Although partitions partially enclosed the multiple-bed wards, there were doors only on the single rooms. Observation was decidedly facilitated for the reduced night shift. The open area around the nursing station was ample enough for it to serve both as a base for the nurses and as a natural gathering point for staff. "As long as basic planning requirements are for observation and for a nurse, particularly a newcomer to the ward, to feel part of a team rather than that she is working in isolation, a layout such as that at Wycombe gets very near the ideal."[16]

Conversely, from the Swindon ward came reports that because the patients could not see the nurses, they sometimes *felt* neglected.

> At night continued observation by nurses was very difficult. . . . Only increased nurse–patient ratios would re-establish the feeling of confidence that nurses and patients were really in touch with each other. Consultants, junior doctors and nursing staff of all grades expressed the view that more nurses were required to staff the wards adequately and some felt that a "Nightingale" ward would be preferable to an understaffed ward of the Swindon plan.[17]

The *Wycombe* ward was equipped with a patient-nurse direct speech communication system! But it was regarded as a complicated extravagance; patients were so close to the nurses' station that it was not necessary to telephone. However, the deep ward

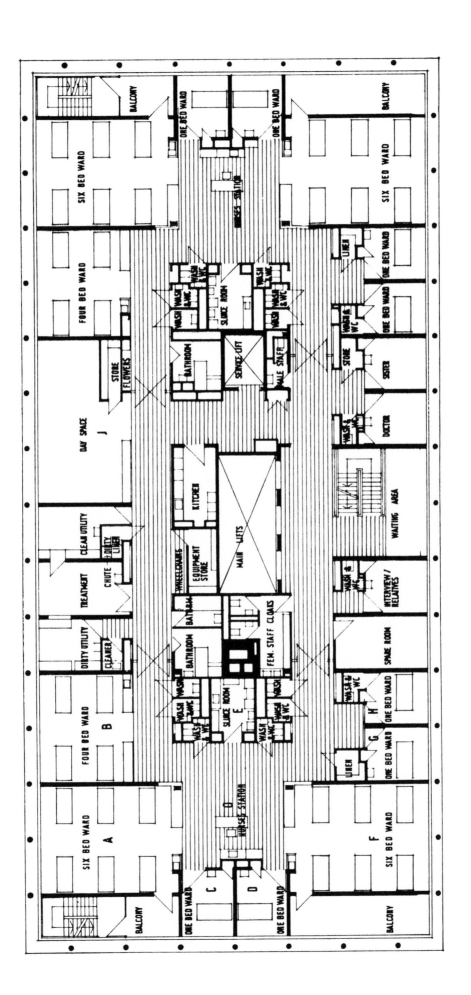

Fig. 225. Plan of a general surgical ward, Wycombe General Hospital (1963–66).

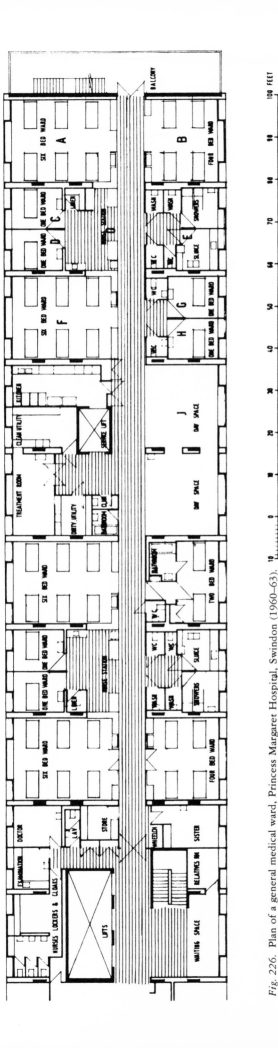

Fig. 226. Plan of a general medical ward, Princess Margaret Hospital, Swindon (1960–63).

did require one worrisome and expensive bit of machinery: air conditioning, at least in the core. For this reason it was considered ideal for one-story buildings, whose interior might be lit and aired by a clerestory,[18] but the government in charge of allocating limited funds for hospital building took a cautious view of the new plan, except in relation to restricted sites such as Wycombe, where the long single-corridor would not fit. "Given their higher capital and running costs, these advantages alone do not constitute a case for the widespread adoption of deep plan wards in this country." "Current costs allowed for hospital planning are not sufficient to provide the sophisticated environment for patient care found at Wycombe."[19] This decision from on high was warmly contested by those who would have liked to put a price on nursing steps, patients' peace of mind, and that invaluable commodity—observability.

The discussion in the literature goes somewhat as follows. The matron of a large London hospital remarks that the double-corridor ward seems the best answer in terms of control and observability (and the moderator parenthetically remarks on the tendency these days to steer clear of the word *supervision*). A hospital planning consultant counters with the key statement that the problem is not to build a few hospitals but to provide a large number of hospitals worthy of the National Health Service 17 years after its inception. "If race-track wards meant a 25 per cent increase in costs, then they were out." An architect reckons that amortized over 50 years (the life-expectancy of a new hospital building), the capital cost is only 6 percent of the running cost, and in this context a capital cost increase of 25 percent does not have that great a significance. The Ministry of Health suggests that future changes in medical requirements and techniques of nursing are likely to be more easily assimilated in wide plans of simple shape than in narrower ones. A hospital management committee approves of the occupancy rates in all wards of smallish rooms: "The admission of both sexes to a single ward has resulted in far better use being made of the beds and has not produced practical difficulties." The evaluation team at work at Swindon and Wycombe offers the reminder that more staff is needed for linear wards, and "expenditure on nursing staff is, therefore, revenue more effectively spent in the deep ward, a point of great importance in times of scarcity of nursing skills." And the director of The Hospital Centre in London underscores the point: "It may be manpower rather than money that will be the determining factor in health service development. . . . One of our topmost priorities in the future must be that of making the best use of our manpower resources."[20]

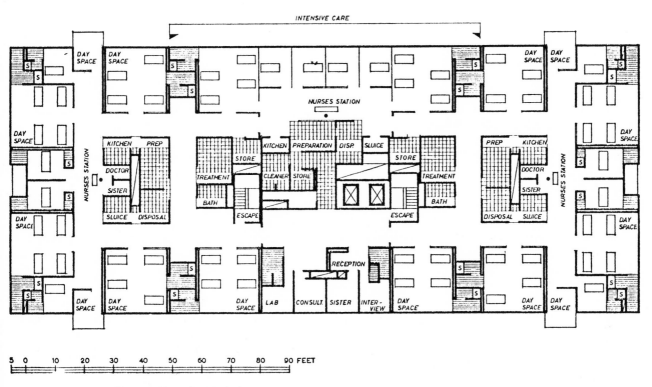

Fig. 227. Plan of the Falkirk experimental ward, Falkirk Royal Infirmary, Scotland (1962–66).

Another innovative plan was that of the Falkirk ward in Scotland (1962–66); fig. 227). This experimental two-story ward was designed to test the deep plan and included a combination of 4-bed and 1-bed rooms, no sixes, and toilets *en suite* in every room—American elements but reasoned through afresh. Two-bed rooms were rejected because the patients might not be compatible, 3-bed rooms tended to become a "two and one" situation, but 4-bed rooms "afforded a corner to each patient, a location demonstrably preferred by most people, for example, in restaurants and trains."[21] One reason for the room toilets and showers was that because both men and women were on one floor the 4-bed rooms had to be self-contained.

Twenty percent of the beds were in single rooms. A conscious effort was made to provide beds for intensive nursing care (this is not the same thing as an intensive care unit) but since the number of acutely ill patients could fluctuate from 12 to 20 percent of the total load, the unit had to be flexibly designed so that beds could be assigned to either intensive or intermediate care. The sickest patients were grouped around the nursing station, and it was noticed that when they overflowed into the intermediate rooms around the corner it was less satisfactory "because the observation of patients is more difficult" (*Falkirk Ward*, p. 43).

The acutely ill were *not* to be nursed in private rooms, which were reserved for infectious, infectable, noisy,

confused, or terminal cases. To the reduced privacy of a 4-bed ward for dangerously ill patients was added glazing on the corridor wall down to mattress level for the sake of maximum observation. In intermediate care areas this glazing was carried down only to nurse-shoulder level (p. 6). Glass partitions with curtaining were provided between rooms as well, but since the curtains were invariably kept closed, this was a sheer waste of money (p. 16). A necessary expense of such a ward was the siting of toilets between the rooms (the corridor wall being glazed throughout). This increased both the length and cost of the building, and once again the official reaction was no: "On the basis of experience gained so far, the Department are prepared to approve deep ward plans in Scotland only on sites where it is impossible to provide linear plans economically" (p. 47). But members of the evaluation committee expressed the view that the design of the Falkirk Ward was a safe basis for planning for the next fifty years (p. 54).

The usual audiovisual aids were installed at Falkirk but nurses found them too complicated and felt they reduced nurse–patient contact; furthermore, they could not be used by patients unable to speak to a nurse, confused patients, or the elderly. "Mechanical systems are no substitute for personal supervision" (p. 6). There is deep distrust of machinery: "The more mechanical and electrical equipment, the more chance there was of failure" (p. 52).

Unfortunately, the deep ward plan beloved by nurses demands artificial ventilation. That warm advocate of deep ward planning, John Gainsborough, admits that the Americans seem to be better at it than the English are. For a long time it was assumed that the American climate with its extremes of summer heat and winter cold necessitated air conditioning even in linear wards, whereas the English climate might possibly not need it even in deep wards. But it was found impossible to ensure a reasonable standard of comfort by windows alone, even in Britain. As soon as you double the corridor you lose forever the cross ventilation so beloved by Florence Nightingale. Or the opposite may apply to an exposed site such as that of High Wycombe, "where to open a window is to invite a minor gale. One can envisage the day, in the not too distant future, when the 'generous windows' will be peppered by those noisy drip dropping Yankee devices—individually packaged air-conditioning units."[22] Without artificial ventilation, toilet areas must always be sited on an exterior wall, lengthening the building and increasing its cost. In Britain's frequently foggy weather, respiratory cases recover much more quickly in a fully air-conditioned atmosphere. And anyway, soon it may not be possible to ventilate some urban hospitals naturally because of the noise problem. But the government retorts: "These measures would be justified only in special situations such as on some restricted city sites or near airports." And what about cost? Full air-conditioning costs three to four times as much as heating the same area.[23]

A prime determinant in the controversy over whether or not to air-condition has not yet been mentioned. With the prevalence of *staphylococcus aureus* in hospital wards in recent decades, infection has once again had to be controlled partially by ventilation devices, for staph is stubbornly resistant to antibiotics. In fact, it was bred as a resistant strain by careless physicians who indiscriminately dosed with penicillin as a preventive measure. A 1962 experiment demonstrated that when one bed is deliberately infected, the organism will spread throughout a 20-bed ward in three hours of normal activity.[24] It was hoped that the move from open wards to smaller units would greatly lessen infection rates, and so it did for a time, but they rose again, heartbreakingly. In 1963 one such move reduced the percentage of infected surgical cases in the ward from 12 to 1.7 percent. "This satisfactory situation did not continue in 1964. . . . The hospital strains . . . reached a percentage of 14 per cent in July and August."[25] Here and elsewhere it is emphasized that the organism is picked up not in the operating room but in the ward itself, from curtains, bedding, air, lesions, or noses. It came to be thought

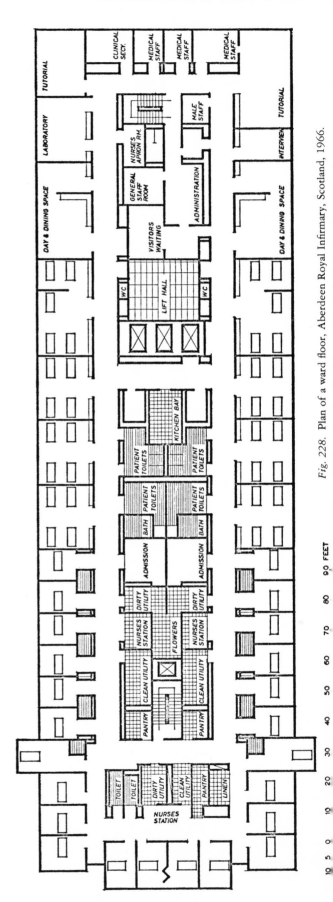

Fig. 228. Plan of a ward floor, Aberdeen Royal Infirmary, Scotland, 1966.

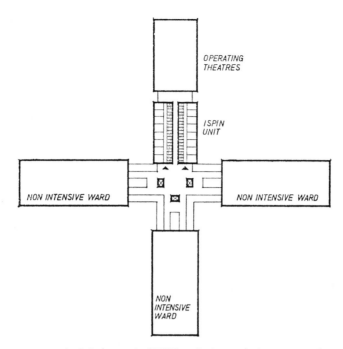

Fig. 229. Plan of Gainsborough ISPIN unit inserted into a cruciform plan.

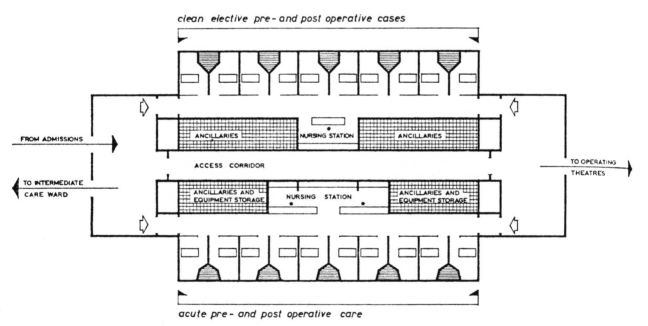

Fig. 230. Detail of ISPIN unit.

wise to operate soon after admission because a patient who had been around in the ward before operation long enough to pick up the organism in his nose might, after operation, infect his own incision. Highly infectious patients such as those with burns could infect a whole ward even from a private room by means of air currents across the room into the main corridor. Such a room had at least to be artificially ventilated under negative pressure.

But why stop there? If artificial ventilation is mandatory to control infection in certain areas, why limit it to those areas? The danger of cross infection throughout the ward is very real. And if to control it the whole ward is mechanically ventilated, why not also add refrigeration? John Gainsborough suggests that English mechanical ventilation is inferior to the American simply because, without refrigeration, the atmosphere feels warm however many changes of air are ensured.[26]

But, comes the retort, again and again and again, air-conditioning costs three to four times as much as heating the same area!

The contemporary British ward plan dearest to the Gainsboroughs' hearts is that of the Aberdeen Royal Infirmary (fig. 228),[27] which was designed according to suggestions of the Aberdeen University Department of Bacteriology specifically to combat cross infection in a surgical unit. No room has more than 4 beds, and 41 percent of the beds are in single rooms. Ten single rooms for intensive nursing care are wrapped around the nurses' station. All lack toilets, which are across the corridor. This stage I ward block opened in 1966. The Gainsboroughs hail these single intensive care rooms as a portent for the future, "as against the pattern of small, noisy and inhumanely packed open spaces for the most seriously ill patients."[28] In the floor plan, 6 single rooms with toilets for infectious patients follow on either side of the service core, and after that, "tailing off," multiple-bed rooms for intermediate care, an arrangement in which the Gainsboroughs see "all that is good in progressive patient care with absolute flexibility as regards male and female admissions." This is, they say, the only plan adequately designed to combat cross infection and the sole plan to have grouped single-bed rooms together at the center of gravity of the ward, with all nursing facilities at hand and full observability.

At the Aberdeen Royal Infirmary, rooms are mechanically ventilated. Air is fed into them directly and 75 percent of it is picked up in the corridor for cleaning and recirculation. The arrangement does not strike the Gainsboroughs as quite safe. They propose what they call an ISPIN unit (isolation, pre- and postoperative care including intensive nursing) with all single rooms to be inserted between the operating room and the wards intended for nonintensive nursing (figs. 229 and 230).

The Aberdeen plan is controversial in two respects: its unprecedented provision for privacy and its commitment to a room of not more than 4 beds (the partition in the 5-bed rooms transforms them into a grouping of 2 and 3). Symposia were held in which the issue of the 4-bed versus the 6-bed room was thoroughly, heatedly, but inconclusively aired.[29] A room with 6 beds saves nurses steps along the corridor, but they have farther to travel once inside it. With 4 beds each patient has his corner, but with 6 beds a patient can more easily opt out of a conversation. Admission of a single patient to a 6-bed room sometimes means moving 3 or 4 others to achieve a suitable grouping, therefore 4-bed rooms are more flexible. A quantity surveyor reported an instance where a 60-bed floor divided into 4-bed wards was found too long for the site. A racetrack layout was

therefore contemplated at 30 percent additional cost, but with the introduction of 6-bed wards instead of 4, the building fit the site, the racetrack could be abandoned—economy triumphed.[30] The response to this example was that if economy dictates reducing standards below a Falkirk level of accommodation, a 6-bed ward with sanitary facilities en suite would be better than a 4-bed that omitted the toilets. In the end, "the symposium did not reach a unanimous view on this matter."

The first stage of the rebuilding of St. Thomas's Hospital, London, as a T-shaped block (1956–66; fig. 231) did limit the wards to 4 beds but, with the exception of one infectious room with its own facilities, placed toilets—none too many—across the single corridor. The new Greenwich District Hospital (1968; fig. 232) is an enormous 4-story square with the interior core broken by three courts to permit light and air and to prevent people from becoming disoriented. The building type had been successfully used for other functions abroad—a factory in Dallas is cited as one of the sources, modern German office buildings as another. Five-, six-, or one-bed rooms run around the periphery of the Greenwich Hospital. The single beds opposite the nursing station have their own toilets, not so the large wards. It is interesting to note that one model for this hospital, the new Bellevue Hospital of New York City, has toilets in every one of the 6-bed wards around the periphery, yet there are relatively fewer single rooms. The irreducible minimum of plumbing in the United States is still an optional extra in Great Britain. Greenwich is remarkable for flexibility: the large wards may have 6 beds in them or 5 and a day space, as the sister determines; those in the middle of each side —that is, at the end of each nursing unit—may be assigned to either unit according to need; and a service subfloor beneath each main floor allows for considerable flexibility of engineering services and hence of the arrangement of rooms and departments.[31] It is also remarkable for having cost a very great deal and it will never be duplicated.

Much of the expense is due to air conditioning. Originally it was hoped that it would be enough to air-condition the center core and that wards along the external walls might be ventilated simply by opening the windows. But natural ventilation would be quite ineffective even in the perimeter rooms of a building of this type. Natural ventilation works in older, more heavily built constructions, in hospitals with higher ceilings and in Nightingale open wards with cross ventilation, but not in small wards with only one window wall. Keeping doors shut to assist the ventilation system meant that a patient–nurse call system with speakers had to be installed.[32]

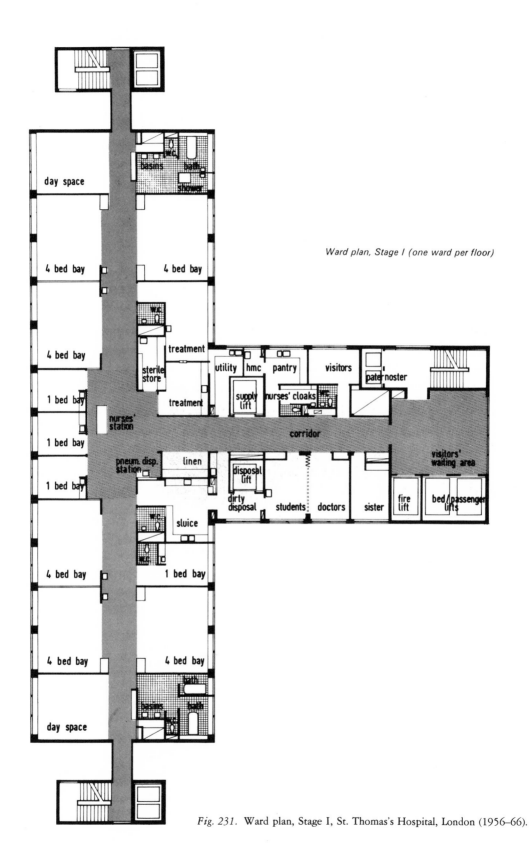

Ward plan, Stage I (one ward per floor)

Fig. 231. Ward plan, Stage I, St. Thomas's Hospital, London (1956–66).

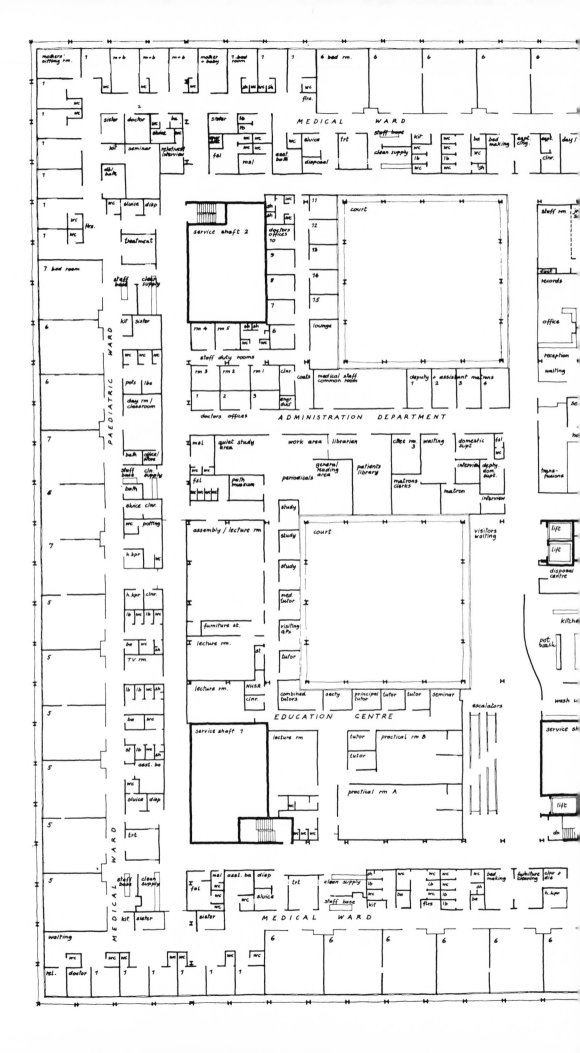

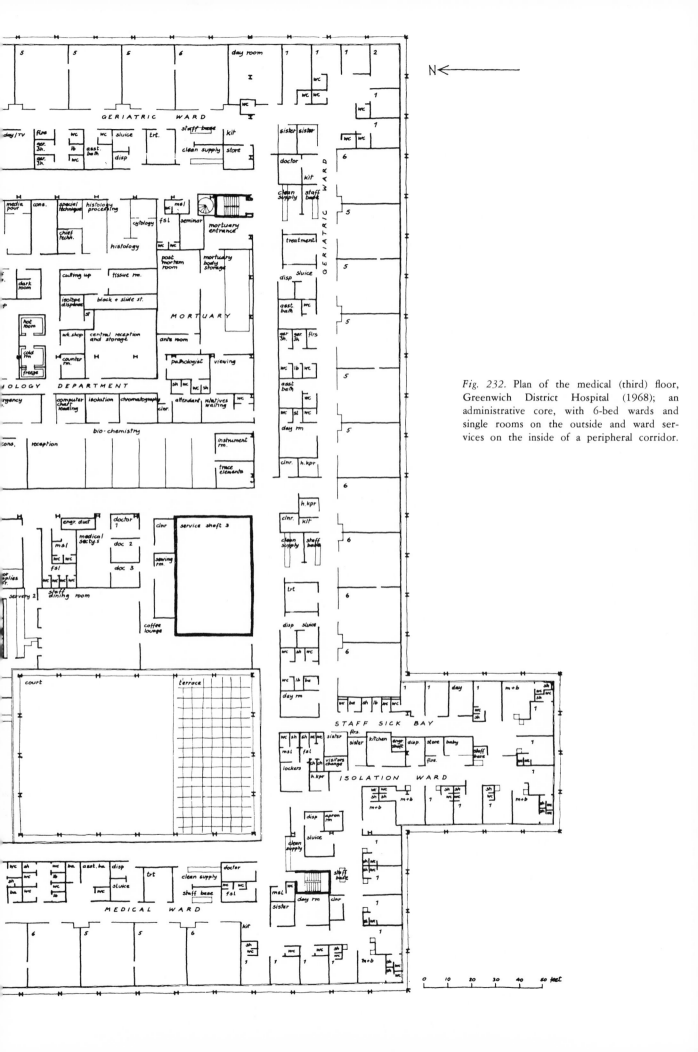

Fig. 232. Plan of the medical (third) floor, Greenwich District Hospital (1968); an administrative core, with 6-bed wards and single rooms on the outside and ward services on the inside of a peripheral corridor.

STANDARD WARD 4

STANDARD WARD 1

STANDARD WARD 3

STANDARD WARD 2

Ward plan, Stage II (four wards per floor)

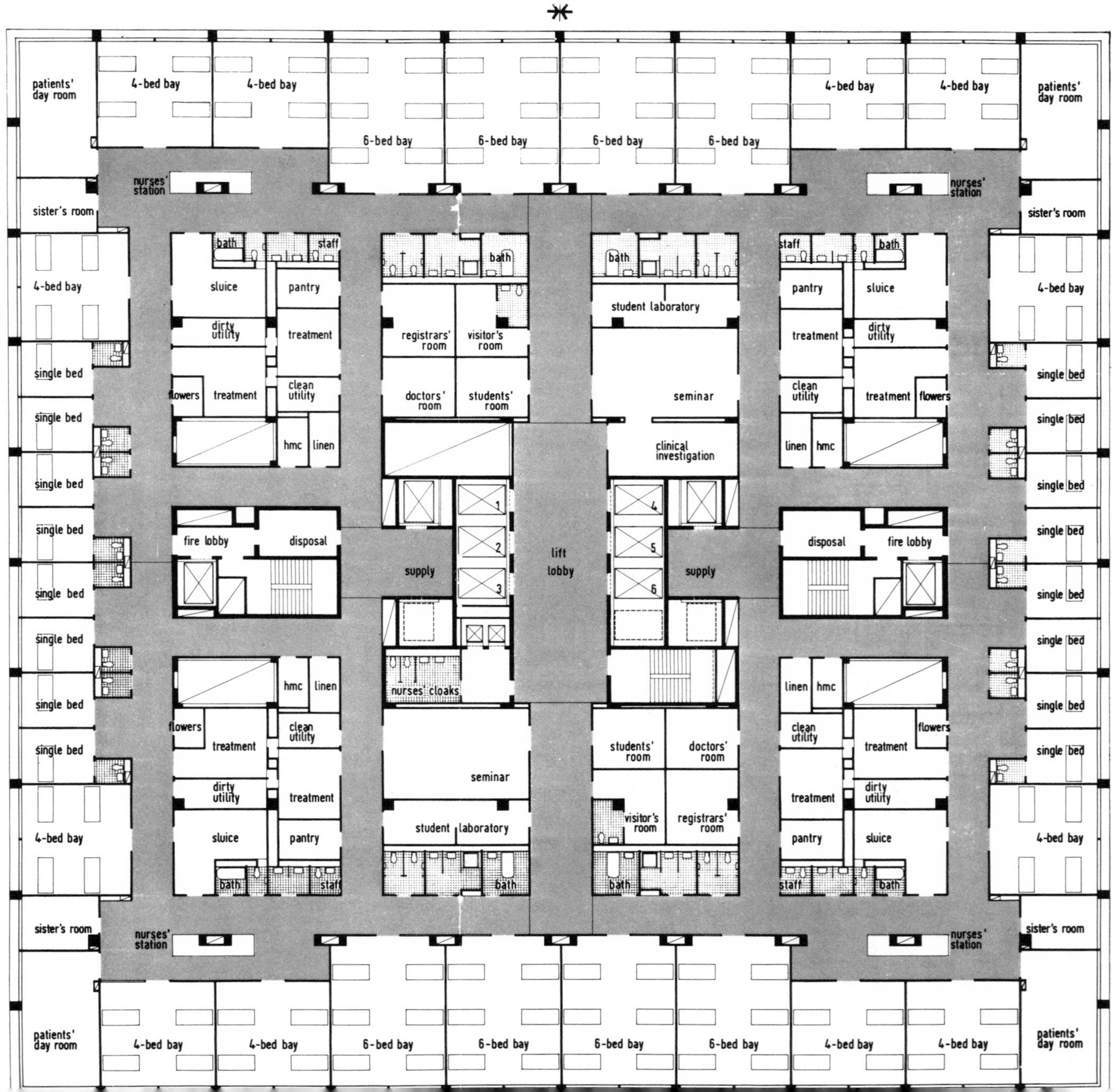

patients' day room

sister's room

4-bed bay

single bed

single bed

single bed

single bed

single bed

single bed

single bed

single bed

4-bed bay

sister's room

patients' day room

4-bed bay

nurses' station

bath

sluice

dirty utility

treatment

flowers

treatment

fire lobby

flowers

treatment

dirty utility

sluice

bath

nurses' station

4-bed bay

4-bed bay

staff

pantry

treatment

clean utility

linen

hmc

disposal

linen

hmc

clean utility

treatment

pantry

staff

4-bed bay

6-bed bay

student laboratory

seminar

clinical investigation

supply

doctors' room

students' room

registrars' room

visitor's room

bath

6-bed bay

6-bed bay

bath

bath

6-bed bay

6-bed bay

registrars' room

doctors' room

visitor's room

students' room

lift lobby

supply

nurses' cloaks

seminar

student laboratory

bath

6-bed bay

6-bed bay

staff

pantry

treatment

clean utility

linen

hmc

fire lobby

disposal

hmc

linen

clean utility

treatment

pantry

staff

6-bed bay

4-bed bay

bath

sluice

dirty utility

treatment

flowers

flowers

treatment

dirty utility

sluice

bath

4-bed bay

nurses' station

nurses' station

patients' day room

sister's room

4-bed bay

single bed

single bed

single bed

single bed

single bed

single bed

single bed

4-bed bay

sister's room

patients' day room

Fig. 233. Standard ward plan, St. Thomas's Hospital, Stage II (plans

The second stage of St. Thomas's Hospital (plans published 1966; fig. 233) will be a 14-story ward block with a 5-story treatment block[33] behind it and a communal block beside it. (Another huge ward block on the other side of the communal building is planned for Stage III. Its design has not yet been determined.) Stage II will have four 28-bed ward units on each floor, divided as at Greenwich, with the floating beds at the junctures assignable to either unit. Intensive nursing beds opposite the nurses' stations are in 4-bed rooms, and the only rooms with their own toilets are the singles for Class B patients a good way down the hall. Intermediate care is given in 6-bed bays without toilets, which are across the corridor. At Greenwich, ward services run clear around the building in a band one-room deep between the corridor that serves the patient rooms and the corridor serving the inner core, where all the other hospital activities are: laboratories, teaching, clinical departments, and even operating rooms. At St. Thomas's the core, unbroken by courtyards, is hatched by cross corridors and will require one of the largest air-conditioning plants in the country.[34]

Much experimentation is going on. The opposite of the compact, urban, air-conditioned block of St. Thomas's Stage II and of all highly mechanized towers

that must be planned to the last detail before building, is Slough Hospital west of London (1966; fig. 234), which rambles all over an enormous lot in one-story L-shaped wards with clerestory lighting. Slough reminds one of early twentieth-century pavilion hospitals in the distances to be traveled; like pavilions, attached or separate, it can be well ventilated by natural means. There is one tower, for the administration (whereas at Wycombe, the wards formed the tower, and the operating rooms and clinical departments wandered afar.) The lot at Slough is big enough to allow for horizontal expansion of each department, if that is what is really needed in such a plan.[35]

The two experimental buildings of Bury St. Edmunds and Frimley (1968–72) employ a single plan varied to suit two quite different sites in order to prove that hospitals whose components are standardized can be built more effectively, cheaply, and quickly. All possible freedom is to be allowed for future changes on the grounds that artificial barriers between departments and functions make for inflexibility and have to be avoided wherever possible. "The structure must get out of the way . . . so that services of all types can travel in any direction both horizontally and vertically without their passage being impeded

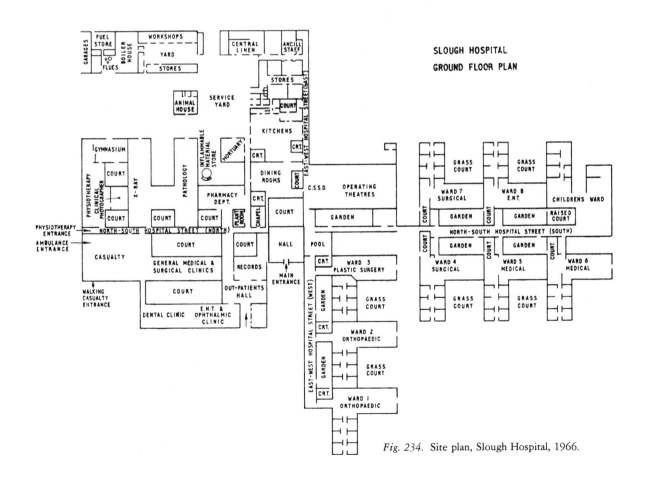

Fig. 234. Site plan, Slough Hospital, 1966.

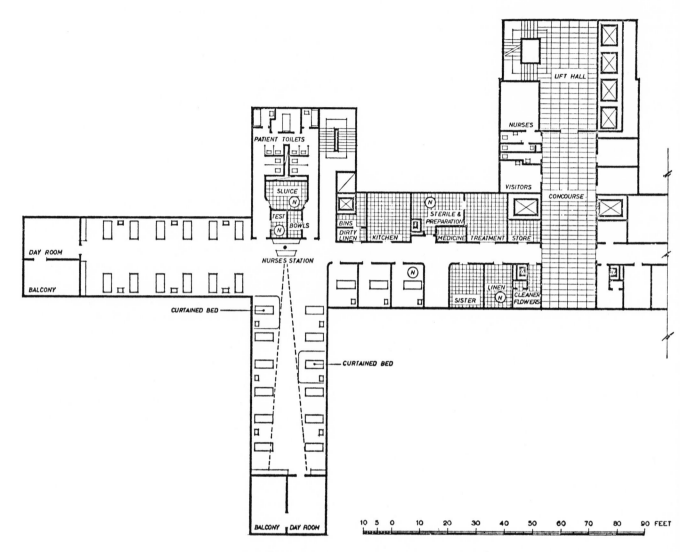

Fig. 235. Plan of the open ward of the new Guy's Hospital (1961).

by structural beams, slabs, or walls." The claim is made for this concept of hospital construction that, laid out along clear and simple lines of communication, it is a direct descendant of the Brunel prefabricated hospital of 1855.[36] Engineering is paramount. Between the ribs of a grid framework, the floors are only 5 cm. thick so that secondary services can be located afterward at any time; only primary services are drawn in on the plan. At Bury St. Edmunds and Frimley, deliveries are made horizontally by ramp from a supply center in the rear. Two-story rambling buildings and an extensive lot with plenty of trees make courtyards seem like patios and restore a domestic scale to hospitals. As for the distances involved, each patient or staff member is to proceed by car to his appropriate access point, the expectation being that "almost the only people likely to have to travel from one extremity to another are the drivers of the supply and disposal floats. Most of the patients and

staff will find that their own personal 'circulation zone' is relatively limited."[37]

In some ways, one of the most surprising postwar British hospital plans was that of the new wards of Guy's Hospital (opened 1961; fig. 235). They are a deliberate perpetuation of the principles of the old Nightingale ward and stand, as Miles Hardie puts it, in splendid isolation. Nothing like them has been built since or was built for many many years before. Each arm of the L contains half the usual ward patient population in 12 open beds with a generous space between them. The balcony is still at the far end together with a dayroom. But the toilets, lavatories, baths, and service rooms are behind the nurses' station, at the crook of the L and toward the corridor, the nurturing stem on which this L-shaped ward depends as the wards of the old St. Thomas's Hospital depended on their main corridor. (The communal building of the new St. Thomas's is intended to replace that main corridor, where everybody met everybody else several times a day, around which the social life of the hospital revolved, and which shattered the isolation of the separate departments.)

With the dedication of devotees to just principles and a lost cause, the nurses at Guy's run these wards immaculately. Although echoing noise is one of the first things one notices going from subdivided wards into open ones, they are kept admirably quiet. The staff swears by them: "The patients at Guy's liked the open wards, the nurses liked them, and the doctors liked them, and if Guy's had to build again in the foreseeable future, they would build in the same way."[38] The administrator called for an official evaluation.

These wards gave excellent observability at night, whereas the staff claimed that a double-corridor ward could not be scanned by one pair of eyes. However, critics pointed out that a nurse tending a patient in one wing of the L could not see what was going on in the other and furthermore that if only three beds were curtained off, a nurse at the nursing station could not see the other beds.[39] The nurses naturally grouped seriously ill patients at the nursing station, but this meant placing them at the center of the thickest traffic. Ambulatory patients were using the dayrooms at the end of the L, which meant a long, tiring walk to the bathroom and contending with not very pleasant traffic to and from the sluice (dirty utility) room on the way. Since these wards were ampler than the standard Nightingale, even the nurses noticed the extra walking. There were not enough toilets. The single rooms could not be supervised and were therefore not used for the seriously ill, for whom they had been intended. Moderately ill patients who were kept in them had no private toilets, their doors were left open for ventilation and supervision, and the kitchen across the corridor made a racket. The chief complaint from patients was that the wards were drafty.

One might think this would finish off the open ward, but no. Like its creator, Florence Nightingale, the open ward takes a long time dying. In 1969 there were still those to rally to its defense:

> It is, we think, difficult to see how a well-curtained properly spaced bed in a large ward is any less private than a bed in the enforced matyness of a four-bed ward—or still worse the cosiness of a two-bed ward with an irritating companion. Perhaps it is time we stopped making assumptions about what we think the patient likes and instead mounted some scientifically oriented consumer research. It might possibly be that we are making the patient pay for something that he doesn't really want![40]

A debate was mounted in the House of Lords on "Hospital patients and privacy rights." "I beg leave to ask Her Majesty's Government whether they will acknowledge the right to privacy in hospital, and in particular the ability to choose to be in a single room, as something to be established as soon as financially possible." Notice that the request is not made in terms of an all-private-room hospital. The Lords were quite aware of the financial state of the National Health Service, but they did put in a plea for a larger percentage of private rooms in the long run. A retired medical man reported that he could never locate a private room for his colleagues, because it was always taken up by some emergency case before nightfall. He refers here to the "amenity bed," and true to his class he is for absolute privacy:

> I can think of nothing worse than a ward that contains three people, except being in a ward which contains two people, because you have to be polite to somebody, and being polite as well as being ill is almost too much to contemplate.[41]

Dr. Hugh Gainsborough, a member of the same social class, favors hospitals of all single-bed rooms if architects can provide them with adequate observation. He dismisses the odd ducks, the traitors, who think differently:

> The arguments presented against such a concept are generally false. Those put forward by respected senior executives who have enjoyed their "slumming" in open wards, the human warmth and company of patients with whom they usually have so little contact, need not detain one. Most of us want absolute privacy with safety.

And he refers us to the paper written by Asa S. Bacon in 1920 presenting the first plan for an all single-room hospital. "This 41-year-old vision has not yet reached us."[42]

Privacy has always been a commodity one must pay for and in Britain too it is available for money. New nursing homes with all private rooms exist for those financially able to support the National Health Service through taxes and to pay so much a day for hospitalization on top of that. "The trouble is that you have to pay a devil of a lot!" as one of the Lords exclaimed. Private insurance is possible; "provident associations" are there to help. The nursing home has the great advantage that one need not drop everything to rush to the hospital for an operation on the day an opening finally turns up. One can schedule the time, which is very much better for businessmen and mothers with small children. One can arrange for nonurgent surgery that overworked surgeons of the National Health Service may never get around to performing.

Nursing homes greatly resemble an American all-private-room hospital: private toilet, telephone, radio, television, air-conditioning, and of necessity the full nurse-call system. Making a virtue of it, nurses in nursing homes praise the way the intercom "has reduced the fruitless coming and going to which they had been previously accustomed."[43]

The Gainsboroughs meditate on how much a paying patient is willing to sacrifice for absolute privacy:

> It is indeed strange that most people who can afford privacy and demand it are willing to be nursed in all serious illnesses in nursing homes or hospital private beds, even though in the former in this country there may be no resident doctor and in all cases there is the alleged danger in single rooms of poor observability. Why is there no outcry against these dangers by the doctors and nurses working in this private sector? One must ask, too, why the Americans continue to use such a large proportion of small private rooms if these are not safe. . . .[44]

We called on the sister in one of the new wards in the Stage I 11-story T-shaped block of St. Thomas's to ask how her nursing in the smaller wards compared with that she had done for many years in the old Nightingale wards of that hospital (at the time, half of them were still in operation). She first spoke of the quiet: "I didn't get used to the quietness here for about 18 months. I could hear the quietness for that long." Then she spoke bitterly of the heat:

> The ceilings are low. I could hardly walk in the heat some days this summer—five times a day I had to soak my feet in cold water. In winter when the heat is full on, there's a very heavy atmosphere. It took me a year to get adjusted—I found I was absolutely exhausted in the evening. When patients are in hospital for a long time, they get headaches. On hot days they fry. The windows are double glass and they open only nine inches —this drives us mad. They were locked at nine inches because of some suicides. We change offensive dressings at temperatures up to 90 degrees. In stage II they are going to install air conditioning. To go to the old wards on a hot afternoon is like going into the country, and winters are just as trying. Nurses go to sleep in report time from the sheer stuffiness.
>
> It is a half-mile journey to the terrace. One can take only those patients outdoors who are really well, because one must leave them there for the afternoon, in charge of the nurse in the nearest ward. I miss the old balconies. They did the patients a world of good. The old wards are very nice. You can sit in the middle and see every

single person in the ward but the two directly behind you, and those two you can hear. And there is the most amazing spirit among patients in the old ward—it is amazing and touching how they help each other.

This communal helping is interpreted away by advocates of increased privacy as follows: "Are the other patients the best people to help in their well-meaning but awkward encouragement? . . . Is it not really that doctors and nurses, perhaps for lack of time or from poverty of empathy or poor training . . . refrain from that five minutes talk at the bedside that could make all the difference?"[45]

The nurse observed that she never wore out a pair of shoes until she came to the new ward. (The subfloor is cement, not wood.) Then she added wistfully:

> If I was asked to go back to the old wards I wouldn't mind. Probably I'd miss this. If you write it down you can convince yourself you're better off here. Everything here is easier, there's more room, you can keep patients separate. . . . Patients have more privacy, really, among thirty than among four. Someone not so very ill can get lost better among thirty. Also, in the large ward it is easier not to get involved. In a four-bed room, in order not to get involved they must walk out to the day-room—if they are mobile.
>
> In the new wards you need a conscious effort to give the patients a sense of your being there. Neglect consists in their not seeing you much. There's a constant conscious effort to keep up the spirit of your being present—you go through the wards frequently to see the patients even though you don't do much for them. If they are well, they love your coming by. If they are not very well, they are only too glad to be looked in on. This sense of your presence used to be unconscious on your part, in the old ward—the patients could just see you and know you were there.

She shook her head. "You tend to think with progress your standards tend to go," she said. "It's a very worrying thing nowadays, training young nurses." We asked her whether the intercom was used very often. "It tends to give the patients a bit of a fright," she replied, "particularly the elderly. It's easier to nip down and give them a bedpan if they want one."[46] She told us that if the call button falls out, patients have a hand bell, and the elderly ones prefer the hand bell to the call system. "Or they can ring up the desk by phone. So they needn't feel they're stuck or isolated at all. When they go to the operating theatre they leave the phone unplugged, then the nurses take their calls. It means a lot more work for us, but then, that's what we're there for, isn't it really?"

PART 3

The Yale Studies in Hospital Function and Design

CHAPTER 10

Research Approaches to Contemporary
Hospital Problems

In Part 1 hospital problems were dealt with historically, whereas Part 2 dealt broadly with their contemporary aspects in the United States and Great Britain. Part 3 is devoted to an examination in depth of how one fairly new, above average, typical ward building—the Memorial Unit of the Yale–New Haven Hospital—works. To the extent possible, its wards were tested and measured. New approaches were devised to the problem of evaluating a hospital ward. This kind of hospital research is a modern discipline that we glimpsed at work in the United Kingdom (the Nuffield studies) and the United States (USPHS studies). It is a type of clinical research concerned with how well a hospital functions. The research method will now be examined more closely.

The ordinary yardstick of architectural measurement will not serve. It must be clear by now that a hospital is not just a building, an architectural project. It is a living organism because no matter how it is built, it is run by people for other people. Individuals use or abuse the building placed at their disposal; patients crowd it; staff workers seize upon facilities cunningly contrived to make their work easier and run them in precisely the opposite way from that intended. The poorest nursing care might conceivably be found in the most meticulously designed nursing wards. "Much as I hate to admit it," the hospital architect James S. Moore once said, "the architecture contributes very little to making a patient well or to patient care." We too admit this. We even believe one could give good medical care in a stable—but that does not mean stables should be built for hospitals.

Once a hospital opens it is never static; it crawls with life because it is used by people, and sick people at that—people with their guard down, helpless, indignant, worried, in pain or anguish, inpatients, outpatients, frantic relatives; people whose humanity is intensified by trouble. The staff has its own inter-relationships, rivalries, and hierarchies. In dealing with human beings instead of building materials or mathematical formulas, precision becomes impossible, prediction difficult. A hospital runs like the croquet game in *Alice in Wonderland*—the flamingos serving as mallets peer around at you, the hedgehog balls run away. Everything's alive. How, then, can one attempt hospital research?

In answering this question a definition of general research must first be established. There are two approaches to general research: basic and applied. Basic research seeks to establish the truth of a certain situation, not caring whether anybody is going to use it or not. Basic research is possible in medicine and the sciences, but in the hospital field the only research that can be called basic is the establishment of a study methodology or refined measurement. Results obtained through the application of the methodology or measurement become applied research when they enable an administrator to operate his hospital more effectively and economically.

The hospital planner Charles Neergaard wrote in 1952:

> Hospitals require a special kind of research for planning and construction. An official central clearing house of information, available to all engaged in hospital design, could give guidance from past experience as to what has and has not worked, what new materials, methods and equipment will do a job better. Know-how and know-how-not are equally important. If each new hospital could avoid the many mistakes from which the old ones have suffered and adopt the features which have functioned with the least maintenance and replacement, the savings would run into millions.[1]

In hospital research as in medical research, the first work was descriptive. One had to find out what actually was happening before any attempt could be made to diagnose, prescribe, and control, just as, in medicine, the disease had to be described before a cure could be sought.

An important early piece of hospital research was the United States Public Health Service *Study on Hospital Design*, published after World War II.[2] The Hill–Burton Act of 1946 had granted money for hospitals to the states, which were in turn to allocate funds to towns. It was then discovered that the architects did not know how to build hospitals. The USPHS therefore sent researchers to the "good hospitals" to measure them, and the researchers went on to do work with room mock-ups in a limited way. For the first time, an attempt was made to standardize hospital measurements. Hospitals had been built with 24-inch doors that would not take a hospital bed. No one ever asked what would be done to get the patient out of such wards in case of fire.

The power of money was employed to enforce these USPHS recommendations because Hill–Burton funds were released from Washington only for plans that conformed. Thus the USPHS plans were copied everywhere, and it was forgotten that they were suggested as minimal standards. Only the single corridor was illustrated—and a single corridor can be very inefficient. Only a certain proportion of single- to multiple-bedded rooms was thought correct: one-third private, one-third 2-bed, one-third 4-bed. This system would not apply in every situation; in the wealthy town of Greenwich, Connecticut, for example, the 4-bed rooms would stand empty.

United States Public Health Service standards are still used in several areas. This work may be called descriptive, but it is good—so good that it offers the hospital designer an easy way out. The danger is that since the volume was first published in 1952, much has changed in the medical field: there was then no cardiac catheterization, recovery room, progressive patient care, meals on wheels, and very little provision was made for outpatients, though today the outpatient department is the fastest growing. The plans were revised (most recently in 1962) to provide a 50 percent increase in laboratory and X-ray department space. Also, fortunately, the USPHS began to allow some freedom in interpreting its standards.

From 1942 to 1945 the Commission on Hospital Care, supported by a grant from the Commonwealth Fund, engaged in relatively bold basic research into the question of how many beds are needed for a certain area. Working from the bed-death to bed-birth ratio and assuming that everything in a hospital is random in its nature, they applied a Poisson distribution with three standard variants to allow for peak loads.[3] They concluded that

> both statistical theory and study of individual hospital data indicate that the extreme limit of occupied beds will not be greater or less than the average daily census plus or minus approximately four times the square root of the average daily census. That is to say, it is unlikely that the need for beds in the course of a year will exceed the average census by four times the square root of that average.[4]

Their recommendation was 4.5 beds per 1,000 population. Few areas could muster so many beds, and the commission, discovering eventually that fewer would suffice, lowered the recommendation to 3.5 beds per 1,000. They then defined the extreme limit of occupied beds as the average census of the hospital plus three times the square root of the census. This was a more sophisticated piece of research than its predecessors because the magic number supplied could actually keep pace with growth, for as population increases, the average census will increase. The formula works out pretty well in the maternity suite since that operates in a genuinely random way; it no longer applies elsewhere. This is another descriptive piece of work; what it essentially says is "Let's find out what's going on now, before we try to figure out what should go on."

Any magic number can act only as a crutch. In the research whose results we present in this section of our volume, we are not concerned with supplying hospitals with magic numbers or absolute units of measurement. Applied research into hospital problems is formidably difficult and often impossible. Much applied research rests upon comparison; whether one design, technique, or piece of equipment is better than another, worse, or just as good. The comparison presupposes knowledge of three things: accepted criteria, sensitive methods of measuring the criteria, and information about factors that significantly affect the measurements. In hospital research, regrettably, we often do not have knowledge about one or more of these items; therefore comparison as a method is usually out of our reach.

Thus we turned to methodology itself. The Yale Studies in Hospital Function and Design were mainly devoted to the three basic elements of research: developing criteria, developing methods of measurement, and analyzing factors that affect the measurements. Only in a few instances was it possible to direct any one of the three elements to research for actual application by hospital administrators. Instead, we offered a methodology whereby administrators can determine their own needs.

Hospital research is complex. In medical research we can divide patients into two categories, give one group a pill, the other a placebo, and note results. But how can we compare a centralized with a decentralized dietary service?

The dietary department, like many other services in a hospital, has been shaped by technical developments. When food was sent up from the kitchen in big cans to be dished out on the floors, the service was decentralized. Then hot plates were devised and a centralized system came in; plates were sent already dished up from the central kitchen. The plates did not keep food hot enough, and heated food carts were invented; reenter the decentralized system: food served from food carts in the floor kitchen. Food packs came in, and the service was centralized: packs were sent up from the kitchen. Now that microwave ovens have been introduced that reconstitute frozen food to precisely the right temperature in less than a minute, one plate at a time, decentralization again seems likely and one might even anticipate hotel service in the hospital: service on demand from the floor kitchens.

Comparative Model

At the Stamford (Connecticut) Hospital it was possible to draw a classic comparison between a centralized and a decentralized food system, for the hospital had decided to switch from centralized to decentralized and ran out of funds halfway through. Both systems were operating side by side. We were thus able to measure three things there: staff cost, desired temperature of the food, and patient satisfaction. Staff cost was established by a comparison of man-hours devoted to the two systems. For desired temperature, a thermometer was plunged into the food immediately before serving and patients were asked immediately afterward—not hours later—"Was the hamburger hot enough?" We ascertained patient satisfaction by questionnaires, though by and large we are very pessimistic about questionnaires. They can be biased one way or another so that even the experimenters do not know that it is a loaded questionnaire. In a double-blind test the medical experimenter really does not know the pill from the placebo. But on hospital matters a questionnaire can be a very sticky thing, whereas a general survey is impossible.

The questions were specific: are you satisfied? Are you dissatisfied? We did not qualify them because some patients simply cannot handle finer shades of meaning. "Fairly dissatisfied"—what will he make of that? We made certain before we began that subjects knew what _we_ meant by _satisfied_ and _dissatisfied_. The same person administered the questionnaire throughout to assure constant ratings. Patients, incidentally, are not annoyed by questionnaires; they are always dreadfully bored and they love anything that amuses them. The problem is not to get into the room, the problem is to get out.

In this study we were indeed able to compare two groups of patients and to record statistically significant differences, the only differences recorded here. A statistically significant difference is one with a low probability of having occurred by chance.

The voice intercommunication study (chapter 14) was based on a criterion of sorts. It was asked at the outset whether the addition of a two-way speaker between the patient and the nurses' station, over and above a simple call light above the door, really lessened the number of steps a nurse had to walk to tend a patient. The unit of measurement was clear: staff nurse trips. The experiment might have been conducted by closing off the speakers on one floor,

letting them operate on the other, and afterward comparing the two floors. But it was felt that not enough was known about how this audible feature was being used by the patient, what influence type of accommodation or the relative seriousness of the patient's condition might have upon it, and how the staff used the system. The present system could still be compared to the way it was when there was only a light, if all calls were analyzed and it was determined which would have required an extra trip had only the light been on. This approach was rewarded by the discovery that the voice intercommunication system is used more for communication between members of the staff than as a patient-to-staff call system, a finding that might have been missed had the study been designed as a straight comparison.

Conceptual Model

It is clear that in an organization as complicated and as poorly understood as the hospital, comparison is an inadequate technique for solving most problems. Ethically and practically, hospital researchers cannot often set up two groups, control and experimental, and compare effects of an experimental variable on the two. So they turn to another kind of comparison: that of actual practice with a theoretical model. This is called operations research, an attempt to set and solve problems by relating them to a theoretical model.

Historically, operations research derives from two fields, industrial management and applied statistics. Industry attempts to improve efficiency by setting up what it calls minimax models, in which production is maximized and costs are minimized. Such a model must be able to define the cost of everything, show whether the cost rises or falls, and what it would cost in terms of dollars if the industry did not possess this particular system or piece of equipment. But in a hospital you cannot consider the savings involved if the hospital could not make oxygen or an operating room available within a reasonable time. As for the contribution of applied statistics to operations research, it will shortly be clarified.

Three types of models have been found useful for hospital research: conceptual, mathematical, and computer models.

A conceptual model is a diagrammatic representation of some abstraction, usually an interrelationship. For example, it can give a picture of the departments within an organization and their relationships to one another or of an institution's work-flow pattern better than a thousand words. However, it cannot quantify or be used to project future patterns—for instance, it cannot state how values change in relationship to an increase in size. To show one example of a conceptual model and emphasize our contention that hospital research is a complicated affair, we append a diagram that attempts to express the relationships among hospital research, medical research, and research in the community (fig. 236).

At the core is medical and nursing research; the outer ring represents research in the community and community facilities, programs, and services; and hospital research has been placed between them. The three fields are anything but static, hermetically sealed, and separate. Medical research develops new drugs and techniques; an increase in medical knowledge cannot help influencing hospital procedures. Like an overtaxed balloon, medical research bulges out into hospital research, and nursing research does likewise. But the pressures work in both directions. Hospital research intrudes into medical research when it tries to determine the clinical effects of hospital care, and into nursing research when it investigates the clinical effects of nurse-staffing patterns. We have used arrows rather than bumps to indicate the influence of medical research on the community. This also is a two-way street: research into the medical aspects of community facilities, programs, and services has an impact on medical research itself.

A distinction must be carefully drawn between hospital research and research in hospitals. Research in hospitals may be defined as medical or nursing research carried out in the hospital (bumps 1 and 2) and using the hospital as its locale, whatever its contribution to medical or nursing care. However many active staff members may participate, it is not truly hospital research, because the primary concern of the investigators is with medical or nursing implications and applications. And, for our purpose, community-based research is similarly limited. Studies in economics, housing, and health needs and services directly or indirectly affect the operation of the hospital. They are vital to its existence and force us as hospital researchers to adjust, redirect, and reevaluate our aims and objectives, but these studies do not aim to solve our critical problems.

Mathematical Model

So much for the conceptual model. A mathematical model is an expression of interrelationship based on the rules of mathematics. It usually takes the shape of a mathematical formula, though it may be expressed in blocks of a certain size. When we chose as a unit of measurement for the Yale Traffic Index (chapter 15) the distance a nurse must travel to tend a patient, the choice of unit was arbitrary, but the derived formula based upon that unit can be applied to any hospital. And hospital efficiency can then be measured by this arbitrarily chosen unit. The frequency of interarea travel (x) can be combined with measured distances (y) to express functional efficiency in terms of a simple mathematical model.

This may not be the only way to measure the efficiency of a nursing floor. We might base a study upon how often the nurse touches the patient or upon any other relevant detail. Whichever unit we chose would be the parameter of this particular design problem. (Design, for a researcher, is the way his experiment is set up to minimize biases and other experimental errors. The design of an architect—building design—is quite a different thing.)

In attempting to measure patient satisfaction with the dietary service, we arbitrarily fixed upon the heat of the patients' food as a unit of measurement. This we could measure, as we could efficiency. We could even measure privacy, but we have never hit upon a formula to measure supervision and control.

In a study not included in this book, of how many recovery rooms are needed in relationship to the number of operating rooms, the technique of comparison was found to be inadequate: a two-to-one relationship would actually have been satisfactory only 27 percent of the days of the study period. The problem can be handled by the use of another mathematical model, this time a regression equation relating individual lapsed times of the one in terms of the other.

A mathematical model also proved useful for solving the problem of how many oxygen outlets are needed on a particular service (another study not reproduced in this book[5]). Here again an average was found of little value. To be meaningful, averages must be supplemented by a clear indication of the upper and lower limits of distribution. Even when they are accompanied by measurements of distribution, that distribution only rarely follows a normal curve; a description of the type of curve involved is imperative if reasonably accurate projection of the curve and prediction of future use are contemplated. The difficulty is compounded by a tendency to equate the average with a 50 percent figure, the median. For example, we studied the oxygen requirements of a certain surgical floor over a year's time and found an average daily census of 63 patients, of whom an average of 0.9 patients received oxygen. The danger is that these figures will be interpreted as meaning that one oxygen outlet on this floor could take care of about 50 percent of the anticipated need (since you cannot install nine-tenths of an outlet). In reality, one outlet would have satisfied the total oxygen requirements of that floor 77 percent of the days of the year. Further analysis also revealed significant differences in oxygen utilization among the medical, surgical, and obstetrical services. In this study, for the first time, the probability of a patient's requiring a service was used as a measurement of need. Such an

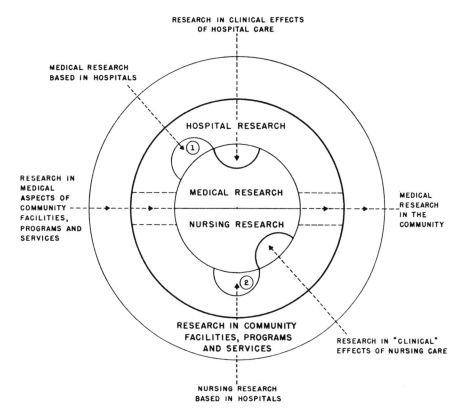

Fig. 236. Diagram expressing the relationships among hospital research, medical research, and research in the community.

expression of prediction would seem to be more valuable to administrators and designers than a flat recommendation because it offers a series of alternatives against which other considerations, such as the cost of installation, may be balanced.

We must emphasize here that neither the recovery room nor the oxygen outlet study provided criteria. In neither did we answer the questions: How long *should* a patient with a certain diagnosis stay in the recovery room? How many patients *should* have received oxygen during the year? Answers to both questions are beyond the competence of the study team. A basic assumption had to be made that the quality of care in the study hospital was high enough and the services provided numerous enough for there to be little difference between patients who should have been given a service and patients who actually received it.

Like a conceptual model, a mathematical model is descriptive; unlike a conceptual model, it is also predictive—by changing the value of x or y you can project what will happen under different circumstances. A valuable mathematical model for solving hospital problems is the queuing theory, known sometimes as the Poisson distribution theory. The aim of the minimax model of industry, it will be recalled, was to minimize costs and maximize production; in the hospital the problem is more likely to be to minimize hours of waiting and maximize services. A classic instance of this in industry is the tool crib, which costs a certain amount in dollars to be manned but which also costs a certain amount in dollars for the

time of the workers standing in line waiting for service at the crib. How many workers should be assigned to the tool crib? Every one standing idle costs the plant money. But every worker with a broken tool who cannot get it fixed immediately also costs money. How many broken tools are there likely to be?

In the hospital, a tool-crib situation is likely to prevail in the emergency room and the delivery room. Broken bones are like broken tools—no telling when they will occur. And one accident in no way affects another; one casualty in the emergency room does not deter in any way the next casualty from coming to the emergency room. Similarly, babies are born with no reference to one another, and, contrary to popular belief, not all are born at two in the morning; there is about an equal probability of their being born at one hour as at another.[6] Accidents and births are random occurrences, and for the prediction of random occurrences the appropriate mathematical model is a Poisson distribution. Indeed, the Poisson model only works when independent events occur at random. Although regulation of emergency or maternity admissions to the hospital is impossible, a Poisson distribution tells us that there are still practical limits to the probable number of patients who will require these facilities at any one time.

Such limits, and the probability of any given number of patients being in the maternity suite at any one time, can be determined with reasonable accuracy through the application of queuing theory. Queuing theory is an extension of the Poisson occurrence model in that it also accounts for the length of time a patient remains in a facility. Queuing theory holds that the number of people in a facility at any one time will follow a certain pattern forming itself around the average number of people in the facility during a given period.

Mathematical prediction by the law of probability may be seen in a very simple form in the fall of a pair of dice. There are 6 sides to each of the 2 dice; therefore there are 36 possible ways for the dice to fall. It is not equally possible to throw each number from 2 to 12. Only one combination of 2 dice produces a 2, only one a 12; but there are 6 possible ways to throw the number 7. If a table of probabilities were drawn up it could be used to predict the behavior of the dice, provided the dice were true.

The basic supposition in mathematical prediction is that the dice are true. Consequently there is an equal chance that any side of either one will end up on top. Random prediction methods are based upon this behavior of dice. If the 2s, 12s, 7s, and all the other numbers produced by the fall of the dice were laid out on a curve according to the frequency of their occurrence, the curve would be bell shaped, the classic curve of averages.

A Poisson distribution differs from this normal curve in certain ways, one of which is a tendency in a distribution with a small mean toward a long tail on the right side of the curve, which indicates a long series of probable recurrences before the vanishing point though the probability grows slimmer and slimmer. E. C. Molina has evolved tables that give the details concerning Poisson distribution once the average number of people in a facility is known.[7] The tail is of only moderate interest to the manufacturer, who is balancing the cost of hours to man his tool crib against the probability of broken tools. He would merely calculate how much time his machinists might spend in the queue before it would pay to add another shopkeeper. But the hospital cannot afford to have a queue of expectant mothers, even though, to prevent a queue from forming in busy periods, the delivery suite may have to be so large that in other periods it is empty a considerable fraction of the time.

We had to run three sets of experiments for the delivery suite because it really consists of three different subfacilities, each with a different average census: the labor room, the delivery room, and the postpartum recovery area. We compared the actual population of all three sections of the delivery suite over a thirty-day period using a Poisson distribution derived from the average number of deliveries by the application of Molina's table. We found sufficient agreement between the two sets of values to be able to say that the distribution of the number of patients in the delivery suite at any one time can be predicted by using a Poisson distribution based on the average number of patients in the unit. The special usefulness of the Poisson distribution is that not only does it describe, it also can be used to predict.

The maternity service is a lovely thing to study because it is so simple and limited. Only a relatively small number of patients can be classified as a "complicated case." If a case is complicated, it is usually transferred to another division. The Poisson distribution is an excellent mathematical model to use in studying the delivery room complex because input is literally random and independent. That is, it may serve as a superior model when all births are natural. Enter the variable. In this context the intruder is not a random happening but the element of planning. What to do about Caesarean sections? What should be done about hospitals that follow a policy of induced labor in a significant number of cases? In both instances, arrival times are set in advance and the beautiful random pattern is smashed. If relatively few Caesarean births occur in the course of a year, you might say of the dice that they are almost but not quite true. But where the combined scheduled Caesarean sections and scheduled inductions account for a large percentage of the total patients of a maternity service, the randomness of arrivals is destroyed and the validity of the model nullified. Another complication of the real world was the radical changes in the length of time women stayed in the hospital after they had their baby. Queuing theory became risky.

Computer Simulation Model

The dilemma leaves us with no alternative but to turn to a third kind of model, the computer simulation model. Before any reliable projection of existing data can be contemplated, we have to find a pattern that will include both the random and the planned in their actual proportions. An institution's life is often complicated. As J. P. Young says,

> Upon close examination it is easily seen that a high percentage of operations research problems involve uncertainty, or a stochastic process of one sort or another. If one turns to mathematical theory, he will in many instances find that there is no theory with which to cope with the problem or at best the mathematical manipulations are too formidable for human undertaking. Even the simplest stochastic problems are limited by the few existing probability functions which can be conveniently manipulated; and far too few real world problems can be classed as simple. Many times, actual operations are based on a network of interlacing and uncertain input—

output processes. Under these conditions, operations research has no choice but to turn to simulation, monte carlo, or gaming techniques, whatever one should choose to call them.[8]

What is needed is a model that can be used for predicting the activity of a mixed system—part random and part scheduled. Even if a mathematical model could be developed to describe this mixed system, the cost of computing the mathematical solution might well be more than the cost of obtaining a solution by simulation. The Yale Traffic Index can be calculated by hand—slowly, true, but it can be done. The computer provides a far faster solution. Our maternity suite calculations (chapter 16) can in all practicality only be done on the computer by simulation. And a simulation model would probably be of even more value to predict the loads of patient facilities where the lack of randomness in patient arrivals is even more marked.

For an explanation of simulation, let us return to the dice. The pair we are handling now is definitely untrue: there is a rounded corner on one, a nick on the other, which influence their fall in a certain manner every time. No general law applies any longer, but probabilities could eventually be worked out to describe and predict the behavior of this particular pair of dice. It will require a very long period of simply throwing the dice and noting results, but probabilities can be derived from the results. The game played out to determine laws of probability for each separate set of dice is simulation, or monte carlo, and to save infinite time and trouble we do such problems on a computer.

For instance, our concern is with the intervals between births in a certain hospital. From them we are going to determine the use of the delivery suite. The only way to get accurate records is first to follow and record, ourselves, the pattern of births over a period of time. In this way we collect a reliable representative sample. If a computer were not to be used, the experience of years would have to be collected and an attempt made to derive from it some laws that presumably would hold true for the service in the future, as long as all conditions remain the same. Using the computer, we must still collect an ample number of reliable observations and from them determine the behavior of the system and the variables influencing the activity we are trying to simulate. This information is fed to the computer. Simultaneously the computer is given a series of instructions about how the activity operates.

The computer is put to work and plays out a huge sample. It can play out an endless number of combinations each of which will be a valid, though not actual, instance of how the service is operating, and as long as all conditions remain the same, each of these hypothetical situations will be valid. It might take a year to collect 5,000 births in a hospital. If 500 are collected with care and fed to the computer, along with the general rules by which the maternity service operates, 5,000 births can be played out in about 5 minutes and observations about the pattern they fall into will hold as true as they would for 5,000 actual births.

Nor is this all. The service can then be altered in certain ways; one or more of the ingredients may be changed and the effect observed during a further run of the computer, which will play out a hospital now operating under a new set of conditions. Patient populations can be made to grow or decrease, proportion of the sexes may be changed, patients suffering from certain ailments may be added or taken away, staff may be altered, any number of other experiments may be tried, and valid results will be obtained. This permits not only prediction but prediction under changed circumstances as well. It saves the trouble of manipulating an actual service—assuming that were possible, as of course it is not. As a rule, the hospital researcher cannot influence the service he is studying at all, let alone in a certain direction. He cannot suggest that a doctor do something or other to his patients so that the hospital researcher will find out something he wants to know. So he sets up a simulated service and manipulates that.

For the maternity study we assumed an infinite number of available rooms; there were thus no waiting times. We found that in the study hospital, 15 rooms would have been required to make sure that no one was kept waiting throughout the year, but the fourteenth and fifteenth labor rooms together would have been occupied only 0.1 percent of the time. We put this information into the hands of the administrator and told him if he wanted to satisfy all loads all the time he would have to provide 15 labor rooms. Every once in a while, maternity cases really stack up. In real life when this happens, however, somebody makes the decision, "Let's move these patients a little faster." There is always some way to handle it on the one or two occasions during the year when all 15 labor rooms are in use. It would seem wiser to reduce the number of labor rooms but build expansion space to be used at need, one labor room that could be turned into a delivery room.

Thus we say to the administrator not "You need six delivery rooms," but "If you supply six delivery rooms, the probability that you will be in trouble is 0.006." The decision is his. He has to live with those delivery rooms, we don't. The simulation also gave us an estimate of the error one could expect if one simply applied Molina's tables to the problem. It was not so large as to make the simplest methodology applicable, provided scheduled inductions were held to a fairly low proportion of total births.

An administrator who has obtained the average number of patients arriving at the delivery suite over a reasonable period of time can, by using Molina's tables, prepare tables of probability for his own institution. The tables would contain enough information for him to judge the adequacy of existing delivery suite facilities. They also offer him a series of alternatives against which he can weigh the adequacy of his staff.

We have no doubt that similar predictions could be worked out for the pediatric floor. We would like to determine the relationship of surgical beds to operating rooms, but there we run into trouble. On the maternity floor everybody comes with the same diagnosis; you need not attempt to judge whether heart surgery is more important than, say, an operation for hemorrhoids. Too many things can happen to operating room patients. Simulation of this service awaits the result of our new research on the effect of the diagnostic mix on the utilization of ancillary services. But for the first time we are able to predict requirements for certain services and spell them out in terms of money. For the first time, we can actually go to a community and say, "Gentlemen, this is what it will cost you!"

CHAPTER 11

A Centralized versus a Decentralized Food Service

wo kinds of food service are usually found in a hospital: centralized and decentralized. If a hospital is ked which is better, it will probably come out in vor of the one it has. Proponents of a centralized od service claim it to be more economical for the ollowing reasons: in a central, well-supervised kitchen e size of portions can be controlled so there will e less waste of food, a single tray-loading service ves money since it takes fewer in help to operate, ace can be reclaimed for much-needed beds if the ursing unit need not allow for a floor pantry. Those ho prefer the decentralized system also have advan- ges to cite, the three mentioned most often being at the patient receives hotter food from a kitchen n his own floor (when the food is delivered by the ietary department), he receives more personalized rvice from a pantry on his own floor, and a decen- alized system is more flexible—there will be quicker sponse to changes ordered in the patient's diet when e pantry is on the same floor.

Such claims are not new. They have been made and ontradicted time and again, as first one side prevailed d then the other. Back in May of 1914, when the ospital was a complex of many low, sprawling pa- lions, *The Modern Hospital* ran an article on this bject in which it was stated:

> By sending the food to the ward in which it is to be served, and having it again well heated if necessary before serving, much better service can be effected. A central serving room in which all trays are served is certainly a great conven- ience, but it is nearly impossible to send trays to distant parts of the house and keep the food hot in transit.[1]

In 1929, when skyscraper hospitals were the newest ing, Dr. S. S. Goldwater had this to say about the roblem: "The number of hospitals that are setting p food trays, especially the trays of private patients, central kitchens, is considerably greater than in 913."[2] Then the electrically heated bulk food truck as invented, and in the March 1948 issue of this agazine we read:

> With an institution whose physical plant is spread over a wide area . . . decentralization becomes mandatory. . . . From the standpoint of economy,

decentralization in the vertical plant is prefer- able. . . . It is possible to reduce the number of employees. . . . The food will reach the patient in much better condition than if it were brought varying distances from a central serving area.[3]

Some new electric trucks are a combination refrigera- tor and warmer: they simultaneously keep hot foods hot on one side and cold foods cold on the other. One such unit, for example, has slots on the left side for 21 individual trays loaded with the cold items for each patient, compartments on the right side for individual hot plates and soup bowls, and space on top for hot water for coffee or tea. The truck is wheeled to the patient's door; then and not before, the hot items are added to the cold ones on the tray. This development, and the widespread acceptance of the idea that the dietary department should be made re- sponsible for serving the tray to the patient as well as preparing the food for that tray, have caused recent opinion to favor a centralized tray service. But who knows what will be invented tomorrow? In the run- ning battle valiantly carried on for longer than the Thirty Years' War, there is little possibility that either side will permanently prove the other side wrong.

At the Stamford Hospital in Connecticut in 1958, as already noted, both services were found operating side by side. When the situation came to our atten- tion, the centralized system was already a year and a half old, so the shakedown period was over; nor had the decentralized system been neglected in the mean- time. Stamford had an excellent dietitian, who de- livered good food under both systems. It is a small hospital, patients expect good service, they pay for it, and they get it. In both systems the maximum orga- nized effort was being put forth.

It was of importance to the study that we were able to find two units on the centralized system and two on the decentralized system nearly identical in physical layout, clinical service allocation, and distance from the main kitchen. Supervision would be the same, of course, since both systems were run by the same dietary department. The food was the same and was cooked in the same kitchen. Only in handling it did differences arise, at the point where it was either ladled into a bulk food truck or served in individual dishes that were then loaded into a hot-and-cold-food truck.

Limiting ourselves to the factors we could measure —patient satisfaction, temperature of food, and staff costs—we determined to test these three hypotheses:

1. There is no difference in patient satisfaction between inpatient units utilizing centralized or decentralized tray service.

2. There is no difference in temperature of food when delivered to the patient between inpatient units utilizing centralized or decentralized tray service.

3. There is no difference between inpatient units utilizing centralized or decentralized tray service in the amount of labor required for each.

One hundred and forty patients were interviewed after each of three meals: 69 from the two centralized, 71 from the two decentralized medical–surgical floors. In the centralized system, 38 patients were on regular diets, 31 on modified diets; in the decentralized system, 36 were on regular diets, 35 on modified diets. There was no significant difference in overall satisfaction with the food between the two types of tray service, but there was a significant difference in the ratings of patients on modified diets. Those on the centralized system rated their meals higher (3.4) than those on the decentralized (3.0). Special diet people are always dissatisfied; they often do not get any salt or are not allowed many foods they are accustomed to. But why this special dissatisfaction with the decentralized service? It seems that on the centralized service, regular and special trays were prepared in approximately the same way, one as tastefully, colorfully, and with as much individual attention as the other. But on the decentralized system, food for special diets was placed in individual casseroles and spooned on the plates by maids in the floor kitchens —it was not very appetizing by the time it reached the patients. So the first hypothesis stands after we allow for a significant difference between the two services in the satisfaction of patients on modified diets.

As for the second hypothesis, no significant difference was found between the two services in regard to patients' satisfaction with the temperature of food. Indeed, what was met with was apathy. Surprisingly few patients complained to the interviewers about the temperatures of any foods. It had been hoped through the question about food temperatures to establish a preferred temperature once and for all, but it soon became evident that patient opinion was going to offer too rough an estimate—if it offered any.

There is a dearth of basic temperature criteria in hospital literature; no two references agree. It is disconcerting to find hospital food service personnel talking about "serving hot foods hot" without being able to say what "hot" means in degrees Fahrenheit. In 1928 Rhoda A. Tyler recommended it be at a temperature of at least 160' F. and preferably at 170' F.[4] But in 1933 Zoe D. Wertmann suggested 130°–140° for meats and 140°–150° for vegetables (including potatoes) and soup.[5] In 1954 in a study limited to vegetables Margaret L. Thomas concluded that 140° would be acceptable to patients.[6] The last two authors made the point that patients "acclimated" to institutional food will not desire it as hot as people do who eat at home.[7]

The only established criteria for temperatures that satisfied us were those for coffee and tea. The average was judged to be 170° for coffee. Since it cools off at an approximate rate of 3.1° per minute, 170° would permit some time for temperature lost. At Stamford Hospital the average temperature of coffee on the centralized service was 169.6°, on the decentralized 175°; the difference is not statistically significant. There was more of a range in temperatures on the decentralized system—from 150° to 196°, or 46°. On the centralized system the range was only 31°, from 154° to 185°.

As for tea, the dividing line between good- and bad-tasting tea is a tea-brewing temperature of 180°, according to West and Wood (1955).[8] In the 80 tea-water temperature readings taken at Stamford Hospital, the temperature fell below 180° only three times. All three times happened to be on the decentralized service, but this is so infrequent that any kind of statistical comparison is impossible. Again, the range was greater on the decentralized system [42° (163°–205°)], compared with the centralized system [22° (183°–205°)].

In measuring temperatures of other foods, we made comparisons only when we had at least four temperatures for each service on the same item taken during the same meal (table 1). In one evening meal the soup on decentralized trays was significantly hotter than on centralized trays, but on another evening there was a significant difference in the temperature of the salmon steak and this time the patients on the centralized service received the hotter food. The second hypothesis stands: there is no difference between one type of tray service and the other in temperature of food presented to the patient. There is only a wider variation, at both ends of the scale, in the temperature of food served on decentralized trays.

Measuring staff costs was more difficult. The first step was to ascertain total direct hours and total direct wages for all dietary department activity and to express them in terms of minutes per meal and cost per meal (table 2). The real problem was to assign total direct-labor hours and costs to one tray service or the other. Staff had not been allocated with an eye to making that task easier. Some were assigned exclusively to the centralized service—those who loaded food trucks, for example. Some were exclu-

TABLE 1. Comparisons in the temperature of certain patient foods between centralized and decentralized food service at Stamford Hospital.

Meal	Item	Average Temperature (°F)		Significant Difference*
		Centralized	Decentralized	
Noon	Clear soup	150.5	136.5	no
Evening	Clear soup	139.1	149.2	yes
Breakfast	Boiled eggs	135.8	134.8	no
Breakfast	Scrambled eggs	127.6	132.0	no
Breakfast	Hot cereal	137.6	128.0	no
Evening	Boiled potato	139.6	141.8	no
Evening	Mashed potato	139.0	141.9	no
Evening	Salmon steak	144.6	126.0	yes
Noon	Braised steak	138.5	132.3	no
Evening	Roast beef and gravy	133.3	123.5	no
Evening	Stuffed pork chop	132.6	134.0	no

* P less than 5%.

TABLE 2. Direct labor cost per meal.

	Period One	Period Two
Total direct labor hours	2,583.50	2,581.00
Total direct labor wages	$3,361.71	$3,362.50
Total patient meals	5,259	5,598
Total employee meals*	1,718	1,715
Total Meals	6,977	7,313
Minutes per meal	22.22	21.18
Minutes of supervising time	5.11	4.76
Minutes of operational time	17.11	16.42
Direct labor costs per meal	$0.4818	$0.4598
Direct cost for supervision	$0.1423	$0.1332
Direct operational costs	$0.3395	$0.3266

* Expressed in meal equivalents.

TABLE 3. Total dietary employees by tray service activity for two weekly periods.

	Period One	Period Two
Centralized tray service only	16	16
Decentralized tray service only	21	21
Centralized and decentralized tray service only	3	3
Centralized tray service and other activities	6	7
Centralized and decentralized tray service and other activities	13	13
Other activities not directly involved with tray service	10	10
	69	70

Hours and Wages by Tray Service Activity

	Period One	Period Two	Period One	Period Two
Centralized tray service only	591.50	599.00	$731.30	$738.98
Decentralized tray service only	629.50	636.25	708.56	711.85
Centralized and Decentralized tray service only	79.25	77.50	85.25	83.20
Centralized tray service and other	297.50	314.00	330.34	352.65
Centralized, Decentralized, and other	606.00	586.50	929.11	907.50
Activity not directly involved with tray service	379.50	367.75	583.15	568.32
Totals	2,583.50	2,581.00	$3,367.71	$3,362.50

TABLE 4. Breakdown of direct dietary hours by activity (period two only).

	Total	Centralized Tray Service	Decentralized Tray Service	Other
Centralized tray service only	599.00	599.00		
Decentralized tray service only	636.25		636.25	
Centralized and decentralized tray service only	77.50	68.13	9.37	
Centralized tray service and other	314.00	98.19		215.81
Centralized, decentralized, and other	586.50	156.86	71.60	358.04
Other	367.75			367.75
Totals	2,581.00	922.18	717.22	941.60
Meals served		3552	2046	
Minutes per meal, direct tray service		15.58	21.03	
Percentage of decrease		25.9		

TABLE 5. Breakdown of dietary hours and wages by activity (for two weekly periods).

	Centralized Tray Service		Decentralized Tray Service		Other	
	Period 1	Period 2	Period 1	Period 2	Period 1	Period 2
Total hours	914.94	922.18	716.22	717.22	951.49	941.60
Meals served	3,339	3,552	1,920	2,046		
Minutes per meal, direct tray service	16.44	15.58	22.39	21.03		
Percentage of decrease	26.6	25.9				
Total wages	$1,151.43	1,162.37	827.54	824.32	1,388.74	1,375.61
Meals served	3,339	3,552	1,920	2,046		
Dollars per meal, direct tray service	$ .3448	.3272	.4310	.4030		
Percentage of decrease	20.0	18.8				

sively decentralized—the serving maids on the floors. The chefs worked for both services and the cafeteria besides. In doing time studies for them, measurements had to be made as to what part of their time went to each service. In table 3 it will be seen how those hours and costs were assigned. Table 4 shows how the direct-labor hours were allocated, both of staff employed in one area and of staff employed in several. Note the larger amount of mixed time in the centralized service. It takes much longer for cooks to serve individual portions on a patient's tray than for them to load many portions onto a bulk food truck. The cost of this extra activity on the part of kitchen staff is often overlooked when the two systems are compared. True, under a decentralized system, food still has to be served on the patient's tray in the floor pantry, but a pantry maid receives a lower salary than a cook. Likewise, a decentralized pantry maid is paid

less than a decentralized tray carrier. Such salary facts account for relatively low savings on the centralized system: although (table 5) it required 26.6 percent fewer direct man-hours during one study period and 25.9 percent fewer during another, the resulting savings per meal for each period were only 20 percent and 18.8 percent, respectively. Nevertheless, costs of patient tray service and number of man-hours of work were both lower for the centralized system.

These results proved the third hypothesis false. There *is* a difference between centralized and decentralized tray service in the amount of labor required for each. If the decentralized half of the study hospital were converted to a centralized tray service, the hospital could expect a 20 percent decrease in man-hours per tray served. Neither temperature of food nor patient satisfaction would suffer. Patients on modified diets would probably be more satisfied.

CHAPTER 12

A Brief History and Description
of the Yale–New Haven Hospital

Whereas the comparison between a centralized and a decentralized food service in chapter 11 was carried out in the Stamford Hospital because of the special situation existing there, the Yale Studies in Hospital Function and Design primarily had as their setting the Memorial Unit of the Grace–New Haven Hospital, now called the Yale–New Haven. A brief history and description of this hospital is thus appropriate here.

The original New Haven Hospital was incorporated by the General Hospital Society of Connecticut in 1826 as the fourth voluntary general hospital in the United States, preceded only by Pennsylvania Hospital of Philadelphia (chartered 1751), New York Hospital (1771), and Massachusetts General Hospital of Boston (1811). When the project faltered for lack of funds, four professors of the Yale medical faculty each pledged a hundred dollars annually for five years (from their salary of a thousand dollars a year) to keep it going. In 1832 the architect Ithiel Town was instructed by the society to construct a three-story hospital "after the manner of the Episcopal chapel of this city."[1] Town proposed the new State House as a model instead, and in 1833 a two-story edifice with basement and columned portico (fig. 237) was built on a hill across the marshes from town to lessen the danger of contagion. There the Yale–New Haven Hospital still stands, across the connector to the Connecticut Turnpike from downtown New Haven.

According to the specifications for the hospital building, exterior walls were to be plastered and finished like Mr. Hillhouse's new house, cellar windows were to be grated like those in Mr. Ralph I. Ingersoll's new house, side lights of the rear doors were to be like Mrs. Whitney's, and—a concession to economy—the glass throughout the building was to be "the best of second quality of New England crown glass."[2] All wards had large windows and were heated by open fireplaces, which led to seesawing of the opposing claims of heat and ventilation. Wood fireplaces ventilated but did not adequately heat in the New England winters. They were thus bricked in and cylinder stoves substituted, which warmed the wards beautifully but suffocated the patients. A hot-air furnace was installed and the fireplaces were reopened, whereupon most of the hot air was found to be escaping up the chimney. The fireplaces were bricked in again, but fuel consumption remained exorbitant. Gold steam heaters were introduced with much the same results as with the cylinder stoves. And so on for the life of this building. It was razed in 1930.[3]

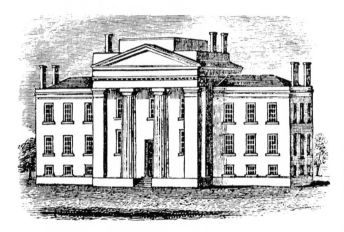

Fig. 237. The original New Haven Hospital building (1833).

During the Civil War, the building was leased to the government to become Knight United States Army General Hospital, in which 25,340 soldiers were treated with but 185 deaths.[4] A contemporary print (fig. 238) shows the central block flanked by long, low barracks and the usual tents for contagious cases. Not until 1873 were two permanent new wards on the pavilion plan added (figs. 239 and 240). The buildings of this hospital (as of any hospital in this country or Europe whose growth extends over more than a century) constitute a microcosm of ward styling. By 1914 there were three pavilions and an isolation building, and construction had begun around the borders of the site (fig. 241). These areas were eventually almost solidly filled in: the old pavilions were incorporated within longer, wider, modernized wings; laboratories, classrooms, dormitories, and a fine library were added for the medical school, and in 1952 the Memorial Unit for new wards was erected on an adjacent lot on a modern X-shaped plan (fig. 242), whose effectiveness for nursing we have tried to evaluate in these studies.

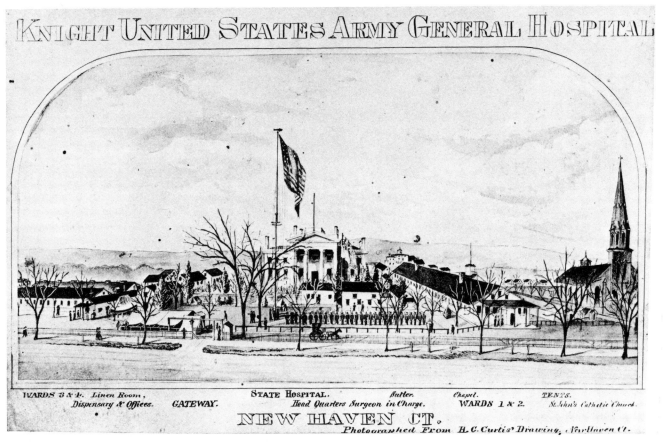

KNIGHT UNITED STATES ARMY GENERAL HOSPITAL

NEW HAVEN CT.

Photographed From H. C. Curtis' Drawing, NewHaven Ct.

| WARDS 3 & 4. Linen Room, Dispensary & Offices. | GATEWAY. | STATE HOSPITAL. Head Quarters Surgeon in Charge. | Sutler. | Chapel. WARDS 1 & 2. | TENTS. St.John's Catholic Church. |

Fig. 238. New Haven Hospital as the Knight Army Hospital during the Civil War.

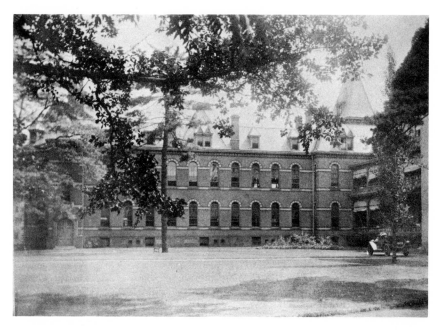

Fig. 239. East wing of New Haven Hospital (1873) as seen in 1913 from the lawn in front of the original columned structure.

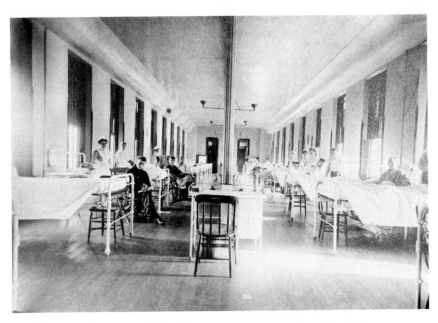

Fig. 240. Interior of 1873 ward, New Haven Hospital, in 1913.

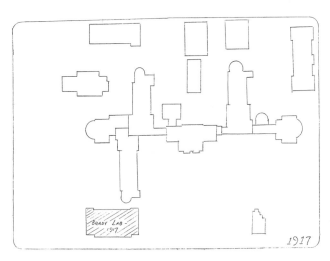

Fig. 241. Site plan, New Haven Hospital, 1917.

The Memorial Unit was originally an eight-story building with basement (see frontispiece; two floors were added in 1971–72). Central supply was in the basement, admissions and laboratories on the ground floor, operating rooms and X-ray department on the second floor. Between the first and second floors was an interfloor for mechanical equipment, original with this building so far as the designers were concerned and devised in order to keep expensive heavy equipment all in one place, easy to find, and much easier to keep in working order. The third and fourth floors were obstetrical, the fifth and sixth were for surgical patients, and the seventh for medical. The eighth had a physical therapy department in one wing of an otherwise undeveloped shell. In 1961 the intensive care unit was added here.

The building was carefully planned, indeed was kept in the planning stage longer than intended. After the laundry was finished in 1949 (a building eventually attached to the rear corner of the Memorial Unit), the builders ran out of funds and found themselves with three more years in which to plan.

The west wings of ward floors were given over to private rooms, 27 on a floor. The east wings were to have 48 beds all in 4-bed rooms, except for 4 singles. This did not work out at all. The original intent was to place 24 beds in each of the gunshot corridors of the **V**, which were to be handled from the nursing station at the juncture as two units during the day and one by night. A 24-bed unit proved not large enough and 48 beds too large, so the complement was cut to 40 and the two extra 4-bed rooms on each floor were joined to form a fine big office for the chief of the service.

Four-bed wards were amply represented in the usual expectation that among three companions a patient would find one who was congenial. There are 3-bed rooms for orthopedic cases solely because of equipment that would be too huge and bulky to fit into a 2-bed room, and all the rest of the rooms have either two beds or one.

The space behind the nursing stations at the crossing of the **X** was undifferentiated in the basement. It was used for admissions on the first floor, for urology and the cystoscopic suite on the second, and on the third for a kitchen; on the nursing floors 4–8 the space was uniformly turned into a floor pantry plus a nursing supervising office and nurses' lounge and toilet.

This, then, was the setting for our studies.

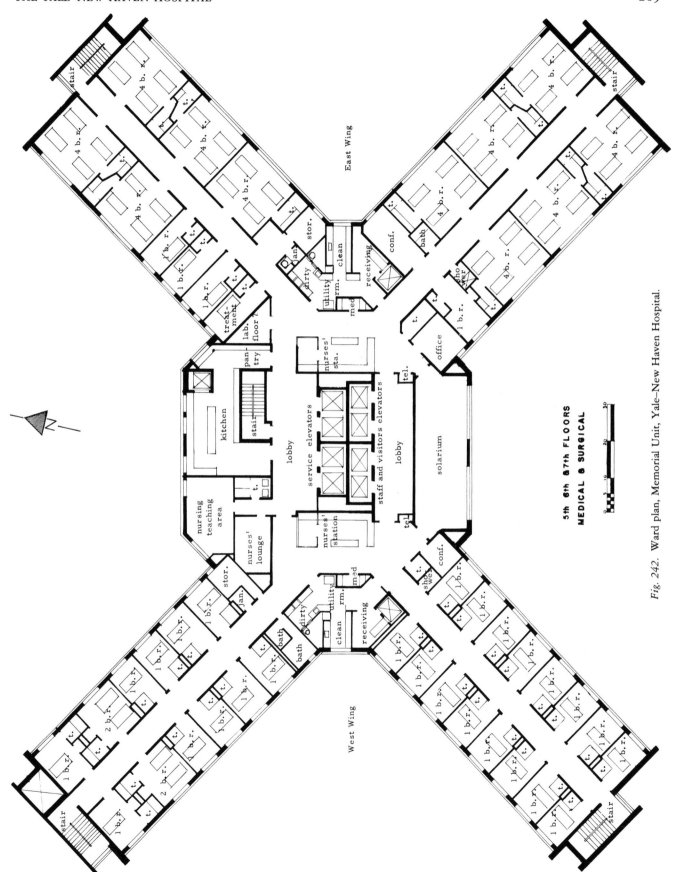

Fig. 242. Ward plan, Memorial Unit, Yale–New Haven Hospital.

5th 6th &7th FLOORS
MEDICAL & SURGICAL

CHAPTER 13

A Patient Interview Study: What Do Patients Like?

Study Method

On cards routinely issued to them upon their departure from the hospital, patients have a good many spontaneous comments to make about the quality of the medical care, the nursing care, and the food they were served. But they say almost nothing about their physical surroundings—so little, in fact, that a special study had to be undertaken and special questionnaires put to them to elicit *some* opinions on this subject.[1]

It turned out that, whereas certain features (the toilet unit and the nurses' call system) were considered very important by patients in all types of accommodations, many aspects of their setup were judged satisfactory simply because that is what was there. By and large, patients considered whatever rooms they were assigned to (so long as they were not actually offensive) adequate and often better than that—good, or even excellent. And they felt exactly the same way about the rooms they had occupied when they were interviewed weeks later at home. Private patients liked one-bed rooms, ward patients preferred four-bed rooms, corner-bed patients enjoyed the corner bed, and so on. From their unswerving enthusiasm for the status quo we learn that from the patient's own standpoint there is no *best* design for a hospital room; once certain basic standards have been met, many designs are acceptable that vary greatly in layout, appearance, and size.

The study was carried out in two hospitals, the Yale–New Haven and Genesee Hospital in Rochester, New York,[2] both quite new, eminently acceptable in design, and above standard in layout and equipment. In all, 505 patients in different accommodations were interviewed, half of them during the summer months, half in midwinter. The interview technique was used because it opened the way to further comment and helped to determine some of the reasons why patients felt as they did. Questions might be asked two ways: "How do you feel about what you actually have in your room?" or "What would you like to have here instead?" It seemed more productive to ask for a specific evaluation than seek a response to some hypothetical arrangement. The patient just could not picture anything else.

With the exception of the follow-up afterward to ascertain whether opinions change, all interviews were conducted while the patient was in the hospital. Testing for significance was done by the chi square test, and in most instances only differences significant in the statistical sense were reported. Two kinds of questions were tabulated, the first a question that could be answered one of four ways: "Yes," "No," "Yes, but," and "No, but." For instance: "Do you prefer being in a private room?" One might say yes, one might say no; one might say, "Yes, but when I feel better I would like company," or one might say, "No, but when I am sickest I want a private room." The "Yes, but" and "No, but" incorporate their own opposites. Answers to these questions were reported as percentages. The other kind of question was an opinion response: "What do you think of the drapes?" Such questions were rated on a scale of 1 to 5. If the answer was rapture unqualified, it rated 1; if strongly favorable, 2; if simply positive, 3. If favorable but with qualifications, it was rated 4; if negative, 5. The critical number is 3, the highest possible figure that would indicate satisfaction on the part of a majority of patients.

For example, patients at the Yale–New Haven were asked, "How do you feel about your room?" The average response to this question was 2.3, which (being less than 3.0) reveals a definitely positive attitude; the planners of this hospital did succeed in providing a pleasing physical environment for patients in the opinions of the patients themselves. The largest number of complaints spontaneously arising were about drafty windows and insufficient ventilation—which brings us to a discussion of hospital windows generally.

Windows

Ironically enough, when we asked patients in the same hospital, "What do you like most about your room?" we received the same answer: the windows. This was true of men and women in every social class and in all accommodations except the administrative singles (a single room for the sickest patients, assigned on need rather than ability to pay) and 2-bed rooms (which at the Yale–New Haven were all converted from deluxe singles, not very successfully). These windows are picture windows, a three-panel unit, 70 inches wide, 65 inches high, and beds are so placed that patients can see out. Very few complained of the windows being too bright or too big; private patients liked the picture windows very much, patients in the 4-bed rooms liked them even more. They reveled in the view—or, expressed mathematically, rated their windows 2.69. As one woman, speaking for many others, put it, the window opened the whole room to the outside and made her feel less a prisoner. Half of those in the rooms with picture windows volunteered the information that they spent a great deal of time looking out the windows and enjoyed the opportunity to do so. The view from most of the windows of the Yale–New Haven is a pleasant one, and during the time these studies were undertaken much interesting demolition and construction went on in the immediate vicinity, which gave patients something to "supervise." The placement of the bed in relation to these windows meant much to them—so much that it altogether determined their opinion of the windows themselves, for in administrative singles, where for treatment purposes beds had to be angled so the patient could not see out the window, the same windows were rated unsatisfactory (3.7)

One must bear in mind that the layout of most hospital rooms leaves the patient no alternative. He lies facing a blank sidewall. Since the door to his room opens away from him, it is impossible to see into the corridor from the bed and he is practically forced to look out the window. Thus the ability to do so becomes extremely significant to him.

An interesting comparison can be made with the single rooms at Genesee Hospital. There the study wing was composed of much narrower rooms with corner beds, the one window being on the same wall as the head of the bed and behind the patient, so he could not see out at all. These patients were oriented completely away from the window and the out-of-doors. They faced the door of their room, which opened toward them, and what they valued was an opportunity to see into the corridor. The center of their interest was the life there; when asked what they liked best about their rooms, they cited seven different items without ever mentioning windows. Patients who presumably were paying for a private room because they valued their privacy kept the door open much of the time, though in so small a room an open door results in utter lack of privacy. They were so involved in what was going on they even complained more about corridor noises than did the patients in the Yale–New Haven. Probably they were more aware of the noise because they were more aware of everything that happened. And yet

they had no quarrel with their windows. When specifically asked, they rated the windows 2.62, a bit more favorable than the ratings on the picture windows! New Haven patients, however, spontaneously cited windows as the feature they liked best, whereas those in Rochester never mentioned windows at all until they were asked. Only 8 patients at Genesee thought the window in back of them too small, only 12 regretted that they were prevented from looking out. Eight patients said they were very glad to be out of drafts, but then again 8 patients complained of a draft from the window behind them.

At the Yale–New Haven, complaints about the picture windows had to do with drafts. An overwhelming majority of those interviewed in the winter said the large windows leaked: "It's as drafty as a World War I prison!" Yet three-fourths of those interviewed during the winter months admitted that they opened their windows for considerable periods of time, and some even said the rooms were kept too hot. Both hospitals were subject to harsh winters, but only 16 percent of the patients in the corner-bed rooms, with their double-hung windows and 25 percent less glass surface, complained of drafts or overcompensating heating. The fixed center pane at Yale–New Haven frustrated many patients in the summertime: "If I see a large pane of glass, I want to be able to open it!"

General Furnishings

Whereas at the Yale–New Haven the one thing patients liked best was the windows, at Genesee Hospital it was the color scheme. It was probably no accident that this was appealing. Placing the bed in one corner made it possible to design these rooms much smaller than most others, and a generous effort must have been made to camflouage smallness by the use of color. Though the room is only 8 by 12 feet, occupants did not seem to resent the curtailment of space nor complain in any way of being hemmed in, although when specifically asked, 90 percent definitely recognized that space was at a premium in such words as "This room is too small to take another stick of furniture!" However, in the larger 4-bed rooms of the Yale –New Haven, 70 percent of the patients wanted no more furniture, or, if any, straight chairs for visitors to keep them off the bed. (A few said they would rather temporarily share their beds than seat the visitors on chairs that would encourage them to stay on endlessly.) A strange finding at Genesee was the perfect satisfaction of 83 percent of the patients with the shelf space provided for books and flowers, which was only the top of the bedside stand. Are flowers not as popular with patients as their visitors believe? The Yale–New Haven offers in addition to a bedside table, an overbed space and a formica window ledge insulated against the heat of the radiators it covers, yet 25 percent of the patients in private rooms complained they still had not enough display space! In 4-bed wards with half as much space per person on the window ledge, only 4 percent were dissatisfied.

Beds

In Genesee Hospital the most popular piece of furniture was the bed. The patients rated it 1.91, very fine with a touch of enthusiasm. Its two distinctive features were the very things they liked about it: corner placement and their own ability to raise and lower the whole bed electrically. Of 150 patients in these high–low beds, only 41 preferred them high; 109 kept them in the low position as much of the time as possible, perhaps because it felt more like home. Twenty-four patients spontaneously offered the information that to have one side of the bed against the wall made them feel more secure.

From the patient's standpoint, a sense of security is the most important thing a hospital can offer. Ernest Dichter's research into "The Hospital–Patient Relationship" led him unequivocally to the conclusion that "the measurement of a successful hospital should not be how modern its operating room and its facilities are, but whether or not it provides the patient with what he most profoundly needs, security."[3] This is essentially why comment cards elicit many criticisms or praises of the medical care, nursing care, and dietary service, which have directly to do with the patient's needs. Such items either reinforce the feeling of security, or they destroy it. When it comes to physical decor, any of a number of possible alternatives is altogether acceptable; what is important is whether the whole hospital experience has been a happy one. If it was, the patient will see no reason to change a single detail, even of the furniture. And when some item of furniture happens to reinforce, by association with home or for whatever subtle psychological reason, his sense of security, then ratings soar and unsolicited praises burst forth, as happened with the corner bed.

The real decision about the corner bed will not be made by patients but by the way nurses and doctors feel about it. We asked patients whether they thought a corner bed was convenient for the nurses. Thirty-three did not feel qualified to answer the question; the remaining 122 were almost equally divided between positive and negative responses. Most of the 66 who thought the location convenient cited the ease with which the bed *could* be moved away from the wall when it had to be. The 56 who demurred usually had gone through some specific experience where the bed *had* to be moved away from the wall to permit intravenous

feedings, treatments of some sort, or a medical examination. A master's thesis concerning itself with this question concludes that the determining factor in the use of the corner bed might be how sick the patient is. The average daily number of bed movements, save for the acutely ill, was found to be no more than two a day, so moderately ill patients would present no problem. But, the thesis concludes, "The acutely ill patient is more efficiently cared for in an island type accommodation with more than a three-foot clearance on either side of the bed."[4]

The matter should be checked more fully. Even with our present knowledge it seems clear that in designing a progressive care hospital, corner-bed location should be seriously considered for the intermediate-care zone.

At the Yale–New Haven the bed was rated a low 2.78, but this is misleading because the great majority of complaints were about the inevitable plastic mattress- and pillow-covers rather than the bed itself. It was said to be too high, and patients came up with all sorts of suggestions—stools, floor grips, ceiling grips, anything—to help them get in and out of bed more easily. Since the studies were completed, high–low beds have been introduced into the unit.

Lounge Chair

The lounge chair was less popular than the bed. Rated at 2.87, it was the least satisfactory piece of furniture at the Yale–New Haven. It is a perfectly undistinguished specimen of chair: leather seat, leather back, wooden arms and legs. Twenty-five percent of those interviewed criticized it for some reason or other. Many suggested a contour chair, of all things, never pausing to consider how they would get up from a contour chair. It is hard to design a chair to fit everyone—people come in different shapes and sizes. In general, patients of a higher class economically and socially tended to be more critical of all the furniture, and this lounge chair especially annoyed them. Thirty-nine percent of them expressed dissatisfaction, whereas only 16 percent of the poorer patients felt that way.

Tables

The overbed table at the Yale–New Haven rated highest of the four standard pieces of equipment in the room with one of the best scores in the questionnaire (2.30). Yet patients had many criticisms to make of it, most involved with how far it could be raised or lowered. It can be raised to 45 inches from the floor and lowered to 29 inches, neither low enough to be used at the lounge chair nor high enough to fit over very fat people in bed or to clear a bed which is lifted for some reason (on shock blocks, for example). The bedside table (rated 2.58) is equipped with a pull-out shelf and two drawers, and a cupboard at the bottom for urinal and bedpan rack. Fourteen patients thought it was not big enough, because they wanted clothes space there instead of in the locker. "They put this damn short shirt on you, and your bathrobe is across the room. It sure keeps you in bed."

Lights

The reading light at Genesee Hospital was thought far better than the one at the Yale–New Haven. The latter, rated 3.26, definitely unsatisfactory, is an incandescent bulb in a bullet-type fixture attached to the head of the bed by a double-jointed swiveling arm without even a spring at the joints. There is no way to manipulate the light from the bed except by handling the metal shade, and although it is a triple shade the outermost layer still gets plenty hot.

Attached to the joint nearest the wall is another bullet-type light fixture, which can be aimed either at the ceiling for general illumination or straight out into the room. The patient has no control of this one, and that is what is the matter with it. He can not reach it to move it, he cannot even turn it on and off. It is operated by a switch at the door, and there were many complaints about *this* arrangement.

Forty-three percent of the patients in Classes I and II found considerable difficulty in reading when these lights were used. (Classes have been assigned here, as elsewhere, according to the Hollingshead Index of Social Position, which considers education, occupation, and, in the case of patients living in New Haven, residence.[5] The highest class is I, the lowest V.) A mere 20 percent of Classes IV and V reported trouble reading, whereas Class III reacted about the same way as Classes I and II. We could only interpret these percentages one way: Classes IV and V do not spend much time reading.

By comparison, the overbed light at Genesee Hospital, rated 2.33, was recessed in the ceiling, focused on the patient's book, and could be controlled from the bed. These patients were satisfied, but in neither hospital did patients have much to say for the general room illumination. This problem is genuine: the patient is lying down, so that it is extremely difficult to design an overhead light that will not shine into his eyes; any light that illuminates at all may be too bright when he wants to drop off to sleep, as patients tend to do all hours of the day or night.

Toilet Unit

In both hospitals, patients rated the toilet unit the third best feature of the room. This finding may be broken down at the Yale–New Haven as follows. In the 4-bed rooms, the toilet unit was the second most popular feature, surpassed only by the picture windows.

Those in single rooms rated it third, after the picture windows and their privacy. Those in 2-bed rooms and administrative singles did not mention this feature at all—and small wonder: these rooms did not, like the others, have modern, prefabricated steel units but closet toilets of the hackneyed hotel type, and, in the administrative single, the toilet also acted as passageway between adjoining rooms. A toilet that looks like any other toilet can easily escape remark, but it is impossible to overlook a complicated installation of stainless steel, more like a trailer or a Pullman compartment. The average rating of the toilet at the Yale–New Haven was 2.40 and includes dissident votes from rooms that did not have the new unit at all; public opinion of the stainless steel contraption was probably much higher. At the Genesee, which had a similar prefabricated unit in every room polled, the score was more favorable still: 2.20. What mattered in both hospitals was that there was a modern unit in the room—shiny, intricate, impressive. There was no significant difference between responses from patients in 1- and in 4-bed rooms. And nobody in either hospital wanted the steel unit changed a bit. The sink was separate from the toilet area at the Yale–New Haven and included in it at the Genesee. In spite of the different locations, 92 percent of the patients at both hospitals said they preferred the sink in its present location.

Both toilet units were very small. The compartment at the Yale–New Haven is only 31 inches wide by 46 inches deep by 88 inches high, and the door (a sliding door to assure every possible inch of use) is narrower than that. Yet only 2.6 percent of the patients returned an unqualified no to the question, "Is there enough space in the unit?" and only one reported claustrophobia. When the sliding door is shut, ventilation operates all the time through an opening in the ceiling leading to a central exhaust system. However, when patients were asked, "Is there enough fresh air in the unit?" 22 percent in summer and 6 percent in winter thought there was not. The unit at Genesee Hospital is likewise ventilated by central exhaust, yet there 98 percent of the patients found the fresh air satisfactory. That unit is a mite bigger—36 by 42 inches—as it must be to include a sink as well. The 86 added square inches (1512 at the Genesee, 1426 at Yale–New Haven) seem to have been felt by Genesee patients as extra air as well as extra space. Possibly the 22 percent at Yale–New Haven who complained of a lack of fresh air were expressing unconscious claustrophobia.

Noise

At both hospitals we asked patients to list the noises that bothered them. From the Genesee group came an odd response to this question: more than half said they heard noises from the next room, more than 80 percent heard noises from the corridor, but only 22 percent said that the noises bothered them. We are at a loss to account for this almost saintly tolerance on the part of the Genesee ill. At first we thought perhaps that, oriented to the corridor from their corner beds, they understood and therefore forgave what was going on. But the two categories of noise by which they were far less annoyed than patients at the Yale–New Haven have nothing to do with keeping informed: the first, patients talking too loudly with their visitors, which a third of those interviewed at the Yale–New Haven complained of, but only 17 percent at the Genesee; the second, the grim sound of patients being sick, which a mere 8 percent at the Genesee objected to, as compared to 20 percent at the Yale–New Haven.

It is perhaps possible to explain this by the accommodations of those patients who complained of noise: everyone interviewed at the Genesee was in a single room. When we asked patients in the 4-bed rooms of the Yale–New Haven, "Does it bother you having other patients in the same room? Are you disturbed by doctors or nurses taking care of the other patients? Do visitors to other patients in the room bother you?" we were told that the chief source of bother was the other patients themselves. Visitors came second, medical personnel third. In many cases, patients said they were so glad to see doctors or nurses coming to care for the other patients, it was a relief rather than a bother to have them in the room.

Medical intrusions bothered patients more during the night than in the day, and so did the other patients' groaning. Yet greater bitterness was felt toward patients who were too well, and talked and laughed and carried on. "The less ill patients joke, sing, and make a nuisance of themselves," said one patient at the Yale–New Haven. More than one lamented that this hospital had eliminated doors to the 4-bed rooms, which were subsequently added due to a new fire regulation. In both hospitals patients were annoyed by other patients' radios and TV sets, especially by the click of the multichannel radio switch, and by the staff and nurses talking and giggling among themselves: "Nurses are insensitive to noise!" "Private duty nurses yap all day long."

Once again the class factor crops up in noise studies at the Yale–New Haven: in all accommodations, Classes I and II were more sensitive to noise and more articulately resentful. In the one- and two-bed rooms, 63 percent of patients from Classes I and II kept their doors shut much of the time, but only 33 percent of Classes IV and V did so. Because, at Genesee Hospital, Classes I and II were mainly in the larger private rooms rather than the small corner-bed singles, we could not find enough members of these classes on the study wing to draw a comparison. It must thus be remembered that not only were the accommodations in the two hospitals dissimilar, but the social class of the patients was also not the same. In both hospitals we found many patients from Classes IV and V. Those at the Genesee were more bothered by noises from the corridors. Unexpectedly, although patients off corridors not yet carpeted heard a lot more noise, they professed themselves no more disturbed by it than the patients who were off a carpeted corridor. There was no greater reaction in single than in multiple-bed rooms; the sensitivity of patients to noise varied only with their social standing, not their accommodations.

Food Temperature Preference

We move now into another of patients' preferences: the temperature at which they like their food. In his article on how to give the patient a sense of security (quoted above), Ernest Dichter observes, "The cold cup of coffee, then, has deep emotional meaning. To the insecure patient it is a sign. Good hot coffee is symbolic of the home away from home, of being welcome. Bad coffee is the perfect symbol that he is a stranger, that he is receiving what amounts to the orphan's negligent care." What is true of coffee in the symbolic sense is actually true of all food—it should come hot, as a sign that the hospital *cares*. All people, in hospitals or out, like hot food hot, and for the hospital patient this is even more important—his meal is not just a break in the working day, it is a major event.

Hospitals should serve food at the temperature patients prefer, if possible and if they can find out what that temperature is. To serve it hotter does no one any good—the patient has to wait to eat, and the hospital is out of pocket unnecessarily: getting food hot costs money in the first place, and keeping it hot until it is served costs more. Where should the line be drawn? In actual degrees Fahrenheit, how hot is hot enough?

Measurements on temperature preference have been made before, some not in hospitals but in cafeteria studies. If we consult those having to do with hospital trays, we find that the recommended temperatures vary as much as 30° for meats, 20° for vegetables and potatoes. These findings not having been published in sufficient detail to permit reevaluation of the data, we ran our own experiment at the Yale–New Haven Hospital.[6]

Patients were chosen at random on the surgical floor. Standing at the door of each one's room, we stopped the dinner tray as it was about to be delivered and took the temperature of the food with a battery-operated thermocouple, so much faster than a mercury thermometer. A needle is plunged into the food; the temperature registers at once on a large dial and is recorded. Immediately after the meal the patient was asked whether he found the meat, the vegetables, and the potatoes too cold, just right, or too hot. In this way, in two successive years, we checked 196 patient opinions on the temperatures of meats, 157 on vegetables, and 147 on potatoes. No marked trays were set up or served—these were routine trays, so the experimenters could not control the temperature of the food in any way.

When the results were analyzed, the responses "just right" and "too hot" had to be treated as one. "Too hot" was said too seldom to permit statistical treatment; serving food too hot was one extravagance this hospital rarely permitted itself. The outstanding finding of our study was the wide range of temperatures patients considered acceptable in all three categories: meat, vegetables, potatoes. Some were satisfied with meats at 100°, some demanded 160°. Some felt potatoes were hot enough at 115°, some rated 175° "just right." And the range of acceptable temperatures for vegetables ran from 120° to at least 175°. This is comparable to the results in the cafeteria study of Blaker and his co-workers, who found the general public liked potatoes and vegetables anywhere from 125° to 165°, and meats from 100° to 170°.

What is the lowest temperature that satisfies everybody? It was found that 100 percent of the patients were satisfied with vegetables in the 165°–169° range or above; 88.8 percent were satisfied in the 160°–164° range. Therefore we recommend a serving temperature for vegetables from 160° to 170°. There was no significant difference in findings for potatoes, so they too should be served at 160°—170°. Patients seem to like their meats a bit cooler. At 150–154°—or above—all patients expressed satisfaction with the meats; however, by dropping meat temperatures only 5° (to the 145°–49° range), one-third were dissatis-

fied. Therefore, ideally the range for meats should be 150°–160°.

Ideally, we say. But other factors must be taken into account. In this chapter, by and large, we have tried to focus on features for which the patient's opinion is a critical factor and to leave for consideration elsewhere those decided primarily by other criteria: appearance, convenience, and efficiency. However, food temperature overlaps on that other area. All else discussed in this chapter—color scheme, furnishings, window design, toilet facilities—may be acquired by initial investment. Since it costs little more to do it right than to do it wrong, it might as well be planned to please the patient from the outset. Food temperature is a matter of constant maintenance as well as proper equipment, and maintenance means continuing expense. At what point in heating food and keeping it hot does giving the maximum satisfaction to the patient cease to pay off?

According to our analysis, 160° for potatoes, 160° for vegetables, and 150° for meats—the bottom of our recommended ranges—would satisfy, respectively, 100, 92.2, and 94.6 percent of patients. Raise each of these temperatures 5°—to the midpoint of our recommended ranges for each item—and 100 percent of patients would be satisfied with all three categories of food. Drop each temperature 5°, and 90.5 percent of the patients will still be satisfied with their potatoes, 77.5 percent with their vegetables, and 84.7 percent with their meats—not a perfect showing, admittedly, but still a creditable performance for a kitchen that must consider other factors besides how patients feel. If keeping temperatures to our recommended ranges would mean employing 50 percent more personnel to deliver trays on time plus a considerable outlay for new equipment, food service administrators might well think it worth their while to drop temperatures 5°. A respectably large percentage of the patient population would still be perfectly content.

CHAPTER 14

Who Really Uses the Patient–Nurse Call System?

For years, hospital staffs at every level have been demanding an improved system of communication between patient and nurse. Supervision, easy enough in the large, open 36-bed ward, became quite another matter in a 36-bed ward that was a complex of 3- or 4-bed rooms, semiprivate rooms, and private rooms. The earliest solution, the installation of a nurses' call bell or buzzer at the bedside, served its purpose well. It was then combined with a light over the patient's door. Then came the idea of transmitting the patient's voice in the way the voice of the boss is transmitted to his secretary in a business office. Thereupon designers installed at the bed a microphone, a clumsy apparatus that never quite assured the patient that his needs were being made known, because it worked only in one direction. In more recent years, the hospital looked into the feasibility of establishing a complete voice intercommunication system, the kind now taken for granted in all up-to-date offices. Could it be adapted economically for use within the hospital to bring the patient into contact with service personnel? Electronic and telephone companies experimented and developed several units the hospital could use. The nurses' call system was being viewed in an entirely new light.[1]

Two basic assumptions, not always compatible with each other, were made in designing the voice communication system, originally intended solely as a patient–nurse call system. The first was that there would always be someone, originally a nurse, at the master station ready to answer the patient's call. The second was that this person could then perform the requested service. But if the nurse was off performing the service, she obviously could not remain in the nurses' station to answer calls. The contradiction led to assigning a specific person (a ward clerk or secretary) to answer calls, at least during the busy part of the day. Thus, another person had to perform the requested service. Communication became necessary between the two to relay the request since the ward clerk or secretary could not leave her post. The call system once used to locate someone who could respond quickly to the patient's needs came to be used to locate personnel and staff for reasons having nothing to do with these specific requests.

The Yale–New Haven Hospital has a complete intercom system with a master board at the control desk showing a light for every room. Furthermore, the patient can be monitored at any time from the nurses' station: the nurse simply presses the button for that particular room. Obviously and necessarily, this "Big Sister is watching you" arrangement goes on independently of how the patient feels about it. (One patient somberly protested, "It's like *1984* when they searched for people!") The nurse can also speak to the patient at any time, either into the microphone of the box at the nurses' station or, if it is a more personal message she does not want other nurses at the station to hear, into a telephone extension. Her voice is received by the patient at two different decibel levels. If she speaks publicly into the microphone, what comes out over the patient's head is reasonably dulcet. But if she speaks privately into the telephone attachment, the loudspeaker becomes a very loud speaker, practically a public address system. "Do you want your bedpan now, Mr. Jones?" Visitors to patients in 4-bed rooms have four times the opportunity to listen in on these intimate exchanges.

Theoretically, patients are supposed to use the audio system to specify their needs and save the nurse a trip to find out what they are because if she knows what it is she can bring it with her. Actually, patients at Yale–New Haven were convinced that not only could their very breathing be heard at the nurses' station (this was true) but that their conversations with nursing personnel could also be heard by patients in every other room (this was false, but you could not make them believe it). "I feel freer to talk if they come into the room," one patient said. "I like a light system, but not a speaker system that goes all over." "I do not want to announce to the world what I want," another patient stated. Some waited for a nurse to come by because they were ashamed to use such a public system.

Theoretically too, the audiovisual system is reserved for communications between patients and nurses. Actually, it is used for locating staff. At the Yale–New Haven there is a paging system at the nurses' station pitched quite low. There is a receiving box, identical with those over the patients' heads, affixed to the wall of the corridor and intended to alert staff in any one of half a dozen adjoining rooms, but this is pitched so low it cannot be heard by anyone in any room and it has thus fallen completely into disuse. As things work out, the head nurse or clerical worker assigned to answering calls and conveying patients' requests to the relevant personnel has not been able to resist using the nurses' call system to page the individual in question. "Is Dr. Kilroy there, Mr. Jones?" Mr. Jones may have been napping, but he is not any longer.

This new use of the system also turned up in our patient interviews. Not that patients objected in principle, indeed at both hospitals involved they gave the nurses' call system one of the highest ratings (2.24 at Yale–New Haven, 1.9 at the Genesee), probably because, for all its clamor and obtrusiveness, it gave them a sense of security, so much more important than convenience. They recognized its potential value and in their evaluation were careful to distinguish between the system as such and the nurses' response to it: "You know they know what you want, even if they don't come."

To determine to what extent the nurse–patient call system was being used as a staff paging system, we ran an experiment at the Yale–New Haven in four in-patient units (table 6). From 7:30 A.M. to 10:00 P.M. all calls were taped. For night observations, an observer was stationed on the floor to note each use of the system, each "call." A call was defined as an instance when a person at one station transmitted a verbal message to a person at another station, and it included answers or discussion, if any, related to the message.

We were able to answer seven pertinent questions.

1. Who initiated the call? We could ascertain that during the day, the time of heaviest activity, the staff initiated more calls than patients did. The opposite was true at night (fig. 243).

2. By whom was the call answered? Ninety percent of daytime calls initiated by patients were answered by the ward clerk. This is of interest. She answered the patients but could not, in most instances, perform the services. She had to pass the requests on to members of the nursing staff, and she used the nurses' call system for that purpose.

3. If a patient initiated the call, how long was it before it was answered? On all but one unit, patient calls were answered in less than one minute (table 7). Remember that this means only the time involved in answering the patient's call, not the time it took to fulfil the request. The average waiting time does not begin to indicate the upper extremes on all units, the very long waiting times even for an answer when temporary nurses were on duty who were completely unfamiliar with the system, when the shift was changing, or when, at night, there were no staff members at the nurses' station. Calls were answered fastest when the ward clerk was on duty and there was a minimum of activity at the nurses' station.

4. What was the purpose of the call? More than 50 percent of the calls were requests for a specific article or service. Which articles or services were involved? Here there is remarkable consistency between day and night (fig. 244). Approximately one-third of patient requests day and night had to do with bedpan and urinal. One-fifth of the day requests and one-fourth of those at night were for medication, mainly analgesics and sedatives. Next most frequently the patient wanted a nurse. This was interesting because the patient preferred not to tell the nursing station what he wanted the nurse for; he just wanted to see a nurse.

Patients in 4-bed rooms utilized the nurses' call system 30 percent less than did those in single rooms. To begin with, there are more chances that a nurse will be in a 4-bed room. Also, perhaps patients in 4-bed rooms help one another to a certain extent.

5. What features in the system were desirable? It really did save nursing steps because all calls for information resulted in a trip saved. All requests for medication saved a trip since the nurse could bring it with her. When bedpan and urinal were already at the bedside and there was a toilet hopper in the room, no trip was saved on the bedpan calls. Nor was there any saving on calls for service around the bed, nor on calls requesting simply "a nurse." However, when we analyze all patient-initiated calls, 42.6 percent during the day and 38 percent at night did save the nurse a trip (fig. 245). If staff-initiated calls alone are considered, almost three-quarters of them during the day and nearly all during the night (true, there were very few at night) saved the initiator a trip (fig. 246).

6. What features of the system were undesirable? During the night, the staff initiated calls mainly to communicate information—pass it along from one member of the nursing staff to another. But during the day, two-thirds of these calls were "page calls," by which we do not mean calls answered and attended to but *unsuccessful* attempts to contact a specific individual. This is an inefficient use of the voice intercommunication system and is bothersome to patients. Page calls accounted for almost one-half of all daytime activity—half of *all* calls made, not simply those the staff initiated. They came not singly but in battalions. If the seeker did not locate the person he wanted in one room, he tried another and another, or spoke in a louder voice through the hall speakers. One call would thus be a string of multiple calls (fig. 247).

7. What additional features were needed? One

TABLE 6. Patient–nurse call system study: length and number of observations, census, and staffing per inpatient unit during day and night observations.

Inpatient Nursing Unit	Surgical West	Surgical West	Surgical West	Surgical West	Surgical West	Medical West	Medical West	Surgical East	Surgical East	Surgical East	Surgical East	Medical East	Medical East	Medical East
Number of day hours observed	14.5	14.5	14.5	14.5	14.5	14.5	14.5	14.5	14.5	14.5	14.5	14.5	14.5	14.5
Average nursing staff	4.6	3.3	3.5	3.4	3.3	3.7	3.9	12.9	9.4	10.3	10.7	9.3	6.3	6.5
Average private duty nurses	7.9	5.8	5.1	5.5	5.1	5.6	9.6	2.8	2.2	3.7	5.5	1.6	3.0	1.0
Number of night hours observed			9.5	9.5	9.5		9.5			9.5	9.5	9.5	9.5	9.5
Average nursing staff		2.2	2.2	2.2	2.2	2.2	2.2			2.4	3.3		3.5	5.2
Average private duty nurses		3.2	3.2	4.8	5.6	7.3	3.5	2.0		0.0	2.0	3.0	3.0	0.2
Bed complement	30	30	30	30	30	28	28	48	48	48	48	48	48	48
Bed census	28	27	28	24	29	25	26	43	43	40	48	45	38	43

PERCENTAGE OF CALLS INITIATED BY STAFF OR PATIENTS
PER INPATIENT UNIT FOR DAY AND NIGHT OBSERVATIONS

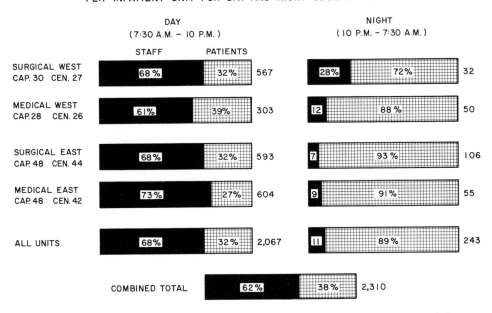

Fig. 243. Usage pattern of the voice communication system, Yale–New Haven Hospital.

PATIENT INITIATED CALLS
PERCENTAGE DISTRIBUTION BY CONTENT

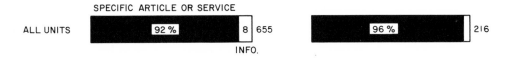

WHAT SPECIFIC ARTICLE OR SERVICE

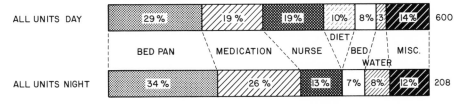

Fig. 244. Content of patient calls by day and night.

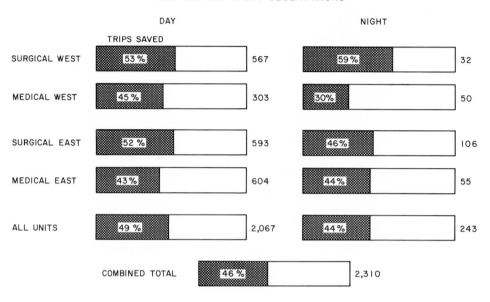

Fig. 245. Trips saved as a result of the nurse–patient call system.

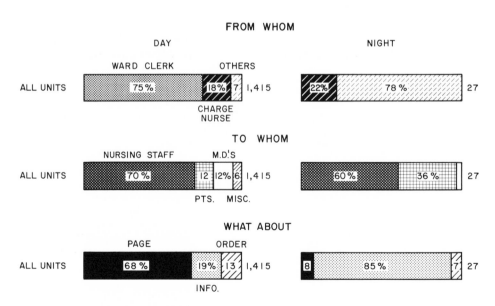

Fig. 246. Percentage distribution analysis of staff-initiated calls in a 24-hour period.

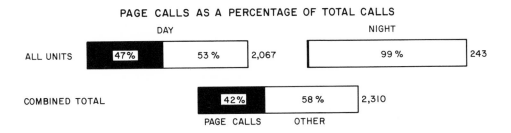

Fig. 247. Page calls (unsuccessful attempts to locate staff) expressed as a percentage of total calls.

TABLE 7. Average time lapse (in seconds) in answering patient-initiated calls per inpatient unit during day and night observations.

	Day	Night
Surgical West	34.7	5.3
Medical West	86.7	103.3
West average	54.2	54.3
Surgical East	46.3	14.1
Medical East	41.3	12.5
East average	44.2	13.3
Average of all inpatient units	49.5	33.8

N.B. These times refer only to the times the requests were answered on the voice intercommunication system and not to the times when these requests were performed.

thinks in terms of a new locating device built into the system to indicate to whoever mans the nursing station that a nurse or aide can be found in a certain room. Would staff remember to flick a light on when entering the room, and off when leaving it? At night, might several floors be combined at a central station, where one operator would be assigned to answer patient calls from all floors and to transfer them to the appropriate nursing staff? This would be a logical extension of the voice intercommunication system once the idea is accepted that it is not primarily a nurses' call system. It is functioning now as an inpatient unit intercommunication system used by staff primarily and by patients only secondarily.

The imagination races on—if a system of remote control could be made to work, and if it solved a number of problems of supervision now badgering hospital personnel, what effect would that then have on the building of nurses' stations in full view and on gunshot corridors?

CHAPTER 15

The Yale Traffic Index

Need for the Study

If one were to show a foreigner, or an American totally ignorant of hospitals, a dozen new nursing units, on which feature would he be likely to comment? He might say of the first, "How good looking!" or of the second, "How very new and shiny!" But after the first half dozen he would probably protest, "How many shapes do these things assume? How elaborate, and how ingenious! You say each one is planned to provide the ultimate in nursing care?" We could show him square units and round units and rectangular units, pinwheels and cloverleafs, low pavilions and skyscrapers, single-loaded corridors with patient rooms on only one side and double-loaded corridors with patient rooms on both, schemes for simple circulation, where there is only one way traffic can go to a room and back, and schemes for redundant circulation with more than one way to get there and more than one way back. We could easily show him dozens of styles. Sooner or later he would be bound to exclaim, "Why don't you make up your mind? Where they're all so different, surely they can't all be equally good! Which one works best? You who are in the business, please tell me: which one is the most efficient?"

A number of people who are in the hospital business have tried to answer this question. How do you go about measuring the efficiency of a nursing unit? One traditional yardstick has been density of beds— so many beds to each ten running feet of corridor. Presumably, the more beds that can be fitted into the space, the less distance nurses will have to travel. Another suggestion is to measure the distance of the bed farthest from the nurses' station. Or the number of beds in relation to area. Or the area allotted to each bed.

Hospital floor plans were rated for efficiency according to one measurement or another, but no two sets of ratings agreed. There was even some confusion over what is meant by the word *efficiency*. Is it functional efficiency, the minimum movement necessary to perform required tasks? Or is it investment efficiency, the cost per patient to build a nursing unit? The two do not necessarily coincide. One can cut corners while building and spend extra every year trying to make an inefficient plan work, or one can invest in a very expensive building and thereafter save on maintenance and nurses' steps. One can build a beautiful and expensive building that proves prohibitively expensive to run. The fourth and of course happiest alternative would be a well-designed structure that did not cost too much to build. How can one tell in advance how efficient a certain floor plan, which looks so functional on paper, is going to be in operation?

The Organization of the Study

The way to determine the functional efficiency of units would seem to be to find a method of measuring the nursing steps each plan requires, since most arguments among architects, hospital consultants, hospital administrators, nurses, and doctors about the relative merits of any plan eventually boil down to how far staff members have to travel in caring for patients. To trace nursing steps is to see how a whole unit functions, not merely one component of it or a small group of interrelated components. The nurse binds the unit together; if we map her travel from patient to patient and from patient rooms to service rooms and nursing station, the path she takes will outline the relationship of each part of the unit to every other part and will graphically indicate the relationship of each part to the unit as a whole.

For the nurse's steps are purposeful steps. In order to care for patients, she must travel from one clearly defined area to another. She may seem to be running miscellaneous errands without discernible pattern but, although each task she performs has something special about it, in the aggregate her movements begin to group themselves by starting place and destination and their frequency can be tabulated. Some nurses are more efficient in their movements than others, but it evens out in the long run. Every staff is made up of real people who possess varying degrees of organizational ability.

The scurryings to and fro of the nurses, and of nursing staff in general, can readily be broken down into trips. We decided to take the trip as a unit of measurement and use it as our yardstick for determining the efficiency of the nursing unit. Data on such movements can be gathered by relatively unskilled observers because the observer is not required to know what task is being performed, only that someone has gone from one place to another. Two or three observers stationed in strategic places can keep track of the movements of as many as fifteen staff members.

Data expressed in terms of trips are concise and can easily be interpreted. From such information can be inferred without much difficulty which areas of the inpatient unit function together and should therefore be placed within easy reach of one another. Since, in relating function to design, it does not matter which way the traffic flows, *to* and *from* can be combined under a single heading called a "link." Important and unimportant traffic links can be identified. This traffic-study approach is often called "link analysis." But we wanted to do more than that. We wanted to evolve a more precise method (within acknowledged limits) of quantifying the convenience, and therefore the efficiency, of nursing units.

A six-month study of traffic patterns was undertaken at the Yale–New Haven Hospital in October 1958 in four nursing units, two surgical, two medical, one of each with 30 and one of each with 48 beds. The observer was set at the nursing station with a clear view of all activity along the V-shaped corridors. Information recorded for each trip was: *Who* made it, where it came *from, to* what destination it was going, and *when*. Because *when* would have had to be broken up into shifts eventually for purposes of interpretation, the job of the observer was made very much easier by doing so at once. Shifts were the regular nursing shifts: 7:30 A.M. to 4:00 P.M., 4:00 P.M. to midnight, midnight to 7:30 A.M. In all, 15 shifts were recorded, 3 each for 4 different inpatient units, and a second set of 3 shifts for one of the units several months later to check results. The shifts were not consecutive. Admittedly, continuous observation for 24 hours would be more desirable than a composite of 3 separate shifts for each unit over a period of a month or more. However, the extra accuracy would have been slight, the strain on the observers very great. In most cases, shifts were processed separately anyhow.

Findings

Figures 248–51 show activity levels, as measured by trips, for the four units during the day, evening, and night shifts. Though color could not be used, the graphs differentiate with sufficient vividness among the staffs: professional and auxiliary nursing, medical, dietary, and housekeeping. Dietary traffic includes the visits of dietitians to the nursing unit as well as

the distribution of meals by dietary maids. Housekeeping activity is confined almost entirely to the day shift and varies a great deal, depending on whether or not major periodic cleaning and/or maintenance work is being performed in addition to the routine daily chores.

TABLE 8. Analysis of total number of trips during the three shifts.

All Personnel: Total 20,251

Unit	Day	Evening	Night
5 West	1,875	832	408
5 East	2,148	1,216	669
5 East	2,411	1,445	660
7 West	2,516	1,158	495
7 East	2,715	1,135	568
Totals	11,665	5,786	2,800
Percentage	51.6	28.6	13.8

Nursing Personnel Only
Total 14,240: 70.31%

5 West	1,311	767	408
5 East	1,308	960	587
5 East	1,578	1,089	626
7 West	1,522	840	422
7 East	1,539	764	519
Totals	7,258	4,420	2,562
Percentage	51.0	31.0	18.0

Nursing activity should be considered as a whole since the ratio of professional to nonprofessional nurses changes so much.[1] Nursing fluctuates less than total activity in volume and in the height of its peaks of activity and depth of its lows. Most other activities are limited to a particular period, usually the day shift, but nursing is a round-the-clock operation, moving by its own laws to an extent that justifies our reading these charts as the record of just two types of activity, independent of one another: nursing, and everything else.

The total number of trips analyzed was 20,251; of these, nursing traffic accounted for 14,240, or about 70.3 percent. For subtotals for each floor, shift, and classification of personnel, see table 8, which shows how important the day shift is in influencing apparent overall traffic patterns, especially when only the total traffic is studied. However, a patient care unit is a 24-hour facility, and each shift should be separately examined to determine the effectiveness of certain locations.

It was decided to use only the 14 major traffic links, which table 9 lists in order of importance. Using the formula $N = n(n-1)/2$, the number of possible links for the 30-bed unit would be 861, and for the 48-bed unit, 465. By lumping patient rooms according to

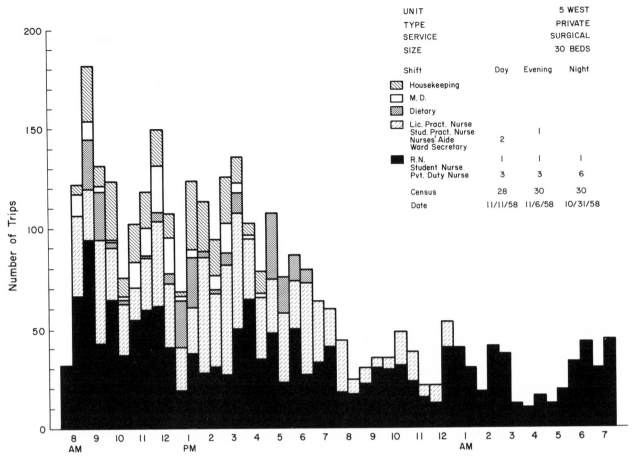

Fig. 248. The Yale Traffic Index: activity level on ward unit 5 West, Yale–New Haven Hospital, during the day, evening, and night shifts.

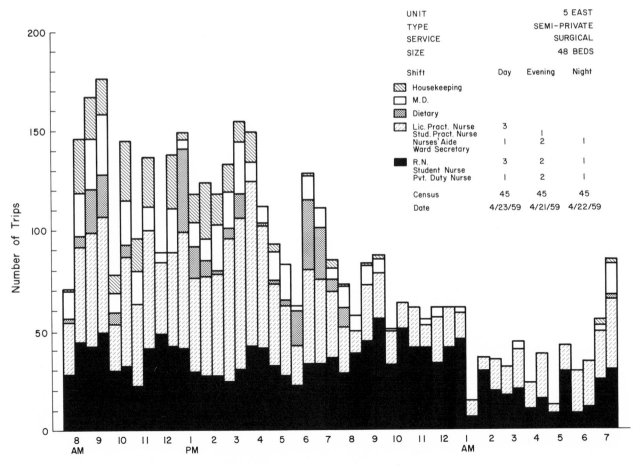

Fig. 249. Activity level, ward unit 5 East.

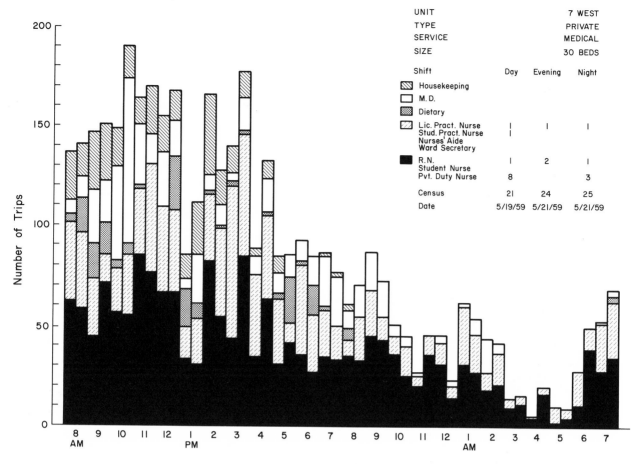

Fig. 250. Activity level, ward unit 7 West.

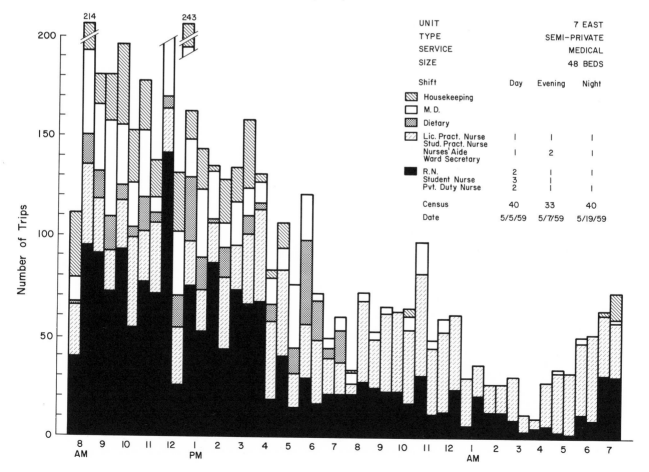

Fig. 251. Activity level, ward unit 7 East.

TABLE 9. Overall cumulative listing of the 14 major links in order of importance.

Rank	Link*	No. of Trips	Percentage	Cumulative Percentage
1	PR–PR	3,672	19.1	19.1
2	N–PR	3,211	16.7	35.8
3	U–PR	2,705	14.1	49.9
4	N–U	1,878	9.8	59.7
5	N–E	1,168	6.1	65.8
6	N–M	1,121	5.8	71.6
7	PR–P	882	4.6	76.2
8	PR–E	714	3.7	79.9
9	M–PR	625	3.2	83.1
10	U–E	482	2.5	85.6
11	U–M	343	1.8	87.4
12	U–P	323	1.7	89.1
13	U–J	220	1.1	90.2
14	N–P	193	1.0	91.2

* Key: PR (patient rooms), N (nurses' station), U (utility room), E (elevator lobby), M (medication closet), P (pantry), J (janitor's closet).

TABLE 10. Differences in traffic patterns between total traffic on the unit and nursing traffic only (first 14 links).

Rank	Link*	Percentage	Link	Percentage
1	PR–PR	19.1%	PR–PR	16.3%
2	N–PR	16.7	N–PR	15.9
3	U–PR	14.1	U–PR	15.4
4	N–U	9.8	N–U	9.9
5	N–E	6.1	N–M	7.0
6	N–M	5.8	M–PR	3.8
7	PR–P	4.6	N–E	3.7
8	PR–E	3.7	PR–P	2.3
9	M–PR	3.2	PR–E	2.1
10	U–E	2.5	M–U	2.1
11	U–M	1.8	U–E	1.9
12	U–P	1.7	U–P	1.9
13	U–J	1.1	N–P	0.9
14	N–P	1.0	U–J	0.4

* See note, table 9 for key.

type, the totals are reduced to 91 and 120, respectively —still far too many to examine and draw direct conclusions from. However, many possible links were either not used at all or used so seldom they did not matter. Also, as might be expected, a relatively small group of links accounted for the large majority of trips. From shift to shift, with one or two exceptions, the 14 links chosen retained their relative importance.

It also had to be decided whether to determine traffic patterns from the total traffic on the unit or from nursing traffic alone (70.3 percent of the total). Table 10 shows the difference between the two. For the first four links there is no conflict. For the purposes of this study it was decided to use the total traffic on the unit to determine the relative importance of traffic links.

Variables

In figures 252–54, it is demonstrated that differences among shifts, services, and type of unit are not significant and need not be allowed for in design. The overall average ranking of traffic links will hold for all types of units at all times and can be used to establish priorities for the relationship of facilities when designing medical or surgical nursing units. Staffing patterns may change from private to semi-private units, bed capacities may vary, but there is no real, fundamental difference in the relationships of functional areas to one another. The key areas, evolved after long years of trial and error, were included in the nursing unit because the nursing unit needed them. The same need will be found in every nursing unit, and relationships among facilities will be about the same from one nursing unit to another.

It is not likely that team nursing would change the pattern. It does break up traffic into smaller subunits and perhaps permits the nurse to travel· less, but nurses everywhere tend to organize their work in such a way as to avoid long trips when possible. It is not always possible. A large part of nursing activity is random, in response to patient calls that cannot be foreseen. Neither in team nor in functional nursing can a completely planned travel routine be adhered to, and thus the effect of team nursing on the ranking of traffic links would probably be relatively unimportant.

Certain other factors influence the volume of traffic: whether patients are housed in single-bed or multiple-bed rooms, whether toilets and lavatories are included in patient rooms or centrally located in the hall. But unless multiple-bed rooms are so vast that one of them can keep a whole team of nurses occupied, there always will be traffic between patient rooms. Grouping patients tends to reduce the traffic somewhat, but the random nature of patient calls will always serve to prevent them from being drastically reduced, no matter how many multiple-bed rooms there are.[2]

Other Considerations

One possible inaccuracy involved in measuring nursing activity in terms of numbers of trips is that to a certain extent proximity generates travel. There was lively activity at the Yale–New Haven, for instance, between the nurses' station and the medicine closet directly opposite; had it been at more of a remove, the nurses would have taken good care to spare themselves many of those trips.

Numbers of trips did not always indicate quantity of services performed. When nurses went to tend four patients in a four-bedded room, they took with them what they needed for four patients, yet this would count only as one trip.

Some trips can scarcely be called functional—trips to search for people or things, trips to pick up a forgotten object, to say something one forgot to say, to make coffee, particularly at night. There are trips that are really nothing but an aimless wandering, but such trips are also part of any system with human components.

The tops of the nursing activity columns best convey the volume of nursing at any time of day—not the total activity columns but the nursing activity columns, and there look not at sheer height alone but also at the fluctuation at the top. At certain periods of the day all the nursing staff on any unit are working at about the maximum rate. How long such periods will last depends on how many patients are in the unit and how much care this group of patients requires. A maximum rate of traffic is sustained much longer on a 48-bed unit than on a 30-bed unit of equally sick patients.

Total traffic was somewhat higher on the medical floor than on the surgical, and professional (not auxiliary) nursing traffic was much higher on the medical floor, probably because emergencies and nonroutine situations are likelier to arise on medical units. There were more trips centering around diet on the medical unit—diet is more important in the treatment of medical than of routine surgical patients.

Four single rooms were set aside for critical or noisy patients on the semiprivate unit, and they received a larger share of the traffic. With this exception, patients were not sorted out so that the sickest ones who required most care and therefore most trips were in any particular rooms. The probability that any room might be the maximum traffic room was thus the same for all rooms. The distribution of trips to rooms being essentially random, we were able to conceive of the category "patient room" as a single

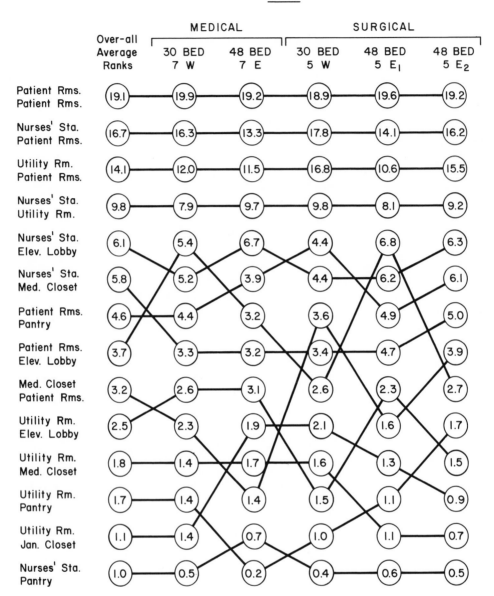

Fig. 252. Differences in relative ranking of the links, day shift.

room, chosen at random and separately analyzed to determine the maximum number of trips in which that one room might be involved. This was a better link than the broader category, "patient rooms," which implies a single area with one entrance located in a particular place.

Traffic from one patient room to another was greatly influenced by the geometry of the V-shaped plan. Having the nurses' station, utility room, and other central facilities at the apex of the V had the effect of dividing patient rooms into two distinct groups. Even when there was a great deal of room-to-room traffic (during the day shift), very little traffic went from one wing to the other. Nurses assigned to care for a particular group of patients never had them scattered in both wings. If the wings of the V are taken together, the average distance between patient rooms is 92.5 feet, but considering each wing separately the average distance between patient rooms is only 31.2 feet. This comes a lot closer to our figure of 29.5 feet as the average distance *traveled* between patient rooms.

The Yale Traffic Index

It was then possible to develop a single index by means of which design schemes for general medical and surgical nursing units could be compared for

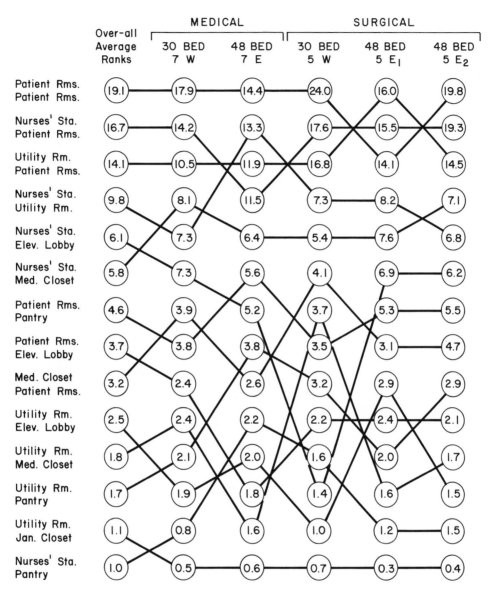

Fig. 253. Differences in relative ranking of the links, evening shift.

functional efficiency. Anyone who must make decisions in building a hospital should have at hand an objective method for comparing optional choices. In deciding among different layouts of the functional spaces of a nursing unit, a most significant criterion should be their relative efficiency. How well do these plans provide for staff traffic? Are related functional areas placed close together? Number of beds per 10 running feet of corridor does not answer either question or, indeed, give anything but the linear density of patients.

Two critical variables, and only two, were involved in developing this index. They were (1) distance be-

tween areas and (2) the relative number of times this distance must be traversed—the most efficient unit being one on which, during any 24-hour period, the minimum total distance is traveled in order to perform the necessary tasks.

It is very easy to determine all distances between areas—except those between patient rooms. From patient rooms to any other functional area the average distance from the entire patient room area may be used since traffic is either uniform or essentially random—uniform for housekeeping and dietary maids, random for nurses whose sickest patient may-be lodged in any one of the rooms. However, the dis-

NIGHT

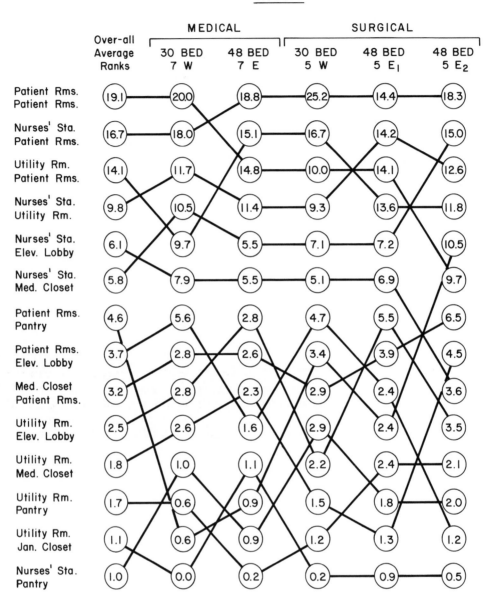

Fig. 254. Differences in relative ranking of the links, night shift.

tances between patient rooms present a real problem because the pattern is neither random nor entirely planned, because it is dependent on both physical layout and staffing pattern, and because there is so much of this kind of traffic. The factors are beyond the scope of the designer. Patient demand and the ability of staff members to plan their own traffic pattern can be neither foreseen nor controlled. For this reason, we propose simply using the minimum average distance between rooms in calculating our index. Minimum average distance is the shortest path by which one could make a complete circuit of rooms in a particular group, divided by the number of rooms.

The number of times a given path was traveled can be represented by the percentage of total traffic it accounts for. We listed the 14 traffic links most frequently used according to the percent of total traffic accounted for by each one; this number was called the a factor. We multiplied the minimum average distance d by the sum of the a factors. The traffic index I_t therefore becomes

$$I_t = \sum_1^{14} d\,(a).$$

Thus far, neither unit size (patient or bed capacity) nor type of accommodations (single or multiple) has been taken into account. It is fairly obvious that an index calculated for a 30-bed unit is likely to be different from one calculated for a 48-bed unit, even assuming the same type of accommodations. In order to compare relative efficiencies of nursing floor designs, the basic index must be divided by the number of patients cared for, N. This gives us I_t/N, a number that will tell us the distance (in feet, meters, yards, or whatever) traveled per patient. This number is useful for deciding nursing unit sizes and types of accommodations.

The Yale Traffic Index Applied

$\dfrac{I_t}{N}$: we at once applied the formula to the nursing units we had been studying. Table 11 shows how traffic index was calculated for the 48-bed semiprivate unit. Table 12 gives the rating for the 30-bed private unit.

We were able to make the Yale Traffic Index much more universally applicable by breaking up the utility room complex, ranking its component parts, and incorporating those rankings in the index instead of ranking the utility room as a whole. The utility room at Yale–New Haven is a single unit. We mounted a utility room study (admittedly with very short links) that made it possible to extend the findings to institutions where utility room components are separately housed. This done, the last real objection seemed to be overcome. A promising new tool had been devised for measuring the efficiency of many different unit plans and, with considerable eagerness, we set out to do so. We took all the old tools along, all the existing yardsticks—number of beds per 10 running feet of corridor, distance from the nursing station to the farthest bed, number of beds per 100 square feet of area—to find out whether any of them agreed with the Yale Traffic Index or, for that matter, with one another.

To compare designs for the nursing unit, we had to make two basic assumptions. The first was that activities performed by nurses are relatively uniform throughout the United States.[3] The second was that with similar facilities, traffic links will assume the same importance independent of plan configurations. We were especially eager to find out whether any basic configuration resulted in consistently efficient nursing unit designs.

Comparisons between units in terms of efficiency generally boil down to a discussion of circulation—that is, corridor length and arrangement. So we decided to classify plans according to circulation: simple (only one path from *A* to *B*) or compound (alternate paths from *A* to *B*; this type is also called redundant). Although corridors in particular schemes may have several branches, circulation is essentially simple so

TABLE 11. Calculation of the traffic index of the 48-bed semiprivate unit at the Yale–New Haven Hospital (5, 6, 7 East). Tabular form for computation.

Rank	Link*	a	d	da
1	PR–PR	19.1	16.8	320.88
2	N–PR	16.7	71.7	1197.39
3	U–PR	14.1	60.7	855.87
4	N–U	9.8	12.0	117.60
5	N–E	6.1	12.0	73.20
6	N–M	5.8	9.0	52.20
7	PR–K	4.6	82.5	379.50
8	PR–E	3.7	74.5	275.65
9	M–PR	3.2	72.7	142.08
10	U–E	2.5	13.0	32.50
11	U–M	1.8	12.0	21.60
12	U–K	1.7	22.0	37.40
13	U–J	1.1	20.0	22.00
14	N–K	1.0	20.0	20.00
				$\overline{3547.87} = I_t$

$$\frac{I_t}{N} = \frac{3547.87}{48} = 73.91$$

* See note, table 9 for key; also K (kitchen).

TABLE 12. Calculation of the traffic index of the 30-bed private unit at the Yale–New Haven Hospital (5, 6, 7 West).

Rank	Link*	a	d	da
1	PR–PR	19.1	11.1	212.58
2	N–PR	16.7	69.3	1157.81
3	U–PR	14.1	36.3	512.25
4	N–U	9.8	12.0	117.60
5	N–E	6.1	12.0	73.20
6	N–M	5.8	9.0	52.20
7	PR–K	4.6	98.5	453.10
8	PR–E	3.7	75.0	277.50
9	M–PR	3.2	72.7	232.64
10	U–E	2.5	13.0	32.50
11	U–M	1.8	12.0	21.60
12	U–K	1.7	22.0	37.40
13	U–J	1.1	20.0	22.50
14	N–K	1.0	20.0	20.00
				$\overline{3222.38} = I_t$

$$\frac{I_t}{N} = \frac{3222.38}{30} = 107.41$$

* See note, table 9 for key; also K (kitchen).

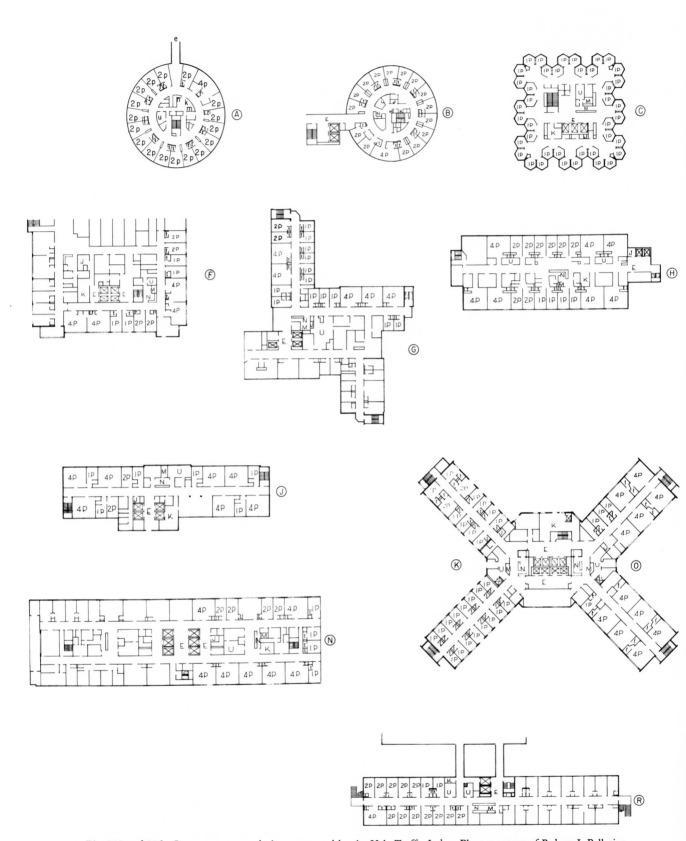

Fig. 255 and 256. Contemporary ward plans measured by the Yale Traffic Index. Plans courtesy of Robert J. Pelletier.

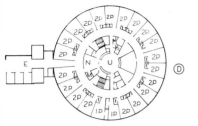

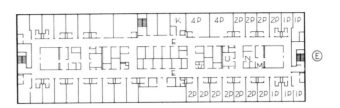

KEY:

N – Nurses' Station
U – Utility Room(s)
M – Medication Storage
K – Kitchen or Pantry
E – Entrance or Elev. Lobby
J – Janitor's Closet
IP, 2P, 4P – Patient Rms. by No. Beds

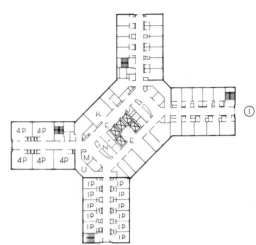

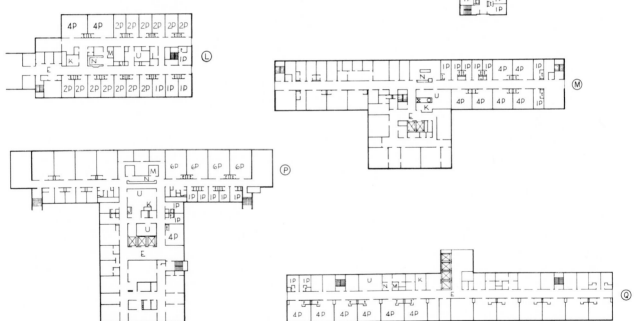

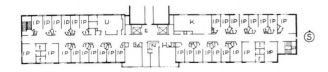

HOSPITAL	CIRCULATION SIMPLE	COMP.	RANK	YALE INDEX	RANK	N. STA. TO PATIENT ROOM·	RANK	NO. BEDS 10 RUNNING FEET COR.	RANK	NO. BEDS 100 SQ. FT.
A		✔	1	2106	1	44	1	2.52	5	0.462
B		✔	2	2215	2	49	3	2.35	3	0.491
C		✔	3	2551	6	71	17	1.35	9	0.396
D		✔	4	2552	7	76	4	2.30	6	0.432
E		✔	5	2677	3	62	15	1.39	19	0.308
F	✔		6	2706	5	68	19	1.29	8	0.410
G	✔		7	3185	13	88	11	1.53	2	0.513
H	✔		8	3233	11	82	13	1.48	14	0.340
I	✔		9	3246	9	80	8	1.90	18	0.326
J	✔		10	3301	10	82	2	2.46	10	0.388
K	✔		11	3315	17	102	18	1.33	16	0.336
L		✔	12	3344	14	88	16	1.38	13	0.352
M	✔		13	3546	16	98	10	1.67	7	0.430
N		✔	14	3609	4	62	14	1.41	12	0.357
O	✔		15	3618	15	97	6	2.13	11	0.364
P	✔		16	3739	8	80	5	2.27	4	0.480
Q	✔		17	3789	12	87	7	1.95	17	0.336
R	✔		18	3986	19	112	9	1.81	1	0.597
S	✔		19	4356	18	104	12	1.49	15	0.339

Fig. 257. Ward plans of Figs. 255 and 256 evaluated by the Yale Traffic Index and others.

long as the branches do not rejoin to form closed loops. Plans in the shape of a straight line, a V, a T, a U, and so forth are usually simple circulation schemes, whereas double-corridor plans, circular plans, and square plans are *usually* redundant circulation schemes.

In figures 255 and 256, the plans we measured are sketched and lettered, and in figure 257 they are evaluated by our index and others. No correlation whatever was found among efficiency criteria. The older criteria, which measure density, do not agree with one another or with the Yale Index.

Our traffic index fairly well establishes that redundant circulation schemes are more efficient than simple ones, especially when nursing units of more than 30 beds are involved. Thirty plans may be too small a sample to draw other detailed conclusions from with certainty, but table 13, which relates the index ratings of the units to their size, demolishes one long-cherished bit of folklore. Inpatient unit efficiency is *not* directly related to unit size. An extreme instance of this can be seen in comparing one design with 26 beds (plan Q) to another with 42 beds (plan C). The smaller

unit was 48 percent *less* efficient than the larger. The variation was caused by a difference in *design*. In fact, within the range of sizes considered, the design of the inpatient unit is the most crucial factor in determining the efficiency of the unit. One double-corridor plan, which would be expected to rank high on the Yale Traffic Index because of its compound circulation scheme, proved even less efficient than any shown in figure 256 for one reason only: the architects placed the nursing station at the head of the unit, near the elevators, thus completely sacrificing efficiency for the sake of being able to control vertical traffic (see Appendix).

Though size is not the determining factor for efficiency of a nursing unit, neither is privacy. Using a privacy index[4] to rank the 30 units by the degree of privacy they offered, we found no correlation with efficiency. Of two plans featuring all-private rooms, which were therefore ranked 1.5 as far as privacy was concerned, one ranked fifth in efficiency and the other twenty-ninth. The two plans offering least privacy to patients ranked tenth and thirtieth in the traffic index. We repeat: design is the thing that dic-

TABLE 13. Ranking of 30 inpatient units
according to efficiency, privacy, and size.

Architectural Type	Circulation	YTI Rank	Privacy Index Rank	Size Rank
Circular	Compound	1	22.0	19.0
Circular	Compound	2	21.0	13.5
Circular	Compound	3	15.0	4.0
Square	Compound	4	26.0	9.0
Square	Compound	5	1.5	9.0
Circular	Compound	6	5.0	29.5
Double corridor	Compound	7	13.0	19.0
Semicircular	Simple	8	14.0	27.5
Semisquare	Simple	9	20.0	25.0
Double corridor	Compound	10	29.0	4.0
D-L* single corridor	Simple	11	6.0	27.5
Square	Compound	12	7.0	2.0
D-L vee	Simple	13	8.0	15.0
D-L single corridor	Simple	14	12.0	9.0
Square	Compound	15	10.0	9.0
D-L vee	Simple	16	9.0	21.5
D-L vee	Simple	17	11.0	4.0
D-L single corridor	Simple	18	23.0	13.5
D-L vee	Simple	19	3.0	23.5
Double corridor	Compound	20	19.0	12.0
D-L single corridor	Simple	21	16.0	21.5
Double corridor	Compound	22	25.0	9.0
D-L vee	Simple	23	27.0	1.0
D-L vee	Simple	24	24.0	17.0
D-L single corridor	Simple	25	28.0	26.0
D-L single corridor	Simple	26	18.0	19.0
Single-loaded single corridor	Simple	27	17.0	23.5
D-L single corridor	Simple	28	4.0	16.0
D-L single corridor	Simple	29	1.5	29.5
Double corridor	Compound	30	30.0	6.0

SOURCE: Adapted from John D. Thompson and Robert J. Pelletier, "Privacy vs. Efficiency in the Inpatient Unit," *Hospitals, 36* (August 16, 1962).
   * Double-Loaded.

tates efficiency, not the size of the unit or the degree of privacy granted to patients in it.

Thus was devised the Yale Traffic Index, an objective measure of efficiency applicable to American nursing units in whatever shape they were conceived. It has helped the designer to know in advance how much he must pay in terms of the amenities for the ultimate in functional efficiency. We put the measuring tool into his hands, with the hope that sometimes he decides in favor of the amenities.

CHAPTER 16

Maternity: Analysis of a Random Service

In the discussion of research approaches to hospital problems (chapter 10), the maternity service was cited as an area of hospital care in which, were all births uncomplicated, a random Poisson distribution might be used to predict occupancy, or, were all births induced, prediction by a pattern of scheduling admissions might be possible. But although most births in the hospital are indeed normal births, one must take into account Caesarean sections; and if the particular hospital follows a policy of induced labor in a significant number of cases, that also destroys the random pattern. Hospitals in general are a mixed system. The maternity service is more random than medicine, which in turn is more random than surgery. Expected occupancy levels vary inversely with the degree of randomness.

Problems of occupancy in a partly random, partly scheduled service can best be approached by simulation on the computer. Because of a more random nature and relatively limited number of complications (cases with serious complications are transferred to another service), the maternity service lends itself to computer analysis. So many contingencies may be expected in other departments that, as yet, we cannot simulate the total patient load on a computer. Maternity therefore may stand for the hospital in the study of a question that has fascinated hospital planners and administrators for years: what is the relationship between size, as measured by average daily census, and percentage of beds occupied? This is not merely a theoretical problem; it has its economic aspect. If the factor of size in small hospitals is in itself the cause for a low percentage of occupancy and consequent high operating costs, this relationship is much more than fascinating and should be understood as a basic determinant of hospital economics.

In investigating the obstetrical service, our purpose was twofold: to demonstrate that its size (as measured by number of patients discharged) affects the average occupancy and to show the effect of size in terms of investment costs and direct costs of operation.

Relationship between the Size of a Maternity Service and Its Average Occupancy

The 33 hospitals in Connecticut with obstetrical service were divided into three groups according to the number of obstetrical discharges: Group I with 2,000 discharges a year (table 14), Group II with 1,000–2,000 discharges a year (table 15), and Group III with fewer than 1,000 (table 16). The fifth column of these tables shows the variation in average occupancy from 70.6 percent in the larger hospitals to 43.6 percent in the smaller ones. Table 17 gives results, which, when subjected to Fisher's Exact Test, reveal that percentage of occupancy in Group III hospitals was significantly lower than in Groups I and II and that percentage of occupancy in Group II was significantly lower than in Group I (with the largest maternity service).

If the data on size are corrected according to average length of stay, a vital factor that might influence occupancy, there is still a significant difference in percentages of occupancy between Groups I and II and between Groups I and III. Only the significant difference between Groups II and III disappears. This information may be found in column 4 of tables 14–16.

Can the data be corrected according to the other factor influencing occupancy, that is, supply of beds relative to demand? This is harder, and prediction is more difficult still. A useful calculation is that the size of each maternity service should equal its average census plus three times the square root of its average census.[1] Table 18 shows the way hospitals in each of the three groups satisfied this criterion. It can be seen that in meeting the criterion there is no significant difference among groups. Twenty-five of the 33 hospitals were within plus or minus 5 beds of the result, and for the entire state of Connecticut the net difference between projected and actual beds was only −13 in a total of 1,150 maternity beds.

Thus from actual data gathered in the 33 hospitals in Connecticut that contain maternity beds, there are indications that the size of the maternity service does have some influence on the occupancy percentage of the service, although the factors of average length of stay and supply of beds relative to demand were not held exactly constant in fixing this relationship.

Simulation is the way to hold these two factors constant. The activity of the maternity service can be simulated and the number of admissions be varied. Because average length of stay and number of beds relative to demand would remain constant for all runs, a direct relationship of size to occupancy could then be determined.[2]

TABLE 14. Selected maternity and financial statistics, Group I hospitals
(more than 2,000 discharges per year).

Hospital	Discharges	Patient days	Average days stay	Percentage of occupancy	Average beds in complement	Beds required using $3 \sqrt{}$ A.C.	Direct cost of routine services	Net gain or loss
I-1	6,275	30,758	4.902	73.3	115	112	$5.20	($1.80)
I-2	5,503	25,356	4.608	73.9	94	94	6.10	4.20
I-3	3,592	14,165	3.943	66.9	58	57	4.33	12.79
I-4	3,503	16,676	4.760	68.2	67	66	7.44	(2.35)
I-5	3,292	13,039	3.961	74.4	48	54	8.60	3.82
I-6	2,685	12,058	4.491	62.3	53	50	6.36	(0.05)
I-7	2,671	12,011	4.497	71.5	46	50	7.13	(1.84)
I-8	2,406	10,727	4.458	77.3	38	50	5.91	2.04
I-9	2,289	9,047	3.952	63.6	39	40	7.22	(2.31)
I-10	2,158	10,608	4.916	72.7	40	45	5.46	1.07
Weighted average			4.493	70.6			$6.22	$1.51

TABLE 15. Selected maternity and financial statistics, Group II hospital
(1,000–2,000 discharges per year).

Hospital	Discharges	Patient days	Average days stay	Percentage of occupancy	Average beds in complement	Beds required using $3 \sqrt{}$ A.C.	Direct cost of routine services	Net gain or loss
II-1	1,949	8,969	4,602	53.4	46	39	$4.71	($1.50)
II-2	1,778	6,771	3.808	64.0	29	31	8.51	1.95
II-3	1,775	7,022	3.956	66.3	29	32	7.67	3.10
II-4	1,725	7,751	4.493	75.8	28	35	8.08	4.14
II-5	1,685	6,759	4.011	50.0	37	31	4.32	(0.99)
II-6	1,609	6,229	3,871	71.1	24	29	6.32	1.47
II-7	1,472	6,416	4.359	53.3	33	30	8.39	(4.26)
II-8	1,393	8,282	5.945	54.0	42	37	6.99	(5.31)
II-9	1,360	6,914	5.084	65.3	29	32	7.05	(3.44)
II-10	1,300	8,155	6.273	79.8	28	37	8.42	(2.36)
II-11	1,210	5,058	4.180	57.7	24	25	4.51	3.88
II-12	1,161	4,764	4.103	42.1	31	24	9.12	(6.82)
Weighted average			4.512	59.9			$6.97	($ .86)

TABLE 16. Selected maternity and financial statistics, Group III hospital
(fewer than 1,000 discharges per year).

Hospital	Discharges	Patient days	Average days stay	Percentage of occupancy	Average beds in complement	Beds required, using $3 \sqrt{}$ A.C.	Direct cost of routine services	Net gain or loss
III-1	987	4,057	4.107	42.7	26	21	$12.68	($13.45)
III-2	906	3,989	4.403	42.9	25	21	6.40	(4.01)
III-3	903	3,426	3.794	40.8	23	19	10.62	(6.82)
III-4	806	3,468	4.303	52.8	18	19	11.40	(4.12)
III-5	764	2,113	2.766	57.9	10	13	12.71	(7.00)
III-6	639	2,814	4.404	77.1	10	16	9.14	.36
III-7	570	2,528	4.345	49.5	14	15	9.09	(7.76)
III-8	458	1,790	3.908	40.1	12	12	6.13	(4.74)
III-9	396	1,689	4.265	46.3	10	11	18.51	(18.08)
III-10	338	1,491	4.411	40.8	10	10	5.66	(5.57)
III-11	329	1,344	4.085	26.3	14	9	13.67	(21.66)
Weighted average			3.856	43.6			$10.55	($ 7.97)

TABLE 17. Distribution of individual hospitals by group, above and below
median occupancy rate (62.3% in hospital I-6).

	Group I	Group II	Group III	Total
Occupancy above 62.3%	9	6	1	16
Occupancy below 62.3%	0	6	10	16
	—	—	—	—
	9	12	11	32

TABLE 18. Number of hospitals in each group with a capacity greater than,
or less than, the average census plus three times the square root of the
average census.

	Group I	Group II	Group III	Total
Capacity of average census + 3 times the square root of the average census.	1	0	2	3
Capacity greater than average census + 3 times the square root of the average census.	4	5	4	13
Capacity less than average census + 3 times the square root of the average census.	5	7	5	17
	—	—	—	—
	10	12	11	33

TABLE 19. Facilities required for maternity service.

Admissions per year	90% Service		95% Service		99% Service					
	Beds	Beds per 100 patients per year	Beds	Beds per 100 patients per year	Beds	Beds per 100 patients per year	Department*			
							LR	PPR	CSR	DR
580	13	2.24	14	2.42	17	2.93	2	1	1	1
1,693	33	1.94	35	2.07	40	2.36	4	1	1	2
2,771	51	1.84	54	1.95	60	2.17	5	2	1	2
3,874	70	1.81	73	1.88	80	2.06	7	2	1	3
5,000	89	1.78	93	1.86	102	2.04	8	2	1	3
5,506	98	1.78	102	1.85	110	2.00	8	3	1	3
6,106	110	1.80	114	1.86	122	2.00	9	3	1	4
7,229	124	1.72	128	1.76	135	1.87	10	3	1	4
8,161	145	1.78	150	1.84	160	1.96	12	3	2	4
9,424	165	1.75	170	1.82	180	1.91	13	4	2	5

* LR = Labor rooms.
  PPR = Postpartum rooms.
  CSR = Caesarean section rooms.
  DR = Delivery rooms.

In order to demonstrate how simulation can aid prediction in this experiment, the input distribution was based on actual figures from the Yale–New Haven Hospital in 1961 (Hospital I-2). The rate of input was increased and decreased while preserving the original relative distributions. From this hospital's records, service times were taken for the facilities involved. Number of beds and number of facilities (labor rooms, delivery rooms, postpartum rooms) were made large enough so that jamming would not occur. The output shows the service that might be expected from any arrangement of facilities. The service level was set at 95 percent with the idea that the remaining 5 percent of patients would be fitted in somehow by providing flexible facilities or discharging convalescents early. Then the cost and efficiency of maternity units could be plotted as a function of the admission rate. Table 19 gives the results of such a simulation run.

Figure 258 presents as a graph the relationship between size and occupancy, expressed as the number of beds needed to serve 100 patients a year. (Differences in length of stay and supply–demand were eliminated.) In maternity services with 4,000 or more births a year there seems to be little difference in occupancy, but below that rate the number of beds needed for 100 patients a year tends to rise, and where there are less than 1,800 births a year it rises more noticeably.

Relationship between the Size of a Maternity Service and Its Investment Costs

Figure 258 also demonstrates that bed investment costs level off at 4,000 admissions a year, but below that number they rise, higher and higher as admissions decrease. Table 19 gives as a function of the admission rate the number of labor, delivery, and postpartum facilities required. For lower admission rates an even higher investment in these facilities is required. Yet the point can be discerned at which size ceases to pay off in terms of lowered investment cost per patient served.

Relationship between the Size of a Maternity Service and Its Operating Costs

Operating costs are difficult to isolate. From available data it can at least be inferred that direct costs per day are more than proportionately higher for maternity suites serving a small population.

Direct cost of routine services for maternity patients, as reported in Connecticut, was used as the cleanest figure obtainable. It is uninfluenced by variables such as interest charges, overhead allocations, and special services. When this cost was compared with hours of bedside care, the correlation was +0.957—close

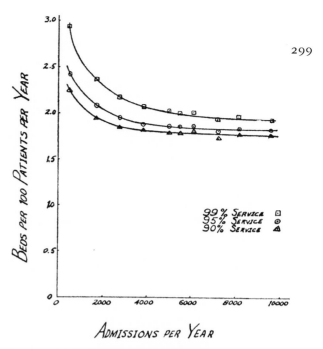

Fig. 258. Relationship between maternity beds required and size of maternity service (for three service levels).

enough that one may suppose that it reflects labor costs involved in the actual operation of the maternity ward.

Of total costs of $37.77, the corrected average direct cost of routine services for the 33 hospitals in Connecticut was $6.94 per patient day. For Group I hospitals, average cost per day was $6.22, for Group II $6.97, for Group III $10.55, a difference between the two extremes of $4.33 a day. Expressed as a percentage, Group III hospitals with the smallest maternity units cost 69.6 percent more per patient day than Group I hospitals with the largest maternity units. These costs are analyzed in table 20 as occupancy was analyzed in table 17.

Although differences among the hospitals within a group are not as marked as in some of the previous tables, there is still a significant difference in costs between Group I and Group III. When this is added to the differences in average groups costs, the evidence warrants the conclusion that size of unit affects not only investment costs but the direct cost of operating the unit as well.

It has been a long time since per diem costs were $37.77 for maternity cases. The figures for 1973 were $139.71 for a maternity and $55.93 for a newborn day. From the point of view of inpatient unit design, however, an even more important fact is that in 1973 the former pattern of close relationship among need, demand, and supply (the maternity service's most unique characteristic) had disappeared—at least in Connecticut. Whereas the Poisson-like model described above was theoretically still sound, its relevance to the actual situation in hospitals was not nearly so clear in 1973 as in 1961. The reasons for this are evident in figure 259, which shows bed capacity, maternity and nonmaternity, and days of care rendered

TABLE 20. Distribution of individual hospitals, direct cost of routine services by group above and below median (median cost $7.22 in hospital I-9).

	Group I	Group II	Group III	Total
Direct cost of routine services				
Above $7.22	2	6	8	16
Below $7.22	7	6	3	16
	9	12	11	32

TABLE 21. Distribution of individual hospitals by group above and below median gain or loss on maternity services (median loss $2.31 in hospital I-9).

	Group I	Group II	Group III	Total
Loss above $2.31	1	5	10	16
Loss below $2.31	8	7	1	16
	9	13	11	32

TABLE 22. Comparison of requirements for one centralized versus three decentralized maternity services.

	Beds	Labor rooms	Postpartum rooms	Caesarean section rooms	Delivery rooms
Required for 1,300–1,400 admissions per year	30	3	1	1	2
	30	3	1	1	2
	30	3	1	1	2
Total facilities for three separate maternity units	90	9	3	3	6
Required for 3,900–4,200 admissions per year	75	7	2	1	3

in each of the two services in Connecticut hospitals from 1960 to 1973. In the nonmaternity service the relationship between beds and patient days is quite clear—particularly so when measured against population growth, represented by the dotted line. The demand for maternity beds, on the other hand, did not keep up with the supply. Two factors were responsible for this. During the first half of the period the average length of time that maternity patients stayed in the hospital dropped from 4.5 to 3.9 days; during the second half, the number of mothers admitted for delivery fell from 55,000 to 39,000. With such a decrease in demand, one could not close maternity beds fast enough.

Total costs per day are made up of many components —too many to reflect the economic relationships among size, occupancy, and costs. Nevertheless,

they can be compared with gross revenue to convey the magnitude of the problem. In 1961 it was found that whereas the average total cost per day was $37.77, the average income was $37.46—an operating loss of $0.31 a day. However, when the hospitals were examined by group a different picture emerged. Group I hospitals (the largest ones) showed an average *profit* of $1.51 per patient day on the maternity service, while in hospitals of Groups II and III the maternity service showed a *loss* of $0.86 and $7.97 a day, respectively (table 21). In 1973 the trend was even more marked. Group I hospitals showed an average gross deficit of $1.45 per patient day on the maternity service, while in hospitals of Groups II and III the maternity service showed a deficit of $13.86 and $29.90 per patient day, respectively. Thus small hospitals not only pay more for a maternity service

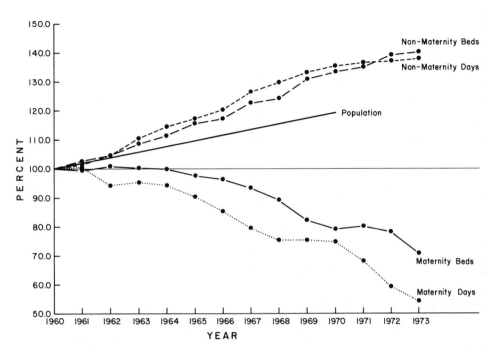

Fig. 259. Percent increase-decrease of bed capacity and days of care rendered in maternity and non-maternity services in Connecticut hospitals from 1960 to 1973.

but they are also less able to recover their costs than larger hospitals.

Discussion and Application

These findings are important for three reasons: (1) they increase our general knowledge of the basic economic behavior of a hospital subsystem; (2) a methodology has been evolved (in this instance a computer simulation) that enables the researcher to study the problem in its pure state, freed from the inadequacies of empirical information; and (3) the results can be applied to hospital planning and administration.

Their most immediate, obvious application would be to the maternity services of the 33 Connecticut hospitals. Thirteen are located in six cities, five of which have two hospitals while one has three. If we compare our predictions of an economically feasible unit with actual experience in the cities where there was more than one hospital, some rather startling results emerge.

In one of the cities there was a Group II hospital with a 37-bed maternity unit. It was economically of marginal size, but because the community had to have the service there was no alternative. Very shortly after World War II, a second hospital was built in the same town with a 10-bed maternity unit. The 37-bed unit had been reduced to 15 beds by 1973, and at last report the larger unit was operating at 64.1 percent occupancy and the smaller unit at 34.1 percent occupancy.[3] The two units were being maintained at enormous cost to the community. It would have been far more economical to concentrate all the maternity beds the town required in the one unit. Predictions of the kind made possible by the simulator would have allowed the direct pricing of alternatives.

At the time of the original study, in another part of the state were three hospitals within approximately seven miles of one another. Each one discharged approximately 1,300 patients a year from its maternity service. Table 22 gives projected requirements of three maternity services with 1,300–1,400 admissions a year. The total facilities required for the three may be compared with the facilities required for a single maternity service with 3,900–4,200 admissions a year. Not only can a substantial saving of personnel be anticipated from one unit that replaces three, but fewer beds, serving a larger population, would result in higher occupancy. In addition, delivery suite requirements for a single unit are significantly less than for three services operating independently. (It is important to stress here that the same level of service is postulated for all of them.)

With information of this kind, unnecessary and expensive duplication of maternity beds in a community can be avoided. The cost of multiple units, especially where duplication results in each of them being of uneconomic size, can be clearly presented to the community. In the case just cited, perhaps if costs had been stated in these terms in advance, different

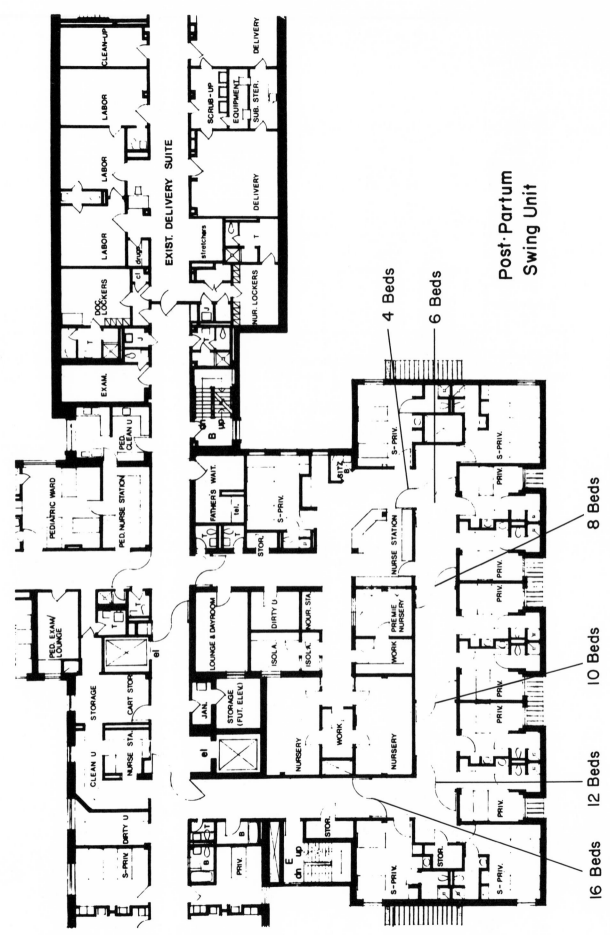

Fig. 260. Early plan for a swing unit. Courtesy Bruce Arniel.

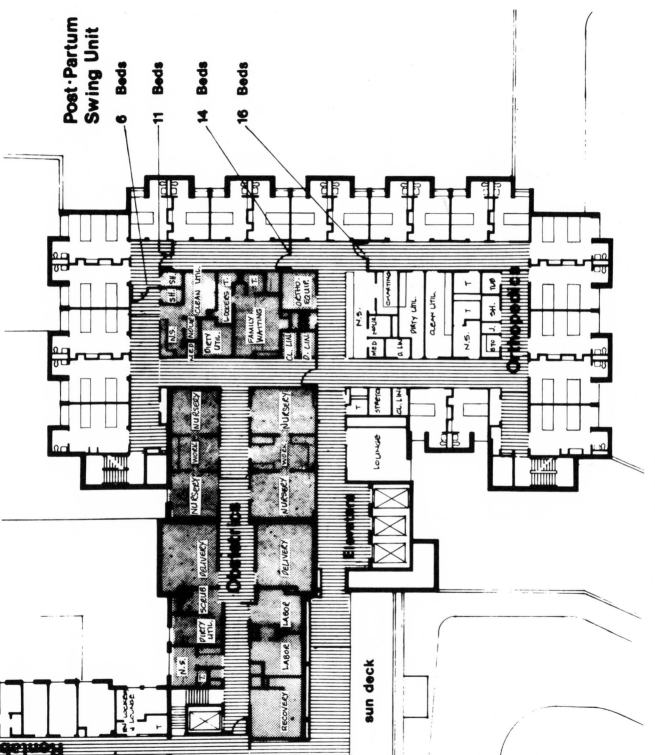

Fig. 261. Plan for a swing unit constructed in 1970.

arrangements would have been made. When coupled with higher direct operating costs in services designed for patient populations of about 1,000 a year, the economics involved seem to us quite clear.

What about a hospital that must have a small obstetrical service simply because it is the only hospital in the community? Can its obstetrical beds be freed from this Poisson-like prison of random demand, low occupancy, and high costs? The legally mandated isolation of obstetrical beds from those on other services not only results in low occupancy for this service but may also result in waiting lines in surgery, for example, because empty obstetrical beds cannot be utilized for surgical patients.

If isolation is required for medical reasons, the cost of the policy is one the community must bear. If, however, a separate system is maintained because of outmoded regulations, this study demonstrates what such regulations cost. Is it not time to inquire into the validity of medical reasons that dictated a practice of not treating nonmaternity patients in the maternity service? Substitution of a mixed input, part random, part scheduled, such as could be initiated by admitting clean gynecological cases, would raise the percentage of occupancy of maternity beds. At a time of wildly rising hospital costs, is it not necessary to consider every possible alternative that might result in more efficient utilization of hospital beds with a consequent decrease in cost per patient day?

One effective alternative available to us even now is to design a "swing unit" that can be enlarged or contracted depending on the maternity service load. The design constraints for such a unit would stipulate complete separation of the staffs involved and of ancillary areas such as utility rooms and nursing stations. Patient rooms must, in other words, not only be redesignated as to type of occupant but arranged so they may be attached to another nursing unit while preserving the integrity of the maternity unit.

Two such units are illustrated, one that has been in operation for some time (fig. 260) and one constructed in 1970 (fig. 261). In the plans the ability to increase or decrease the number of maternity beds is indicated by corridor doors that may be opened or shut, defining the limits of the maternity unit. It should be noted that the newborn nursery does not change; in both units it is located in a cul-de-sac unaffected by changes in maternity bed assignment.

In these two units computer-based information was translated into design—into a plan allowing for an optimum of the two design determinants of efficiency and a sanitary environment. We strongly feel that computer models of the kind described in this chapter can and should play an important role in hospital planning. The benefits to be derived for both planning and operation can best be appreciated when we contemplate the magnitude of the sum allocated in our economy to these services.

CHAPTER 17

The Economics of Privacy

The practice of allowing a private room for medical or economic reasons (for certain types of illness or because the patient can pay for it) has been referred to again and again in this book.[1] But the issue, always controversial, of how much privacy the hospital patient is to be allowed has become increasingly complicated. The degree of privacy often describes the financial relationship between patient and hospital; it may also indicate the patient's medical sponsorship. The terms *private, semiprivate,* and *ward* were extended to apply to different patterns of medical care rendered to the different classes of patients. This classification led to an uncomfortable feeling about patients who were not in private rooms, as if placing all patients in private accommodations would assure one-class care to all.

A recent example of the way economic and medical considerations are linked with the patient's accommodation is found in Duff and Hollingshead, *Sickness and Society*:

> Three types of accommodations are provided for inpatients: ward or service, semiprivate and private. Remarkable differences exist among the three types of accommodations. . . . The (private) rooms are bright and tastefully decorated, furnished with a single bed, a lounge chair, and a reading table; there are outlets for lamps, television and telephone. The general impression is one of light, airiness and quiet. . . . The semiprivate accommodations have 60 percent more beds in the same floor space than the private accommodations . . . the ward accommodations are crowded with equipment. and people, sick and well.

After this bleak description, it is heartening to learn that the medical outcome of hospital treatment for the study patients was unrelated to type of accommodation.[2] The description reflects, however, the attitude of many in the hospital field about the comparative desirability of private, semiprivate, and ward accommodations.

In the early 1920s, Goldwater and Bluestone listed indications for assigning service (i.e., ward) patients to a private room whatever the cost might be. Of eleven indicators for privacy, nine were medical, as follows:

1. Dangerously sick cases
2. Mental and nervous diseases
3. Special diseases, such as acute goiter
4. Communicable or suspected contagious diseases
5. Foul dressing and discharge cases
6. Cases of uncontrollable pain
7. Cases of concentrated treatment, such as tracheotomy
8. Absolute quiet cases in which all stimuli should be controlled
9. Early postoperatives[3]

The list provides a measure of medical and hospital progress in the past forty years. Although communicable or suspected contagious diseases are still admitted to private rooms for the most part, now they are not so numerous nor do patients have the same diseases. Thanks to the discovery of antibiotics and other new health modalities, few patients with pneumonia, turberculosis, typhoid, malaria, syphilis, and so forth are found in hospitals today. The present shortage of nursing personnel and the introduction of huge, expensive, effective machines for monitoring and resuscitation have changed our attitude toward the need for private rooms for the dangerously sick. These patients are now accommodated in intensive care units (often just the opposite of a private room) in multiple-bed wards where even the sexes are mixed. Tracheotomy cases are not so frequent as they were. Postoperative patients go into the common recovery room and coronary patients into coronary care units. As for mental and nervous disorders, with the wide acceptance of milieu therapy, special psychiatric units have been formed in general hospitals and 4-bed wards are favored for many psychotic and neurotic patients, who to some degree assist and monitor one another.

In 1959 we attempted to determine the number of oxygen outlets required in the patient units of each service of the Yale–New Haven Hospital.[4] Data gathered during the study year revealed that far more oxygen was administered to patients in single rooms on the semiprivate floors than to those in multiple-bed accommodations. Although fire hazard was a major reason for assigning oxygen users to private rooms, the patients who needed oxygen were usually sick enough to require a private room for medical reasons in any case. On the basis of our maximum figure for oxygen use alone, an estimated 20 percent of the patients on the medical floor and 10 percent of those on the surgical floor should be in single rooms. To these percentages must be added, of course, single rooms needed for isolation cases on each floor. The increased importance of postoperative infections has increased the need for single rooms to prevent contagion. However, the number of patients requiring private rooms for medical reasons is not high enough to justify a recommendation of all private rooms in every general hospital.

Social Indications

The two types of cases on the Goldwater–Bluestone list requiring privacy for social reasons were disciplinary cases such as prisoners and "social reasons cases, such as patients of unusual sensitivity." These social indicators seem to have been formulated not only about fifty years ago but in a different country. The problem today is not that certain cases require more privacy than others but that society demands more privacy for all. No longer does one try to identify social conditions in which privacy is a form of treatment; today many patients consider privacy a desirable amenity in itself.

To this general tendency toward increased privacy must be added the fact that hospital planners and programmers—medical staffs, architects, and administrators—come from the wealthier classes, Classes I and II of the Hollingshead index,[5] and bring to the question of the social desirability of privacy the bias of their class.

The Economic Arguments for Privacy

The economic argument for privacy rests on two assumptions: that a higher occupancy level may be expected in all-single-room units and that fewer patient moves will be required when every patient is initially placed in a one-bed unit. These two advantages are thought to more than offset higher investment costs arising from the increased square footage needed for all-single-room units and possible higher operational costs resulting from increased travel distances for the staff.[6]

The common assumptions are exemplified in an article by Herbert McLaughlin, who states that

> fewer beds are required in private room units than in semiprivate configurations to serve the same number of patients. This statement reflects an occupancy rate of 85 percent in semiprivate rooms, a high average, and an occupancy rate of 94 to 97 per cent in the single . . . rooms, a reasonable and easily attainable figure in our experi-

ence. . . . Since our comparison was based on a relatively high occupancy of 85 per cent in the semiprivate unit, a large number of bed changes per day can be projected.[7]

He assumes that something inherent in semiprivate accommodations results in lower occupancy and that significantly more moves will be experienced than in private-room units. These two assumptions will be examined in this chapter.

The argument for providing all-private rooms holds that if each room is an individual unit, any type of patient can be admitted to any room. Moving patients from room to room, a costly procedure, will be kept to a minimum. Patients with contagious diseases can be accommodated instantly; no one need worry about matching temperaments, and sex differences, in particular, will no longer prevent maximum occupancy. Although this argument is theoretically sound, the questions really are: How much is occupancy increased with the provision of all-private rooms, and is the increase high enough to offset the increased investment and possibly increased operating costs of all-single-room units?

To answer these questions and analyze the economic problem experimentally in a real-life situation, one would have to admit two groups of patients with the same desire and need for privacy to the two kinds of accommodations involved: one of all-private rooms and the other identical in its layout except that the beds are provided in a mixture of single, double, and 4-bed rooms. In the multiple-bed rooms the patients would obviously have to be either all male or all female, which would automatically determine the difference in occupancy rates of the various configurations of beds. Records would be kept on the number of patients preferring or needing privacy who could not be so placed and were admitted to a multiple-bed facility. Additional data would be recorded on the number of times a patient was moved from one type of room to another to consolidate patients of the same sex. The cost of moving a patient would then be added to the cost of lower occupancy (if any) in the multiple-bed facility to determine the economic differential between private and multiple-bed rooms. Volume of input would also have to be considered, that is, the number of patients attempting to gain entrance to the two different kinds of bed configurations (single and multiple). The ratio of those admitted to those desiring admission, as well as the bed occupancy percentage, would determine the effectiveness with which the two patterns were meeting the need. For example, it might be found that at 70 percent occupancy there was no difference between the number of patients seeking admission and those actually admitted, but at 90 percent the difference might be large. High occupancies must mean that some patients cannot be admitted to one or either of the bed systems.

The Patient Room Simulator

Such a series of experiments would obviously be impractical in real life. Even assuming it were possible to admit the same population or matched populations to two or more bed configurations, the undertaking would be expensive and time consuming and might well interfere with the normal functioning of the nursing units or with the diagnostic and therapeutic activities for which the patients were admitted. An inpatient unit simulator was therefore utilized to reproduce this experiment as closely as possible.

The computer generates a group of patients with selected characteristics: sex, desire for a certain type of room, or need for a single room. Two bed capacities of equal size (in this instance, 151 beds) are then specified, one with all-single rooms, the other with a given combination of single- and multiple-bed rooms. Patients are presented for admission to the hospital in a Poisson (random) distribution, with an average number of admissions per day specified for Sunday through Thursday and with a lower average number of admissions for the other two days. (Friday is assumed to be 85 percent of normal, Saturday 80 percent; these figures reflect actual experience at the hospital over weekends.) If possible, these patients are then admitted to beds. How long they occupy the beds is specified by a distribution of actual hospital lengths of stay. When patients are discharged it is at the beginning of the day, reflecting actual discharge patterns, and new patients are admitted immediately.

It takes 55 minutes of computer time to set up a program, which then requires 4 minutes to run, presenting, admitting, processing, and discharging 34,000 patients. After this first run the variables may be changed, increasing or decreasing the patient load and offering different mixes of room arrangements, and the new program is processed by the computer in the same way.[8]

Our simulation runs were designed to explore the behavior of the system at three values of patient load—with the proposed number of patients 25,869, 29,465, or 33,172—and with five mixes of room arrangements ranging from 4.6 percent of the patients in single rooms to 100 percent in single rooms. Each run simulated 5 years' operating experience. A 35-day rollback was allowed; that is, the simulated unit was allowed to fill up for 35 days before any measurements were taken, so that all results were recorded when it was operating to capacity. For each simulation run the computer collected, stored, and reported the following data:

1. Total number of patients presented, whether or not they could be given a bed. This statistic represents the proposed load on the system. For the first run, the total number of patients desiring to be admitted was designed to produce approximately 80 percent occupancy. In two subsequent runs their number was increased by approximately 14 percent each time in order to determine whether the relative pattern of bed use would persist under crowded conditions.

2. Total number of patients admitted, that is, actually placed in beds. This number is always less than the number of patients seeking admission, and the difference between the two is increased as a greater load is placed on the system. The ratio of patients admitted to those presented in a measure of the degree to which the facilities satisfy the demand.

3. Number of service failures. This number represents patients who could not be admitted for one of two reasons: because there were no beds available for any patients (inevitable service failure) or because there was no bed available for a particular patient, though there were empty beds in the system (system service failure). By definition, there can be no system service failures in a hospital with all-single-room units, since any empty bed can be filled by any patient. A mere comparison between single-room units and multiple-bed rooms according to their percentage of occupancy is not nearly as sensitive and meaningful as a comparison between their total service failures, that is, inevitable failures plus system service failures. By means of the differences in service failures, the number of patients not treated in one system can be compared with that of patients not treated in the other.

4. The average percent occupancy per year over the five-year simulation run.

5. The number of patient moves required to place an admitted patient in a bed. At this stage the program does not take into account transfers at the patient's own request, nor does it consider moves made necessary by a change in the patient's condition.

Because our purpose was to report the economics of occupancy, unrelated to medical conditions or social preferences, in a wide variety of bed configurations other statistics gathered during the runs are not reported here. For instance, we have omitted the number of times a patient desired a specific room but was not able to get it because we assumed that preferences were not so strong that a patient wishing one kind of accommodation would refuse admission to another if the preferred type was not available. This information, however, was included in the simulation in the form of subroutines to facilitate the planning of specific units based on probable patient preferences in specific hospitals.

Findings

Results of the simulation runs were examined first to ascertain the direct implications of the data and then to explore the dynamics of the simulated runs with different inputs. The most obvious finding, as shown in table 23, was the very slight difference in percentage of occupancy for the different mixes of accommodations. When every patient was admitted who could fit into the five different mixes of room arrangements, the difference in average occupancy between the least favorable arrangement, the unit with 4.6 percent single rooms, and that with 100 percent single rooms was only 0.37–0.39 percent during a 5-year simulated experience under three different loads. This would mean additional income from 203 or 204 patient days a year out of a capacity of 5,115 patient days. It is indeed so small a difference that it would be dangerous to plan on being able to satisfy a given demand with fewer beds that are all in single rooms. Using the United States Public Health Service standard[9] of approximately one-quarter of the beds in single rooms (found in table 23 as the third run at each load), the average difference would be only 0.08 of occupancy, which means that 45 patient days a year would be gained in an all-single-room unit.

Two other interesting measurements of bed utilization are the number of moves necessary and the number of service failures. They too are surprisingly low for mixed units where at least 25 percent of the beds are in single rooms. Not until the last run, at 95 percent occupancy, do the moves become very noticeable, and even then they average less than two a week. As for total service failures, the difference between all private rooms and 25 percent private rooms amounts to less than one failure a month until the very highest occupancy has been reached.

When the dynamics of the system are examined under varying patient loads, it becomes clearer why an 80 percent occupancy rate is considered ideal. At this load there are relatively few service failures; most patients who wish to be admitted can be accommodated. (In actual hospital experience, an average 80 percent occupancy usually means high occupancy during selected months of the year and lower occupancy in summertime. Waiting lists or queues resulting from the months of high demand can be cleared during the slow months.) At 89 percent occupancy, with 151 beds all in private rooms, 77 patients a year have to be turned away; at 95 percent occupancy, with the same number and arrangement of beds, more than one patient a day cannot be accommodated.

Discussion and Conclusions

As indicated above, the number of patients presented to the simulator was generated by using a Poisson distribution with three different means: one for Sunday through Thursday, a lower value for Friday, and a still lower value for Saturday. It is not unrealistic to assume three means for many medical and some surgical services, the clinical services in which we are primarily interested. In the obstetrical service, input depends on the pattern of practice, on whether or not the staff is decidedly committed to elective inductions. (The influence of elective inductions on the input of the maternity service has been dealt with elsewhere.)[10] In pediatrics, mixing sexes in a multiple-bed room does not limit bed usage to the same extent as on adult floors.

In view of the sizable number of elective surgical cases, it may be argued that surgical input is not entirely random or Poisson but might best be described as part scheduled and part Poisson. This may indeed be true for some hospitals, where in order to determine the extent to which admissions are affected by bed and operating room availability, the scheduling policy in allocating beds and operating times must be examined. Most operating room schedules are set up on a FIFO (first in, first out) basis. A more rational grouping of cases (for example, by how long the operation takes or postoperative facilities will be required) should bring about a more efficient use of beds, staff, and operating room time. Both the inevitable and system service failures indicated by the simulator might be minimized and higher bed occupancies achieved as the result of a less random scheduling of the operating room.

The number of patient moves generated by the simulator may seem unrealistically low, until it is remembered that the only moves represented are those required to consolidate patients of the same sex in order for another patient to be admitted—no moves for medical or social reasons. Thus until the last two or three beds are emptied, no moves are made at all, and even then only when the empty beds are in a room occupied by patients of a different sex from that of the patient who seeks admission. Such moves represent but a small fraction of the total patient moves observed in a typical hospital. Data on the reasons for patient moves are scarce; they are influenced by the way beds are assigned to the clinical services and by whether or not the hospital is committed to progressive patient care.

A study at the Yale–New Haven Hospital[11] involving 268 moves on the medical and surgical services revealed that 120 (44.8 percent) of the moves were transfers to and from the intensive care unit or danger list rooms, while another 85 (31.7 percent) were changes from one room to another of the same size. In other words, 76.5 percent of the patient moves

TABLE 23. Five-year simulation with varying loads and room mixes: service failures, percentage of occupancy, and number of moves.

	Proposed load 25,869				
Percent of 151 beds in					
Single rooms	4.6	12.6	25.8	51.0	100
Double rooms	63.6	58.3	42.4	38.4	
Four-bed rooms	31.8	29.1	31.8	10.6	
Admitted	25,726	25,821	25,847	25,851	25,853
Total service failures	143	48	22	18	16
Inevitable service failures	13	13	14	10	16
System service failures	130	35	8	8	0
Percentage of occupancy	78.77	79.07	79.15	79.15	79.16
Number of moves	11	5	6	2	0

Proposed load 29,465					Proposed load 33,172				
4.6	12.6	25.8	51.0	100	4.6	12.6	25.8	51.0	100
63.6	58.3	42.4	38.4		63.6	58.3	42.4	38.4	
31.8	29.1	31.8	10.6		31.8	29.1	31.8	10.6	
28,942	29,035	29,043	29,063	29,079	31,104	31,137	31,116	31,167	31,199
523	430	422	402	386	2 068	2 035	2 056	2 005	1 973
255	287	273	293	386	1 255	1 306	1 403	1 499	1 973
268	143	149	109	0	813	729	653	506	0
88.71	88.97	89.03	89.06	89.10	94.82	94.91	94.94	95.09	95.19
181	160	145	68	0	648	593	452	227	0

were for reasons completely apart from the type of accommodation the patient occupied. During the period of the study there were 20 transfers from single- to multiple-bed rooms and 29 from multiple-bed rooms to singles. Patients who changed from private to multiple-bed rooms were those in the danger-list singles understandably eager to get better and return to their own first accommodation, or those who left a private for a 4-bed room probably for financial reasons. Patients changing from multiple-bed rooms to singles were primarily discontented occupants of the 2-bed rooms (converted singles in this hospital, and consequently somewhat crowded and undesirable) or those probably not admitted at the outset to the arrangement they preferred. It was informally reported that a fairly large number of transfers from multiple- to single-bed rooms were due to the fact that the private rooms had telephones whereas the others did not. Patients are always being shifted to and from the intensive care unit for medical reasons, whatever their original accommodation.

More studies are needed on the reasons for and cost of patient moves to determine the effect of type of accommodation upon them. The simulations reported upon here explore but one aspect of the problem. Other areas must be investigated, such as patient-initiated requests for moves and the institution's decision to transfer a patient.

Operating costs cannot be used as much of an argument on either side. A difference in staffing costs has not been demonstrated between all-private-room units and multiple-bed units of the same size and with the same patient mix.[12] No one can deny that corridors are longer in a unit of all single rooms in any form, including the circular. But in comparing units of differing design, it is not at all clear that there is much, if any, relationship between this aspect of the design and the probable distance staff members must travel. "Design is the thing which dictates efficiency, not the size of the unit or the degree of privacy granted the patients in it."[13]

Are there, however, possible operational economies inherent in multiple-bed accommodations? In chapter 14, the study of the nurse–patient call system, it was demonstrated that patient-initiated requests from occupants of 4-bed rooms were 30 percent less frequent than from patients in the single rooms.[14] Why was this so? Were some calls from private-room patients motivated partly by a desire for company? Was there more chance that a nurse would already be in the 4-bed room to fulfill patients' requests without the necessity of their ringing for her? Was the informal group of patients providing services to its members that would be rendered by nurses to patients in single rooms? Another real possibility is that patients from the lower socioeconomic strata are less demanding and require fewer services than members of Classes I and II, who are the ones more likely to be in single rooms.

Less important operational economies, though more concrete and thus easier to specify, inhere in the multiple-bed units. Because there are fewer square feet per bed, basic utility costs (heat, light, and power) will be less for each patient admitted; housekeeping costs will be reduced even more since some of this lower square footage is in patients' toilets, areas particularly difficult to clean.

It is possible that in the future, high occupancy may actually be impeded by the lack of flexibility of miniature single rooms with less than a 3-foot clearance on either side of the bed head. The utilization review mechanism is directed to the proposition that the hospital bed, that most expensive of community health resources, must more and more be occupied by patients who absolutely require it. Every bed must therefore be designed to provide efficient, effective care to patients suffering from a wide variety of medical conditions that will necessitate more and more complex equipment at the bedside. Bunk beds and cater-corner beds do not allow enough room for these complex arrangements.[15]

We must conclude that the optimal mix of private and multibed accommodations in a ward cannot be expressed as a simple universal percentage, depending as it does on medical, social, and economical factors. The USPHS recommendation of 25 percent of beds in private rooms should be regarded as a minimum. Thereafter the proportion of each type of bed arrangement to the others will vary with the specific mission of the institution, the characteristics of its patients, the organization of its clinical services, and the therapeutic philosophy expressed in them. The influence of most of these determining factors can be quantified and applied in a specific situation, and the simulator described here used to predict the results of alternative patterns and various mixes of accommodations.

PART 4

Progressive Patient Care

CHAPTER 18

Toward a Progressive Patient Care System of Hospitals

Dynamo and Virgin

In a superb study, *The Railroad Station, an Architectural History* (New Haven: Yale University Press, 1956), Carroll Meeks traced the evolution of a specific building form from purely derivative to functional, from its origins in the 1830s until there were simply no more railroad stations being built. The United States is still sprinkled with derivative forms, for example a horizontal box of a station in Waterbury, Connecticut (1909) to which was affixed the campanile of the Palazzo Pubblico of Siena. By the time functional and internal traffic problems were solved effectively and efficiently in the design of the railroad station of Cincinnati, Ohio (1929), the passenger station was no longer really needed. These edifices are now being put to other uses or are made the sites for superimposed buildings as was the Grand Central Station of New York City. This is not to say that an urban transportation center should not be designed in the future. It should not, however, be devoted to one mode of transportation but rather serve as a center for a complete urban transportation system of railroads, rapid transit, buses, airport limousines, helicopters, taxis, private automobiles and must also allow space for travelers on foot. It would be a transportation systems terminal, not a railroad station.

There are genuine similarities between the design development of the railroad station and the hospital. As the older, more complex institution, the hospital has gone through many more phases over a longer period, but temples and cathedrals, town houses, and barracks did not evolve into a functional form until the twentieth century. Earlier, one might have come upon a functional form here or there—or a part of one—but the institution was not thought of in terms of one recognizable functional form until the present century.

It is true that the hospital is now viewed as a functional form, although a reasonably acceptable understanding of the give-and-take among its design components is not yet achieved.[1] We have seen how each component was blended into the design: sanitation, ease of supervision, privacy, and efficiency. We have watched priority given to first one design component, then another, depending on how the social role of the hospital was conceived at that period and more recently on the requirements of scientific medicine.

In earlier chapters this work traced the development of the inpatient unit in terms of its design components and reviewed attempts to achieve an optimal mix of the components within a unit of a given shape. In planning the Memorial Unit of the Yale–New Haven Hospital, for example, the attempt was made, by a judicious mixture of design components, to design a ward that would answer the needs of the largest number of patients most of the time they were hospitalized. It was hoped that the two different plans —a west wing composed almost entirely of 1-bed rooms and an east wing composed of 4-bed rooms with only three singles—would meet the requirements of all patients admitted to this hospital. Admittedly, there was an important, nonfunctional differentiation based on the patient's ability to pay. A patient might choose a single room if he desired and could afford to do so. But all such arbitrary schemes, however cleverly mixed, do not optimize the design components related to the patient's degree of illness at a given point in time. For instance, for the sake of privacy much supervision and some efficiency must be relinquished, a situation that holds for all patients electing a private room. Modern technology permits a degree of supervision with privacy through the use of remote monitoring devices. Nevertheless, it is still true that the four components cannot be optimized in the same inpatient unit, that emphasis on one means deemphasis on another. It is now recognized that it is dangerous, inefficient, and expensive to base the design and staffing of an inpatient unit on the average needs of patients during their hospital stay.[2]

Therefore we have had to open up the nursing unit, burst it open one might almost say, and make of it at least four different kinds of units, within or outside one hospital, that offer varying degrees of care. In each unit the design component to be emphasized is the one important to the patient in the current stage of his illness. Supervision can deliberately be optimized when he is very ill, privacy when he is getting better. This cannot be done within a single area even with the most earnest attempts to design for all contingencies. It calls for four or more separate areas individually designed; that is, a *system* of inpatient units within the hospital, each specifically tailored to the patient's needs during a particular stage of his illness. By splitting the hospital into systems we can have a human hospital when humanness is necessary, a scientific hospital when life-saving heroic force is necessary. Both virgin and dynamo, in Henry Adams's phrase, can be served. But a virgin and a dynamo require to be housed in very different kinds of inpatient units.

The process does not stop short within hospital walls. A system of related institutions must be set up outside the hospital but affiliated with it. But to assemble them and give each one its function, we must first very clearly define the primary role of the hospital proper, which is curative. Other social roles historically associated with the hospital—expensive rest home, overendowed old-age home, or diagnostic center for patients forced to be temporarily horizontal—must be rationally assigned to other kinds of institutions: continuing-care centers, home-care programs, or ambulatory-care centers such as group practice units affiliated with the hospital but not necessarily occupying the same building. There are indications that society is beginning to do just this, and indeed is forced to do it—not because of any change in the basic way of doing things but by the increased expense of a hospital day. In part they result from a revolution in medical technology and new breakthroughs in the practice of medicine. However comforting it might be to society to continue in the old patterns, neither this nation nor any other can afford hospitals that perform functions that need not be carried out within a hospital.

Utilization Review and Progressive Patient Care

Two specific indicators (admittedly as yet ineffective) of an imminent change in the hospital's role are utilization review, a term written into the Medicare law, and progressive patient care, which to a limited extent is already operative in some United States hospitals. The goal of utilization review is said to be to place the right patient in the right bed to receive the right treatment for the right period of time. So far it is a crushing disappointment, and its effect on length of stay or placement of patients in the proper institutions has been minimal. However, the problems are primarily technical; there are indications that within five to ten years the kind of decisions required will be made on a specific diagnostic basis by physicians or a medical staff. When their judgments can be supplemented by quality control mechanisms and methods to determine the right placement for each patient, there will be no excuse for not constructing a system of hospitals to provide the facilities.

Progressive patient care is not a new concept. Manchester (Conn.) Memorial Hospital, the first progres-

sive patient care hospital, opened three units for acute, intermediate, and self-care on April 1, 1957. On August 1, 1958, a fourth was added for continuation or long-term care by Edward J. Thoms, administrator of the hospital and author of the concept. Then the United States Public Health Service proposed a fifth care zone, home care.[3]

When first introduced, the concept of progressive patient care swept the hospital establishment like a fever, assuming for its followers the qualities of a mystique. Much emotion was generated pro and con. Opponents claimed that progressive patient care cut the patient up into little pieces, hampering greatly any continuity of care. In their headier moments they pictured patients being tossed from one bed to another within the hospital, with no patient remaining in one locus for more than a couple of hours. It is true that the system has therapeutic and economic defects. The same nurses and physicians cannot follow a patient from one stage of care to another, which does result in a loss of emotional continuity for the patient and of educational continuity for the medical staff. It is said to be difficult for staff or relatives to locate the patient from one day to the next. Worse yet, however, economy of operation and staffing has yet to be proved for these units. The first costs were figured on the basis of the hospital cost to the patient, a calculation that lost sight of the fact that many private nurses, who had been paid for by the patient, would no longer be used. The hospital itself pays for equivalent nursing in intensive care, which calls for enough staff at least to balance economies of staffing in the ambulatory unit.

Progressive patient care depends on the proper implementation of four principles. The first is triage: at the time of entering the hospital each patient will be admitted to the kind of unit he requires. The second is close monitoring of his condition throughout his stay so he may be transferred immediately to the unit he requires as his condition changes. This presupposes that patients can be categorized, and indeed during the early stages of progressive patient care much time was spent on developing a patient classification system. The third principle is that inpatient units can be designed to care for patients in the different stages of their illness. And the fourth, closely related to the third, is that each unit so designed can be staffed with the particular mix of professional and paraprofessional personnel who can best treat the patient during that stage of his illness.

Application of these four principles results in the patient's progress through a series of graduated hospital care zones according to the classification of his needs. Although patient movement is the central tenet of progressive patient care, remarkably few studies have examined the dynamics of that movement. Answers must be sought to such questions as, What are the characteristics of the transfers from one zone to the other, and Can individual hospitals use patient-flow information as a basis for deciding the number of beds to be allocated to each zone in accordance with the characteristics of their anticipated patient load?

To What Extent Are Progressive Patient Care Patients Moved?

A recent review of about 15,000 admissions to the Manchester Memorial Hospital traced the patients through the system.[4] The first fact to emerge from the study was that patients do differ very much in their requirements for different types of care on admission. Twenty percent of the Manchester patients were admitted to the intensive care unit directly, 57 percent were admitted to the intermediate care unit, and 19 percent were admitted to the self-care unit. About 1 percent were admitted to each of the following: the continuing care, coronary care, and psychiatric units. So progressive patient care may be said to have the potential to respond to the different needs patients

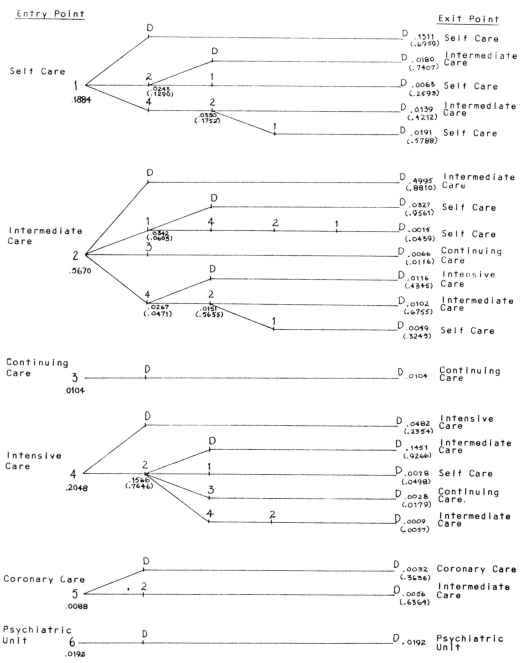

Fig. 262. Paths, frequencies, and conditional probabilities of progressive patient care at Manchester (Conn.) Memorial Hospital.

present when they are admitted to the hospital.

Patients' movement through the system depended a great deal upon which zone they were admitted to in the first place. For example, 20 percent of all patients were admitted directly to the intensive care unit, and of these, 77 percent moved to other regions within the hospital (fig. 262). But 57 percent of all patients were admitted to the intermediate care zone, and of these, 86 percent never left it. In all six zones of care, 71 percent of the patients never moved from the zone to which they were admitted and were discharged from that zone. Thus there was no movement for 71 percent of the patients even in a progressive patient care hospital. Another 22 percent of the patients only moved once during their total hospital stay, which means that progressive patient care, in the sense of more than one single shift during a hospital stay, really affected only 7 percent of all patients. This is a totally different picture from the one frequently summoned up of patients in continuous motion from one floor to another, not knowing who their nurse or doctor is during the transition.

Although this experience in one hospital does give a pattern of transition from one care zone to another, it should not mislead us to expect the same progression of cases in other hospital settings. This particular progressive patient care experience was influenced by the kinds of patients now being treated in the smaller community hospitals of this country. It did not explore the possibility of different kinds of hospital appendages, since no decision was ever made as to whether or not the patient should have been in the hospital in the first place. No preadmission facilities outside the hospital were available at the study institution to determine whether, for example, with selected diagnostic workups available in group practice, the pattern of progress would have been the same. In spite of the fact that there was an active utilization review committee at the hospital at the time, no really critical examination of the necessity of the patient's remaining in the hospital was undertaken and this factor was never measured by any of the newer utilization review techniques. The pattern of movement was based primarily on standard accepted practice and does not in any way represent the transition matrix that might be found were newer modes of treatment instituted.

Furthermore, the number of beds in the institution dictated to some extent the transition probabilities. This was particularly true in the continuing-care section, which at the time of the study was very limited and filled most of the time. Had more beds been provided in this zone, there might have been more admissions to it, particularly from the intermediate care zone.

Planning for Progressive Patient Care

In determining the number of beds required in each type of service in a progressive patient care hospital, it is necessary to take into consideration constraints on total investment and operating costs. It might also be considered necessary or desirable to define certain minimum levels of service in terms of patients accommodated for each type of bed. To plan effectively in this situation, two kinds of problems must be solved. First, the capability, in terms of occupancy and services, of any arrangement of the facilities for any patient mix must be predicted. Second, given this prediction, the best arrangement must be determined according to some predetermined criterion or set of criteria. Then the first problems must be solved again to ascertain whether the prediction is still valid for the allocation found in solving the second problem, and so on until two successive solutions yield the same result.

The formulation of a general progressive-patient-care planning system that allows for the probable differences between one hospital's experience and another's, as well as for changes in a single hospital over time, was attempted in a recent paper.[5] Progressive patient care does give a logical framework on which to construct such a system and thus is an extremely valuable innovation. To give body to the progressive patient care system, two things are now needed. First, a series of institutions outside the hospital must become part of an institutional medical care system ready to accept patients before or after admission to hospital, so that the true demands for hospitalization, based on medical reasons, can be ascertained. Second, a sensitive indicator for patient needs, a patient classification system, must be instituted so that an inpatient unit designed to fit each classification can be objectively and rationally programmed. For this kind of programming, all previous concern for privacy, which was nonessential in its origin and linked to social class, must be abandoned because all four design components, including this one, are to be applied for medical reasons. Or privacy must be formally and deliberately set up as an expensive design limitation.

There are indications that now we may indeed be able to do this. For the first time, in selected instances, we are beginning to approach at least the outside limits of supervision. We know that the nurse must get to the patient in a coronary care unit within four minutes. This medical fact sets the limits for the size of, and distances within, a coronary care unit. It is hoped that as we gain more and more experience with critical measurements like this one, we will be able to design inpatient units with greater logic and accuracy than before.

CHAPTER 19

Progressive Patient Care Writ Large

Acceptance and Development of the Progressive Patient Care Concept

In progressive patient care the patient is viewed as needing a spectrum of services from very intensive to a benign neglect calculated to propel him toward assuming responsibility for his own care once more. It was much easier for hospitals in the United States to visualize the extreme ends of the spectrum and take action than to differentiate among services in the middle area and decide what to do about them. Consequently it is not surprising that the modality first seized on by most hospitals was the intensive care unit.

In 1970, 48.8 percent of short-term general hospitals in the United States had an intensive care unit.[1] Intensive care was further subdivided in large hospitals, where one often finds one or more of the new specialized units for coronary care, newborn care, stroke intensive care, renal dialysis, or a hyperbaric oxygen chamber.[2] Not to be outdone, many psychiatric departments have installed a crisis intervention unit. The most phenomenal growth among specialized intensive care units has been that of the coronary care units. The formidable task of planning the units and educating staff for them was a specified high priority of the early Regional Medical Program (Public Law 79-239). In 1968, 42 percent of the hospitals in the United States had in operation some kind of coronary care unit.

Hospitals adjusted most comfortably to the intermediate care zone since it was none other than the old familiar nursing unit and required little or no change in hospital planning, operation, or the traditional concept of patient care. Individual differences between hospitals began to be seen in their handling of the self-care units, which, in the absence of a sufficient number of patients too sick for outpatient treatment yet too fragile for discharge, were frequently adapted to treat cases of minor surgery that required at most a couple of nights' hospitalization, and for this function they were renamed minimal care units.

But over time, the most profound changes took place in the area of long-term care. In most instances this continuing care was scarcely ever proffered within hospital walls. Here is where progressive patient care spilled out of the hospitals. Patients were discharged to their own homes or to nursing homes. Then Medicare legislation demanded transfer agreements between hospitals and nursing homes and placed the hospitals on notice that closer formal relationships between components of the continuing care system might be expected to follow. In addition, Medicare defined a new kind of long-term institution called an "extended care facility," conceptually somewhere between a general hospital and a nursing home, which was to offer not only extended-care beds but also other required services, such as physical and occupational therapy. Too often there were only the beds. Hospitals themselves were slow in installing these basic services: in 1967, only 55 percent reported a physical therapy department, and a mere 12 percent offered occupational therapy. The whole chronic-care system faces further changes of major proportions. Probably another kind of extended care facility should be required as well, a social care institution, a kind of rest home with nursing supervision. Patients for the most part ambulatory, who are fragile rather than ill and who require some kind of medication and dietary maintenance, can be cared for in this type of institution at considerably less cost than in a nursing home.

Home care was renamed ambulatory care and accepted by Medicare as a reimbursable form of treatment. Of all the areas of progressive patient care, this is the one most neglected by hospitals. In 1967, only 5 percent claimed to have a home care program affiliated with their institution. It is difficult to understand why the concept of ambulatory care in an organized outpatient setting was not considered an important component of progressive patient care. For the first time the links are being clearly identified between ambulatory care as given in hospital outpatient departments and the emergency room and the care given in the inpatient sections of that hospital (fig. 263).

Thus the single zone of continuing care, conceived of as within the hospital, in actuality became two zones for extended care and nursing care, both outside the hospital. The one progressive patient care hospital became a progressive care *system of institutions* including the hospital proper, several kinds of long-term facilities, and a home care program.

Surely the next step must be to strengthen arrangements among them. Only by bringing the constituent institutions to their full strength, avoiding duplications, and improving the communications between them and the quality of care offered by each one, can we make sure that the patient will be in the right institution at the right time for the right length of time.

In describing the future trend of hospitals, their planning, design, operation, and management, we would use just one phrase: progressive patient care writ large. We mean by this an increase in the number of care zones, but much more important than this is the shift from thinking in terms of a progressive patient care hospital to planning a progressive patient-centered medical care system. The technique evolved in progressive patient care hospitals of reviewing each patient's need for a bed within a particular unit may be carried over to the system of hospitals. Within extended care facilities, patients should be reviewed periodically to ascertain whether they are really in the kind of institution they require and are receiving the care they need.

Milieu Therapy

If this goal could be realized, one might even anticipate a more active therapeutic role for the ward itself in treating the patient. Thus far the concept of milieu therapy has been used only in the general hospital in a few very specialized settings, such as psychiatric wards, rehabilitation units, and rooming-in obstetrical units. Because more and more admissions to the general hospital are for acute episodes of chronic diseases, it is important that the period of hospitalization be used not only to cure the episode but also to educate the patient to prevent such relapses. In the case of a hernia, for example, the disease is cured in the hospital; patients do not have to learn to live with it. But in many acute conditions, patients must be trained in groups to care for themselves when they leave the hospital. These people are up and down, not necessarily bedridden. However, they cannot be trained in single rooms. They must help one another and learn from one another; the job cannot be done by merely lining them up in wheelchairs and lecturing to them.

The model for milieu therapy is the rooming-in maternity unit, where in groups of four the patients learn from one another, new mothers from mothers who have had other children, or a new mother on her first day from a mother who has already seen and tended her child for two days. In all milieu therapy, combining professional support and patient interaction results in a better outcome, and the patient retains more of what has been learned. This makes of the nursing unit a positive therapeutic modality designed to contribute as much as medicine does to the ability of a patient to deal with a problem. The approach is quite different from bedding a patient down in a convenient locality where somebody can do something to him and where the patient is not actively contributing to his own healing or that of other patients. Such a setting will undoubtedly affect the prevailing attitude toward privacy, which is determined by social class.

Milieu therapy requires interaction in a small group; patients of a 24-bed unit cannot interrelate in this way. It is not for all patients but mostly for those who must come to terms with their own illness and can gain from the experience of other patients coming to terms with the same or similar conditions. It probably cannot be accomplished in the acute ward of today but could be carried out in a continuing-care unit either inside or outside the hospital, for example, in a restructured continuing-care unit.

Costs Trends Affecting the Design and Utilization of the Inpatient Unit

The economic factor is the force that must and will lead to a progressive patient care system of medical care institutions and will radically affect the various kinds of inpatient units that must be designed. The American public was once quietly respectful of medicine or enthralled by its impressive advances. That day is past. People are now dismayed and angered by their own personal encounters or by reports in the mass media. They still acknowledge the scientific capability of medicine, but too seldom do they see that capability translated into action—and they have good reason to protest. Medical care is often unavailable: general practitioners are vanishing, and the extraordinary superspecialized services, widely publicized, relieve only a few people in one or two locations. Medical care is frequently unreliable—there are some quality measurements in medicine but few real quality controls, most decisions are made and acted upon independently, and within the care process there are no checks to satisfy the general demand for consumer protection. These two deficiencies are very threatening, but the most dramatic aspect of medical care, crying out for some kind of immediate action, is its high and rising cost. This too becomes threatening when people go without care because they cannot or will not pay for it. Though an increasing proportion of the nation's medical bill is being paid by government at all levels, federal, state, and local, and by voluntary or private health insurance, more than one-third of such expenses, totaling $60.3 billion in the fiscal year 1969, is still paid by consumers directly. Most patients make out-of-pocket payments for drugs, long-term institutional care, dental care, and visits to doctors' offices and doctors' visits to their homes. Payments are related to costs of care delivery; it is therefore through the examination of costs that we may arrive at a more rational approach to payments.

The two most difficult problems are the increased cost of new programs in a labor-laden industry and the search for the type and particularly for the size of institution that will be most responsive to the needs of patients and specified communities. For instance, in Connecticut's short-term hospitals nonobstetrical patient day costs are still climbing at the rate of more than 14 percent a year. This trend of the past eight years is considerably higher than the 5–6-percent increase of the early 1960s. Cost per maternity day has climbed faster than nonmaternity, and that of a newborn day has tripled over the past ten years. The state's experience is not unique, and a national increase in costs is not limited to short-term hospitals.

Two tables give the evidence: table 24, national expenses per hospital patient day and patient stay, and table 25, relative increase of expenditures for hospital care when compared with total medical care. These cost trends are dramatic evidence of a significant rise in real expenses per unit of hospital service—whether measured by expenses per day, expenses per average length of stay, or relative expenditures for this component of the total for medical care. They fail to answer the question of how much of the cost rise is due to expansion of scientific medical care and how much to increased salaries for employees, to new personnel, to inefficient internal operation, or, finally, to faults within the total institutional care system that lead to inefficient and ineffective use of a hospital bed.

Returning to Connecticut, if cost figures are matched with utilization data, another dimension is added to the problem. Not only did the cost of, a nonmaternity patient day increase by 148 percent during the 1960s, but also the service units used increased by 37.7 percent. We now have people paying more per patient day, *and* they are using more days. Because the population of this particular area increased by only 19.6 percent during the decade, the figures mean that each 1,000 citizens of the state used 93 more hospital days per year in 1970 than in 1960. Satisfied demand is increasing at a faster rate than the population and seems related more to the number of beds available than to the introduction of Medicare or Medicaid, which changed the method of payment for them. This conclusion bears out Roemer's law: It does seem to be true that the chief indicator for treatment in the hospital is the existence of an available hospital bed.

During the same period in Connecticut, maternity

TABLE 24. Absolute value of total national expenses per patient day and per patient stay in nonfederal, short-term general and other special hospitals (1948–1973).

	Per Patient Day	Per Patient Stay
1948	$13.09	$114.35
1949	14.33	119.39
1950	15.62	127.26
1951	16.77	138.73
1952	18.35	148.00
1953	19.95	158.47
1954	21.76	169.67
1955	23.12	179.77
1956	24.15	186.11
1957	26.02	198.13
1958	28.27	214.67
1959	30.19	235.66
1960	32.23	244.53
1961	34.98	267.37
1962	36.83	279.91
1963	38.91	299.61
1964	41.58	320.17
1965	44.48	346.94
1966	48.15	380.39
1967	54.05	448.62
1968	61,38	515.59
1969	70.03	581.25
1970	81.01	668.42
1971	92.31	738.48
1972	105.21	831.16
1973	114.69	894.58

SOURCE: *Guide to the Health Care Field* (pertinent issues).

days decreased, but maternity beds in the state did not adjust to the decreased demand. A sizable portion of their increased cost was due to their lower occupancy while the same separate staff was being retained to man them, in accordance with state law. The facilities and staff had to be large enough to respond to sudden peaks in the random, independent input. In this case the increased cost problem is an internal one; economies of scale are not being realized. The solution would obviously be to merge underutilized services as regional units rather than to maintain multiple small separate units.

Alternatives to Present Hospitalization Policies

There are two solutions to the problem of increasing hospital costs: either lower the cost of the product or buy fewer units of it. The product is patient days. We do not mean to disparage the possible effectiveness of the first approach when we urgently recommend a decrease now in patient hospital days to be effected through a reexamination of the whole system of

TABLE 25. Total (in millions of dollars) and per capita consumer expenditures for health services and supplies by type of expenditure.

	1969			1970		
	Total	Percentage	Per Capita	Total	Percentage	Per Capita
Hospital care	$10,378	30.5	$50.56	$12,964	33.4	$62.51
Physicians' services	8,877	26.1	43.25	9,690	24.9	46.42
Dentists' services	3,589	10.5	14.48	4,041	10.4	19.41
Drugs and appliances	7,819	23.0	38.09	8,319	21.4	40.11
Nursing home care	742	2.2	3.61	1,186	3.1	5.72
Other expenditures	2,652	7.7	12.92	2,650	6.8	12.78
Total	$34,057		$165.92	$38,850		$185.65

1971			Percentage Increase
Total	Percentage	Per Capita	Per Capita 1969–1971
$14,472	34.1	$69.08	37
10,688	25.2	51.02	18
4,400	10.3	21.00	45
8,779	20.7	41.90	10
1,314	3.1	6.27	74
2,824	6.6	13.48	4
$42,477		$202.75	22.2%

SOURCE: Adapted from Dorothy P. Rice and Barbara S. Cooper, "National Health Expenditures, 1929–71," *Social Security Bulletin*, January 1972.

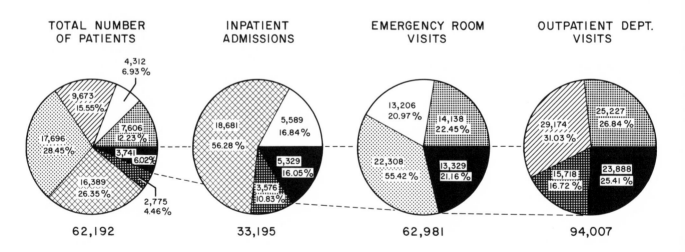

Fig. 263. Diagram showing relationships between inpatient and ambulatory care within one hospital.

medical care delivery. This will bring about (among its other accomplishments) a change in the future design of inpatient units, and (hopefully) will decrease the necessity of building so many of them, at least within hospitals.

The number of inpatient days may be decreased in two ways: first, by having the medical staff monitor whether a patient should remain in the hospital (utilization review); second, by promoting comprehensive health care outside the hospital so that fewer patients need be admitted at all, or if admitted, they should receive a considerable part of their medical workup outside the hospital. Thus we return to a progressive patient care system. A physician considering his patient's need for hospitalization must be aware of alternative arrangements that will assure him that the patient 'will receive proper care. One expedient depends on the other. As hospital inpatient days are reduced by an effective utilization review, the use of its ambulatory services increases. One Connecticut hospital even replanned its future building program as the result of such an experience and invested its capital expansion in outpatient facilities instead of inpatient beds. In this case, operating costs were reduced on the expensive inpatient day, and capital expenditure on new beds was decreased as well.

The effectiveness of utilization review is enhanced by a patient-centered, statewide information system available to physicians performing the review. This system would be able to merge the patient's medical and financial records for the period of his hospitalization, it should review the patient's use of the hospital according to selected diagnostic characteristics that lend themselves to the identification of an unusual occurrence, and it must have the capacity to identify this unusual occurrence before the patient is discharged from the hospital.

Blue Cross has begun pilot projects in home care, another substitute for an inpatient bed. Selected patients during the end days of their hospitalization may not be sick enough to need a hospital bed but would require a formal, supervised treatment program in their homes were they to be discharged. With home care supplementing utilization review, considerably fewer inpatient days can be expected per 1,000 population.

Such developments are exciting but do not go far enough. The *total* system of medical care delivery must be reorganized to provide hospital-type services outside the hospital. Prevention must be added to services so that many diseases can be detected and treated before hospitalization is required. Dr. William A. MacColl has demonstrated that patients receiving medical care through prepaid group practice programs require 40 percent fewer days in the hospital than patients insured through Blue Cross or commercial insurance.[3] Since the likelihood of decreasing the cost per patient day by 40 percent is extremely remote, promotion of group practice and prepayment of medical care in comprehensive health care settings should become, in our present dilemma, the very first recourse.

Group practice has many advantages. The one true quality control we have in medical care—interdependent decision-making—is greatly facilitated in an organized setting. Because of the complexity of their trade, all physicians must occasionally consult with others before they proceed to test or treat a puzzling case. In conventional solo practice this may be inconvenient for all concerned and costly for the patient. In organized, prepaid group practice the consultant may be only one door away with no financial barrier between. Furthermore, available consultants may include the full gamut of medical and paramedical specialists. All kinds of information and several independent judgments can be brought to bear on the patient's problem, and there is an opportunity for a number of people to detect mistakes before it is too late.

Prepayment is an important feature. Although at present most insurance coverage encourages hospitalization by not paying for any other type of care, comprehensive prepayment for a set sum pays for all care received whether patients are hospitalized or not. Since a hospital bed is known to be the most expensive component of the medical care system, there is an incentive to keep people healthy. The fee does not act as a barrier between the patient and his doctor, so that serious disease is likely to be discovered early and treated relatively inexpensively. Were health insurance coverage to include out-of-hospital or ambulatory care, these financing arrangements plus the provision of ambulatory care facilities would take some strain off hospital emergency rooms and outpatient departments that now expensively provide services they were not designed to deliver. This does not mean that expenditures for medical care would decrease, but it does mean that more people would receive more services than they do at present, perhaps at about the present cost level.

The recent trend toward interhospital mergers may result in economic savings and improved quality of care. The same trend can be observed in manufacturing and nonmedical service industries. In the case of hospitals there have been some indications of economies of scale and of the obvious advantages to be had from eliminating duplication of services. The new technology contributes to the trend. Rapid processing of information (for instance, laboratory test results) renders a laboratory in each hospital less critically important. Also, people have the uncomfortable, though never really documented, feeling that large hospitals do a better job of patient care than smaller institutions with more limited resources because of their sophisticated support services or more stringent professional standards. Shared services and a centralized administrative bureaucracy tend to create larger and larger hospitals.

There may be advantages in large-scale institutions. It is possible, however, that the most economic size would lead only to further depersonalization of patient care. In another context Hannah Arendt writes:

> The disintegration processes which have become so manifest in recent years, the decay of many public services, of schools and police, of mail delivery and transportation, the death rate on the highways and the traffic problems in the cities —concern everything designed to serve mass society. Bigness is afflicted with vulnerability, and while no one can say with assurance where and when the breaking point has been reached, we can observe, almost to the point of measuring it, how strength and resiliency are insidiously destroyed, leaking as it were drop by drop from our institutions.[4]

Hospitals are not free from this danger; indeed they are probably more vulnerable to it because of their intensely personal services, which involve multiple decisions by professional, administrative, and service personnel. The issue of centralization versus decentralization is being debated at the very time when monitoring and controlling the quality of medical care in this country's hospitals have become of primary importance to all of us. So far, what little quality control and monitoring there are take place within the hospital walls. Comparative performance data between hospitals are simply not available.

Hospital Pressure Groups

Soaring costs in the hospital during the past decade may partly be explained by the newly discovered scientific techniques implemented in its intensive care units. The machinery and nursing skills involved in saving lives in such units are almost prohibitively expensive. Such services are duplicated in every hospital with any pretensions. But who is to say no? Not the patients, whose lives depend on them. Not the physicians, who are primarily concerned with the scientific excellence of their hospital. Not the administrator, whose pride these units are. And yet it is time and past time to evaluate the situation objectively, to try to find out why a comprehensive health service is so difficult to achieve. We may begin by analyzing concerned groups within the hospital

(patients, physicians, administration, and other interested parties) and outside it (its board of trustees, community, state, and nation).

The hospital as now organized must respond to four identifiable social groups within the community that supports it. The first group is the providers of medical care, physicians of the community who comprise the staff of the hospital but who, with few exceptions, carry no responsibility for its management. The patients, clients of the hospital, make up the second group, which is not as formally organized as the first. They exert pressure directly but more often make their wishes known indirectly through the medical staff or the board of trustees. Society as a whole exerts pressure through federal or state governments or quasipublic organizations. And, finally, specific minority groups are beginning to demand, in addition to patient care services, employee training and educational opportunities.

The groups have different views of the role of the hospital and consequently often apply pressures in opposite directions. The patient–clients may demand expanded medical services, while state agencies concentrate on the escalation of hospital costs. Teaching hospitals are responsive to the stipulations of one provider group: physicians of the medical school faculty. Urban hospitals whose original clients have emigrated must redefine their rules in relation to the needs of a core city and must do so with depleted or relocated medical staff. This interaction takes place in the absence of an overall medical care delivery system, and there is no accepted definition of the hospital's role within that system. Services are duplicated; costs soar.

The provider group has until now dominated hospital planning and program development. It is made up of three subgroups: physicians or medical staff, trustees and the administration, and hospital employees.

The physicians are primarily concerned with translating recent medical advances into services for treating their patients. Never before has the medical staff of a hospital had such dramatic opportunities to save or prolong life. The physician considers himself the principal developer and user of these techniques and is quite likely to wish them at hand, regardless of their cost or the probability of their use over a period of time. Special care units, characterized by random input and rather unpredictable peak demands, are as a result often occupied by very few patients. Also, they represent new services added to the existing ones, which themselves may not have been needed. They are expensive to construct and even more so to staff because they usually operate under the supervision of highly paid professional and technical personnel. As each new program is developed, the number of full-time physicians—radiologists, pathologists, anesthesiologists, cardiologists—increases. This added personnel then exerts more pressure on the hospital to allocate hospital resources to new scientific advances.

The governing body of the hospital (in a community hospital its board of trustees) must so distribute its limited money, manpower, and materials as to keep the hospital viable. Under inconsistent pressures from all sides, the allocation process will be political rather than rational, defensive rather than positive. Careful control will be aimed for through the delicate balancing of pressure groups.

Meanwhile, professional and technical hospital employees demand that their wages and perquisites be raised to equal those in industry and comparable nonmedical service organizations. Since hospitals are a labor-laden industry (about 75 percent of hospital expenses are labor costs), the unit of service, the patient day, is bound to go up in price as a result.

The concerns of the clients, that is, the patients, are usually only indirectly communicated to the hospital. True, they "vote with the feet" by coming to the emergency room in ever-increasing numbers and are thus transforming a former accident service into a first-line general medical care facility. The exact reasons for the increase in utilization of the emergency service are not clear. They probably include unavailability of a private physician, lack of a family doctor, or in some cases actual referral by a private physician to this source of care. Here and in the outpatient department, patients have direct access to services. Elsewhere it is rather difficult for a patient to make use of them without a physician's intervention. And as mentioned above, client pressures are conveyed by the medical staff to the hospital in the patient's name.

Society refashions the hospital as an instrument of current social policy. Recent federal and state legislation has broadened the role of the hospital and reshaped its social responsibility. Medicare and Medicaid express a new governmental concern about the cost of care and, hopefully, its quality. Formal patient-centered quality effectiveness measurements are now required by the Medicare utilization review, and the concept is to be extended to Medicaid patients as well. Comprehensive health planning is more than a statement of each citizen's right to high-quality medical care; it is an attempt to bring the consumer's concerns into the health planning area and thus make hospitals and other medical care agencies more responsive to their communities' needs.

Black and Spanish–American groups in the large cities have demanded patient ombudsmen in hospital emergency rooms and outpatient departments, minority representation on the board of trustees, and above all the responsiveness of hospitals to their concerns as they perceive them. This is not the same as a demand for equal treatment. The treatment itself is being questioned, whether given to one or more racial groups. In the past, in-service training for technical, semiprofessional, and professional jobs has offered minorities an opportunity to move upward. The educational effort will be expensive if it is to be more than an apprenticeship program. Should the patient be charged for these costs, or should the community assume financial responsibility for hospital educational programs as it has for college programs?

The hospital, provider oriented, is finding it very difficult to deal with these demands. Hospitals have not yet discovered how to give their constituents a voice in management, and there is an uncomfortable feeling that to do so may result in severe constraints on administration.

But for too long now, hospitals and, in particular, hospital inpatient units have been designed and operated separately and apart from the society they serve. The new hospital and the new inpatient unit as well must be designed to serve their constituency in ways far more active and flexible than in the past. Perhaps we should think of hospitals, as we had to learn to think of railroad stations, as centers—in this case, for medical care and with the difference that it would not all take place within one building. One can visualize wildly diverse patient treatment units integrated within a total care system.

The single system should be conceived of as regional, rational, responsible, and responsive. The problem facing the American hospital today, deceptively simple to phrase, is this: How can the hospital contribute to a rationally integrated, comprehensive medical care delivery system? The answer is as brief and direct, though not easy to implement. The hospital's role within the system must be to meet the needs of the patients it serves and not the interests of the providers of medical care. Let it cease to balance delicately its four constituencies, and deliberately and actively involve itself in the larger system.

Appendix

To make sure that our index would prove a dependable yardstick, we devised one more test. We ran a follow-up study at the Vassar Brothers Hospital in Poughkeepsie, New York, whose nursing units are about as unlike those of the Yale–New Haven as any could be. Vassar Brothers is circular (plan D) with patient rooms on the periphery and all service areas in the central portion inside a circular corridor. There are numerous ways of passing through the central service areas to shorten the distance to patients' rooms or between service areas. A single corridor connects the unit to the elevators and the rest of the hospital. If the traffic pattern *there* were found similar to that of the Yale–New Haven, the Yale Traffic Index should apply to any nursing unit scheme in the United States.

At the outset we foresaw that certain differences in services (not in layout) would affect the pattern:

1. Vassar Brothers has a centralized-tray-service dietary system. Hot and cold tray trucks, carrying 20 meals each, are delivered to the floor and located at four points in the corridor. At the Yale–New Haven, trays are made up in a service pantry on each floor and delivered to the patients' rooms by dietary maids on small open tray carts holding a maximum of four trays. We assumed that the system at Vassar Brothers would result in far fewer trips between patient rooms and pantry but more trips in the patient-room-to-patient-room link.

2. At the Yale–New Haven each room toilet had bedpan-washing facilities. Although every room had a toilet at Vassar Brothers, only those designed as isolation rooms contained bedpan-flushing facilities; all other bedpans were emptied in bedpan washers in two small subutility rooms. At Vassar Brothers, therefore, a new link was expected in the pattern: the patient-room-to-subutility-room link.

Six shifts, a total of 8,712 trips, were observed at Vassar Brothers Hospital. In table A1, the 14 most important traffic links there are compared with those established at the Yale–New Haven during 15 shifts (20,000 trips). Great similarity is seen, and a few pertinent differences. The most important links retain their significance in nearly the same rank and with, in each case, nearly the same percentage of traffic. The greatest relative change in percentage of traffic and rank order occurs in the pantry–patient-room link (seventh at Yale–New Haven, tenth at Vassar Brothers). This was foreseen; we now know the precise extent of the effect of a centralized dietary system.

Two new links assumed importance at Vassar Brothers Hospital, where one link that had seemed important at Yale–New Haven did not emerge. The new links at Vassar Brothers were between the subutility room and the patient rooms, and between the nurses' lounge and the nurses' station. No separate subutility area was included at Yale–New Haven,

TABLE A1. Comparison of the 14 most important traffic links at Yale–New Haven Hospital with those at the Vassar Brothers Hospital, Poughkeepsie.

Yale–New Haven 15 shifts 20,000 trips			Vassar Brothers Hospital 6 shifts 8,712 trips	
Rank	Link*	Percentage	Link*	Percentage
1	PR–PR	19.1	PR–PR	20.7
2	N–PR	16.7	N–PR	14.3
3	U–PR	14.1	U–PR	14.3
4	N–U	9.8	N–U	11.3
5	N–E	6.1	N–M	8.0
6	N–M	5.8	N–E	6.8
7	P–PR	4.6	E–PR	3.5
8	E–PR	3.7	N–NL	2.1
9	M–PR	3.2	M–PR	2.0
10	U–E	2.5	P–PR	1.6
11	M–U	1.8	U–E	1.5
12	P–U	1.7	P–U	1.3
13	U–J	1.1	M–U	1.2
14	P–N	1.0	S–PR	1.2
			P–N	0.9

* See note, table 9 for key; also NL (nurses' lounge), S (subutility room).

where toilets and hoppers were provided in every room; hence, though the same activity took place, it took place inside the patient rooms and was not observed. The nurses' lounge, however, is another matter. A lounge does exist at Yale–New Haven but relatively distant from the nurses' station and not under its control; moreover, the lounge is shared by two inpatient units. Nurses at Yale–New Haven were observed stowing away purses, cigarettes, and so forth in informal nooks and crannies about the nurses' station, treatment rooms, and conference rooms, and they used these areas together with out-of-sight portions of the utility room for smoking and talking. At Vassar Brothers Hospital the more convenient location of the lounge encouraged its use as planned.

A link existed between the nurses' station and the medication closet at Yale–New Haven whereas at Vassar Brothers no such link was recorded—for the simple reason that the medication closet at Vassar Brothers is *inside* the nurses' station. In both hospitals the two areas were very close together. Traffic between the medication closet and the nurses' station was actually a good deal heavier at Vassar Brothers

because the closet there was quite large (large enough for two people) and contained some work counters, whereas at Yale–New Haven it was so small as to seem crowded for one. At Yale–New Haven it was necessary to take syringes apart in the clean utility station and to hold and sort medication tickets in the nurses' station itself.

However, the basic traffic pattern in the two hospitals was sufficiently similar to support the conclusion that the pattern of traffic was not affected by the *shape* of the unit. Differences could be accounted for by factors of size and proximity (the amount of space in the medication closet, for example) and certain administrative decisions (whether or not to serve centralized meals). The index is not refined enough, and there is some doubt that it can ever be so, to subject future comparisons to the tests of conventional statistical criteria. But it would seem from this comparative study of two very different nursing floor plans that the index should be modified to increase the importance of the medication closet–nurses' station link and that an alternative index should be devised for evaluating units that utilize a central tray service.

Endnotes

CHAPTER 1

1 George Rosen, *Madness in Society*, pp. 116–17.

2 Ekrem Akurgal, *Ancient Civilizations and Ruins of Turkey*, Istanbul, 1970, pp. 108–09.

3 Erich Boehringer, "Pergamon," *Neue Deutsche Ausgrabungen im Mittelmeergebiet und im Vorderen Orient*, Berlin: Gebr. Mann, 1959, p. 156.

4 Mario Tabanelli, "Gli Ospedali delle Legioni Romane, lungo 'Limes' Germanico ed Orientale," *Atti del Primo Congresso Europeo di Storia Ospitaliera 1960*, Reggio Emilia, 1962, p. 1259. The so-called House of the Surgeon at Pompeii (first century A.D.) could also be distinguished from a typical Roman house plan only by surgical instruments found in an inner room. The literary sources attest to a workshop in the doctor's home, called an *iatreion*, a kind of outpatient clinic for treatment of and operations upon the ambulatory poor by physicians who were sometimes supported by a tax upon the community. It likewise seems that a few patients unable to return home afterward were cared for by the physician in his house, again not in a special structure built for the purpose but in the regular guest rooms (Theod. Meyer-Steineg, *Kranken-anstalten im griechisch-römischen Altertum*, p. 8).

5 Rembert Watermann, *Ärtzliche Instrumente aus Novaesium*, Köln, 1970. We owe this reference to Professor George Rosen.

6 Meyer-Steineg gives the average depth of patient rooms at the second military hospital of Carnuntum as more than 5 meters (p. 41), of the outer row of patient rooms at the *valetudinarium* of Novaesium as the same (p. 43). Hence our 15-foot estimate of depth. The rooms differed greatly in width.

7 Meyer-Steineg, *Kranken-anstalten*, p. 43.

8 For the reference we thank Professor J. Gribling of Amsterdam.

9 About a hundred years ago an excavated basilica in Porto was actually identified as this hospice, but it is now thought to be a church of Saints Peter and Paul (P.-A. Février, "Ostie et Porto à la fin de l'antiquité," *Mélanges d'archéologie et d'histoire* 70 (1958): 316–17).

10 F. A. Wright, ed., *Select Letters of St. Jerome*, Loeb Classical Library, vol. 262, London: Heineman; New York: Putnam, 1933, 323.

11 Anne L. Austin, *History of Nursing Source Book*, p. 90.

12 F. Cabrol and H. Leclercq, *Dictionnaire d'archéologie chrétienne et de liturgie*, Paris; Letouzey et ané, 1907–53, 6 [1925]: 2760. Rowan Greer, "Hospitality in the First Five Centuries of the Church," *Medieval Studies* 10 (1974): 29–48, brings together other pronouncements on the subject from the Church Fathers.

13 Information about Turmanin has been drawn chiefly from the two volumes of Georges Tchalenko, *Villages antiques de la Syrie du nord*, a reference we owe to Professor Harald Ingholt. Professor Dieter Jetter is not satisfied with the identification of this structure as a *pandochaeion*. There are no texts, only the ruins, and even they are being quarried for housing materials by local inhabitants.

14 This thought was given us in discussion with Professor Jetter.

15 Tchalenko, *Villages antiques*, 2: 19. Richard Krautheimer (*Early Christian and Byzantine Architecture*, Baltimore: Penguin, 1965) seems to favor the possibility that the "convent building" was actually used to house members of the convent (pp. 70, 108); however on p. 111 he refers to *both* dormitory and pilgrim's hostel as individual parts of conventual buildings. Since at Turmanin there was only one such building, it could not have served as both. Tchalenko, although admitting that "it is impossible to imagine, in our conception of monastic life, the use of these buildings," sees them as hospices, for if the monks had inhabited them "one would be forced to believe that their lives were not passed in isolation but in communal living at all times." Might this have been a community of cenobite monks?

16 Charles Jean Melchior de Vogüé, *Syrie Centrale*, Paris: J. Baudry, 1865–77, 1: 138.

17 Tchalenko, 2: 46. He suggests that the skill in stonecutting acquired while preparing these absolutely indispensable cisterns made it possible for the inhabitants to build, with the crudest mechanical aids, such monumental structures as the conventual building of Turmanin. It should be remembered that there was neither native wood nor clay in the region; limestone was the only building material.

18 Ibid., p. 156.

19 René Sand, *Advance to Social Medicine*, p. 70.

20 G. C. Pournacopoulos, "A Brief History of Hospitals in Greece in Ancient Times and the Middle Ages," *Atti del Primo Congresso Europeo di Storia Ospitaliera 1960* (n. 2), p. 1036.

21 E. Jeanselme and L. Oeconomos, *Les oeuvres d'assistance*, pp. 11–19.

22 For this point of information we thank Dr. Charles H. Talbot.

23 Walter Horn, "La Maquette d'après le plan de St. Gall," p. 395. This is a description in French of a new conjectural model of St. Gall Monastery by Walter Horn and Ernest Born. Nearly the same text appeared in German as "Das Modell eines karolingischen Idealklosters," in *Karl der Grosse, Werk und Wirkung*, ed. Wolfgang Braunfels, Aachen, 1965, pp. 402–10 and figs. 124–25. The definitive three-volume work by Horn and Born is to appear in 1975: *The Plan of St. Gall, a Study of the Architecture and Economy of, & Life in a Paradigmatic Carolingian Monastery*, University of California Press, Berkeley–Los Angeles. Our approach to the St. Gall plan was suggested by a series of lectures given by Professor Horn at the Metropolitan Museum of Art, New York, May 1969. It is difficult to thank him adequately for the extraordinary pains he took in reviewing this chapter.

24 Kenneth J. Conant, *Carolingian and Romanesque Architecture 800 to 1200*, p. 298.

25 Horn and Born, "Sanitary Facilities," in *The Plan of St. Gall*, vol. 2, part 5. 18.

26 Estimated on the basis of available wall space—12 beds if ranged single file, about 20 if staggered as in the monks' dormitory ("Novitiate and Infirmary," in ibid., vol. 1, part 3. 2).

27 Justin McCann, ed. and trans., *The Rule of St. Benedict*, London: Burns Oates, 1952, p. 91.

28 Privies for the master's room and the room for dangerous illness in the infirmary cloister seem to have been omitted inadvertently because this is the only deviation from the

absolutely symmetrical scheme of the two cloisters with their common church. Note the warming arrangements for the *pisalis,* or conversation room, which are identical to those of the pisalis in the great cloister: a fireplace outside the walls and free-standing chimney some distance away from it make it necessary to assume hypocaust heating, a flue conveying the heat of the fire under the floor to the outside chimney [Robert Willis, "Description of the Ancient Plan of the Monastery of St. Gall," *Archaeological Journal* 5 (1848): 91].

29 Horn and Born, "Medical Facilities," in *The Plan of St. Gall,* vol. 2, part 5. 10.

30 Cf. n. 27.

31 Horn, "On the Author of the Plan of St. Gall," in *Studien zum St. Galler Klosterplan,* p. 118.

32 The Rahn model, reproduced in *Dictionnaire d'archéologie chrétienne,* 6: 90.

33 In territories of Holland then occupied by German tribes. Walter Horn refers us to H. T. Waterbolk, "The Bronze Age settlement of Elp," *Helinium* 4 (1964): 96–131. For a brief discussion of this house type see Horn, "On the Origins of the Medieval Bay System," pp. 2–23. For some outstanding medieval examples: Walter Horn and Ernest Born, *The Barns of the Abbey of Beaulieu at its Granges of Great Coxwell and Beaulieu-St. Leonards,* Berkeley–Los Angeles: University of California Press, 1965. The problem in determining prototypes for vernacular architecture is that private houses and humble service buildings are not made to last. Then as now, for every stone church there were hundreds of wooden shelters; the timber vanishes, and we derive a false impression from the predominance of stone ruins. Iron age houses have been excavated in bogs where the woven reed partitions between posts still stood in some cases shoulder high.

34 Horn, "On the Origins of the Medieval Bay System, p. 8.

35 Horn, "La Maquette," pp. 398–99 (see above, n. 23).

CHAPTER 2

1 Kenneth J. Conant, *Cluny, Les églises et la maison du chef d'ordre,* p. 63.

2 As Conant informed us in a letter of Aug. 7, 1969.

3 Conant, *Cluny,* pp. 110–11.

4 To give due credit and to satisfy and delight those who would know more about Cluny, we quote the relevant passages from Dr. Conant's letter referred to above:

The Community was bled in shifts—no sorrow, because the infirmary diet was richer, and included meat, which in the old days was not served in the refectory. It is suspected that the monks thought of the *minuto* as a godsend because it gave them a vacation from the ceaseless round of ceremonies. At Cluny, in addition to the usual liturgical round, the whole psalter was sung every day. You can see that it would be natural to make the infirmary resemble the (second floor) dormitory for these folk. I believe that the wards of 1043 were on the ground, but in 1082 there were wards for about 24 sick monks at the upper level, when the Community numbered about 270. The Community was essentially a bachelor singing society on a healthy vegetarian regime. There was, in the late period, a staff doctor. . . . In earlier times the abbot slept with his monks, but about 1100 a palace was provided where the abbot and great visitors could be cared for; and as time went on the high officials of the abbey came to have apartments for themselves and their staff, which reduced the pressure on the infirmary. However, there were distinguished personages, magnates, bishops, abbots, and even one king who retired to Cluny. The tendency was to set them up in small establishments of their own,

which probably show up in the multiplying dependencies of the infirmary, where they benefited from the relaxed liturgical and dietary regimen.

It was expected that each monk would bring a dowry to the monastery (once the austere early days were past). But this meant that many were professed who essentially wished a retirement home, and Peter the Venerable lamented this practise, which sapped the religious vigor of the house, for it was really contrary to the immemorial Benedictine ideal. I have caught myself wondering whether the great groundfloor hall of the infirmary of 1132 was not a sort of clubroom, with its four fireplaces; the sick or bled would be quartered, naturally, in the balconies, which could take 80 to 100 of them. The plans show great openings at the end of this room; I must suppose that there were wooden protective walls (not shown, for the plans show masonry only)—with doors, of course, and possibly demountable. I recognize a few rooms—wards—at the upper, and perhaps at the lower level. And somewhere there was always a kitchen for the special fare—also a chapel, to avoid casual groups in the Lady Chapel of the Cloister, which had an important liturgical program.

5 Cf. Robert Willis, *The Conventual Buildings of the Monastery of Christ Church in Canterbury,* pp. 158–73.

6 Ibid., p. 86.

7 Ibid., p. 54.

8 Ulrich Craemer, *Das Hospital als Beautyp des Mittelalters,* p. 29.

9 Willis, *Conventual Buildings of . . . Canterbury,* p. 54.

10 Jean Fromageot, "Persistance d'une fondation du XIIIe siècle à travers les ages," *Mémoires de la Société pour l'histoire du droit* no. 26 (1965): 248.

11 We were so informed by the late Professor Bernard Rochot of Tonnerre. He and Dr. Fromageot generously furnished much information about the hospital.

12 E. Viollet-le-Duc, *Dictionnaire raisonné de l'architecture française,* 6: 109–11. We do not reproduce yet another time Viollet-le-Duc's mythical drawing of the queen looking down into the cubicles from the balcony. No one knows how beds stood in the cubicles nor how many patients each bed contained.

13 François Amiot, *History of the Mass,* New York: Hawthorn, 1959, pp. 92–93.

14 L. van Puyvelde, *Un hôpital du moyen âge et une abbaye y annexée,* p. 37.

15 Robert Herrlinger, "Das Johanniter-Hospital zu Rhodos," *Die therapie des Monats* 13 (1963): 97; on the hospital at Rhodes, see especially Albert Gabriel, *La Cité de Rhodes,* vol. 1, chap. 3.

16 Grace Goldin, "A Walk through a Ward of the Eighteenth Century," pp. 129–32.

17 Alphons Bellesheim, *History of the Catholic Church of Scotland,* London: Blackwood, 1887, p. 185.

18 Guido Pampaloni, *Lo Spedale di S. Maria Nuova,* Florence, 1961, pp. 19–20.

19 John R. Spencer, ed., *Filarete's Treatise on Architecture,* 1: 139.

20 Salvatore Spinelli, *La Ca' Granda,* p. 83.

21 Ibid., pp. 128, 132.

22 John Howard, *The State of the Prisons in England and Wales,* p. 122.

23 Cf. Spinelli, *La Ca' Granda.* pp. 108–09. A more recent volume is Liliana Grassi's summation of many years' work on the Ospedale Maggiore, *Lo 'spedale di poveri' del Filarete, storie e restauro.* University of Milan, 1972; plan 24 shows the arrangements of the fireplaces on each right wall as seen from the altar. Hansgeorg Knoblauch, "Uber den Kranken-Raum," *Der Krankenhausarzt.* May 1974, p. 14, calculates Filarete's bed

placement from the vestiges of the small cabinets and privy doors between beds.

24 Spinelli, 134–37, drawing upon a reliable account of 1508 by Giacomo Gelino, a hospital deputy, breaks down the components of this hospital system as follows:

The Ospedale Maggiore proper was to be reserved as far as possible only for patients with acute maladies, curable or incurable, that is, "of a kind soon ended, either by health or by death." Nowadays we would call it a short-term acute hospital.

(1) The first of the confederated hospitals, San Lazaro, was for patients suffering from cancer and similar ailments.

(2) Brolo took in chronic cases (not including cancer) and old folk. It received foundlings—exposed children picked up in the streets—and baptized them, maintaining a staff of wet-nurses to give them nourishment immediately thereafter, and then sent them to private homes in the country at hospital expense until they were four years old.

(3) San Diogini, (4) San Simpliciano, and (5) Sant'Ambrogio also took in chronic cases (not including cancer) and old folk.

(6) San Vincenzo was for mentally ill men, quiet or disturbed.

(7) San Celso was for mentally ill women, quiet or disturbed, and received the foundlings at the end of their fourth year. At the age of eight to ten, the boys were sent to other hospitals to learn a trade.

(8) Santa Caterina was for mentally ill women, quiet or disturbed, and also took in the brighter foundling girls, to make nuns of them "when the spirit touched them, or marry them into a better state of life according to the ingenuity and virtue which appears in them."

(9) Donna Buona was for mentally ill women, quiet or disturbed, and for girl foundlings "who revealed themselves of lower origin," as well as for infirm or aged women. Girls not married off (the dowry was given by the hospital) remained in the hospital "under grave and prudent matrons, where they continually spun gold, worked silk, linen, and similar occupations, from which they earned money."

To this system we should add the great Lazaretto, built in 1488 as the result of a special bequest to the Ospedale Maggiore for plague patients.

25 Spencer, *Filarete*, 1: 138.
26 Ibid., p. 141.
27 Dr. Egill Snorrason adds that the dilemma was not uncommon, that in northern Europe *until 1750* rich people were buried inside churches under the paving, making for a dreadful smell even in cooler climates, and that the custom, and smell, came to an end only with the triumph of rationalism.
28 *La Ca' Granda*, pp. 248–51.
29 "Das Hospital Real de Dementes in Granada," *Krankenhaus* 6 (1962): 228–29.
30 John Howard, *An Account of the Principal Lazarettos in Europe*, p. 58; see also his *Prisons*, p. 122.
31 Quoted in Jetter, "Das Mailander Ospedale Maggiore," *Sudhoffs Archiv fuer Geschichte der Medizine und der Naturwissenschaften* 44 (1960): 75.
32 J. P. Pointe, *Histoire topographique et médicale du grand Hôtel-Dieu de Lyon*, Lyon, 1842, p. 79.
33 Jetter, "Hospitäler mit Kreuzformingen Grundriss," *Atti del Primo Congresso Europeo di Storia Ospitaliera 1960*, p. 643.
34 Robert Herrlinger, "Die Lazarete der beiden Furttenbach," *Atti del XIV Congresso Internationale di Storia della Medicina*, Rome, 1954, 2: 711.
35 Ibid., fig. 6, p. 710.
36 Jetter, *Geschichte des Hospitals* (in notes, always vol. 1), p. 79.

37 Herrlinger, "Lazarette," p. 700.
38 *Encylopaedia Britannica* 18 (1969): 557.
39 *Management of the Poor*, p. 2.

CHAPTER 3

1 Camille Enlart, *Manuel d'archéologie française*, 60–61. The remainder of the passage is relevant:

The persistence of this device may be traced through the Middle Ages. . . . Interior divisions were modified according to need, and rich personages travelled with their "rooms" of tapestry. . . . Woodwork partitions had the advantage of isolating better than curtains, while not taxing the beams of the floors below and offering the possibility of being moved without difficulty and great expense if the arrangement of the rooms was to be changed. Partitions not as high as the big walls also existed, forming either alcoves to shelter beds, or frames in front of the doors to shut out drafts.

2 *Introduction to Contemporary Civilization in the West*, New York: Columbia University Press, 1946, 1: 137.
3 Justin McCann, ed. and trans., *The Rule of St. Benedict*, pp. 71, 127. For this note our thanks to Professor Rowan A. Greer III.
4 Dankwart Leistikow, *Ten Centuries of European Hospital Architecture*, p. 29. Professor Walter Horn supplies us with the following additional sources:

An early important documentary study of St. Mary's Hospital in Chichester is C. A. Swainson, "The Hospital of St. Mary, in Chichester," in *Sussex Archaeological Collections*, vol. 24 (1872), pp. 41–62. New material was added to this account by Henry Press Wright, *The Story of the "Domus Dei" of Chichester* (London, 1885) and by the editors of *The Victoria History of the Counties of England, Sussex* vol. 3 (London, 1907), pp. 100–02. J. Cavis-Brown, "An Old English Hospital," *The Newbery House Magazine*, vol. 10 (1894), 342–51 is an abridged summary of Swainson's and Wright's findings and does not make any further original contributions to the history of St. Mary's. An instructive little guide book, *The Hospital of the Blessed Mary, Chichester*, was published in 1955 in Chichester by Canon A. C. Powell.

5 Gustav Schaumann, *Das Heiligen-geist-Hospital*, p. 488.
6 Cf. above, chap. 2, n. 4.
7 Dieter Jetter, *Geschichte des Hospitals*, p. 37.
8 Francis Thomas Dollman, *Examples of Ancient Domestic Architecture*, London: Bell and Daldy, 1858, 1: 9.
9 Information accompanying a print published Aug., 1789, "The Hospital of St. Cross, near Winchester, Hampshire," in the Wellcome Library, London.
10 Dollman, *Domestic Architecture*, 1: 12.
11 Because of its relevance to hospital building in the form of smaller units, we quote in full the passage dealing with fourth- and fifth-century monastery forms in the East from Richard Krautheimer, *Early Christian and Byzantine Architecture*, Baltimore: Penguin, 1965, p. 70:

For the great majority of monks, the eremetical and hence anarchitectural life gave way by the middle of the fourth century to new rules: either a *lavra* system in which the monks, living in individual hermitages, would gather on feast days at a common centre for services and meals; or a coenobitical system (from *koinos*, meaning common and *bios*, life) in which the monastic congregation lives together in a compound composed of living quarters (cells), a dining-room (refectory), a kitchen, a guest house, and an oratory or a church. Both systems were developed in the course of the fourth century, the *lavra* in Palestine, the *coenobium* in Egypt and Asia Minor. By the early fifth century, monasteries are found all over the Eastern part of the Empire and regular conventual buildings develop in place of the villas, country houses, or clusters of hovels which had served the first coenobitical congregations. Distinct from episcopal residences and from parish houses containing offices and living quarters for the secular clergy, these conventual buildings vary in plan according to specific monastic custom or local building tradition. Cells, refectory, and church may form a cluster of rooms, as in Upper Egypt (Aswan, convent of St. Simeon); they may be loosely arranged around an open area, as in northern and eastern Syria and sometimes in Asia Minor; or they may form a tight rectangular block, enveloping an inner courtyard, as in southern Syria; again, the various chambers may be attached in a row along the flank of the church, as at Tébessa in North Africa. Different as they are, all these conventual plans become standard within the confines of larger and smaller architectural provinces.

12 *Encyclopaedia Britannica* 5 (1969): 340A.

13 Enlart, *Manuel*, 1: 48.

14 Jetter, *Geschichte*, p. 50

15 Salvatore Spinelli, *La Ca' Granda*, p. 120.

16 Alessandro Manzoni, p. 386. The term *lazaretto*, originally (1549) used in English to denote a house for the reception of the sick poor, especially lepers (*Shorter Oxford Dictionary*, 1950, p. 1117), has nothing to do with Lazarus, as might be supposed. It is an Italian dialect form of *nazareto*, from Santa Maria di Nazaret, a church in Venice that maintained a hospital (*Webster's Seventh New Collegiate Dictionary*, p. 475). John Howard in his *Account of the Principal Lazarettos in Europe*, p. 26, applies the term to plague quarantine stations at harbors, for goods as well as people, and differentiated from hospitals as such, though similar. Dr. Egill Snorrason informs us that a *lazaret* in Sweden today is a general hospital, in Denmark only a hospital for soldiers.

17 *The Betrothed*, p. 493.

18 Ibid., 482–85.

19 *Madness and Civilization*, first three chapters *passim*, but see especially pp. 7, 45.

20 Henry C. Burdett, *Hospitals and Asylums of the World*, 1: 88.

21 "Die Anfänge der Irrenfürsorge," pp. 222–23. The quotations are from the Reverend Louis Dwight, a Boston prison reformer, 1827.

22 John Conolly, Introduction to *The Construction and Government of Lunatic Asylums*, p. 24.

23 Samuel Tuke, Introduction to *Description of the Retreat*, p. 18. All page numbers refer to the Hunter and Macalpine facsimile edition.

24 George Rosen, *Madness in Society*, p. 163.

25 Foucault, *Madness and Civilization*, p. 45.

26 Rosen, pp. 162–63.

27 Reginald Blomfield, *A History of French Architecture*, London: G. Bell and Sons, 1921, 1: 131, n. 4.

28 Pierre Vallery-Radot, *Paris d'autrefois, ses vieux hôpitaux*, pp. 206–07.

29 Marthe Henry, *La Salpêtrière sous l'Ancien Régime*, p. 28.

30 Ibid., pp. 29–32.

31 Vallery-Radot, *Paris d'autrefois*, p. 114.

32 Henry, *Salpêtrière*, p. 32.

33 Preliminary stages of the advanced engineering concept

had been worked out at the Hôpital St. Louis. See below, pp. 146–47.

34 The source lists this gouache as *Un coin de la cour des 'Paisibles' à l'Hôpital Bicêtre*. Architecture aside, it cannot represent Bicêtre, which was for men, because the patients are female. The well-dressed males in the center of the painting are undoubtedly spectators. We have inserted a cross and an arrow on the plan of the loges of the Salpêtrière (fig. 57) to indicate where we believe the artist was stationed when he executed this painting. The architecture in it seems to correspond with fair accuracy to the layout of the plan, the loges of Bicêtre being quite different (cf. fig. 61).

35 Paul Bru, *Histoire de Bicêtre*, pp. 158–60.

36 Ibid., p. 258, n. 2.

37 Some of the towns are enumerated in Jetter, "Die Psychiatrischen Krankenhauser, ans Anstalten besonderer Art," p. 213.

38 Philippe Pinel, *A Treatise on Insanity*, pp. 175, 216.

39 The pavilion form is discussed below, chap. 5.

40 J. E. D. Esquirol, *Mental Maladies*, p. 78.

41 Jetter, *Geschichte*, p. 86.

42 Paul Bonenfant, "Hôpitaux et bienfaisance publique dans les anciens Pays-Bas, des origines à la fin du XVIIIe siècle," pp. 187–88.

43 Erna Lesky, quoted by Jetter, "Psychiatrischen Krankenhäuser," p. 209. Jetter adds the following evaluation: "If the Narrenturm, the asylum section of the Vienna General Hospital, was already discredited a few decades after its opening, this was primarily a result of the fact that it was impossible to change it to conform with later methods of psychiatric treatment. Its strong walls even now remind us of the principles of force behind that state charity, which did not count on the possibility that even a dangerous madman might be curable. Therefore it is understandable that this remarkable building was never imitated and had to be generally rejected."

44 *Lazarettos*, p. 68.

45 Jetter, *Geschichte*, pp. 122–23.

46 Jetter, "Psychiatrischen Krankenhauser," p. 207.

47 Jetter, "Der Planung der Schlesiger Irrenanstalt (1817)," *Sudhoffs Archiv fuer Geschichte der Medizine und der Naturwissenschaften* 45 (1961): 127–40; "Psychiatrischen Krankenhäuser," pp. 198–222; *Geschichte*, pp. 205–08.

48 See Jetter's discussion of them in *Geschichte*, pp. 209–26.

49 Ibid., p. 224.

50 Edward G. O'Donaghue, *The Story of Bethlehem Hospital*, pp. 202–03.

51 Howard, *Lazarettos*, pp. 139–40.

52 T. Rowlandson and A. C. Pugin, *The Microcosm of London*, with text by John Summerson, London: King Penguin, 1947, p. 19.

53 C. N. French, *The Story of St. Luke's Hospital*, London: William Heinemann, 1951, pp. 37–38.

54 Tuke, *Retreat*, p. 39.

55 Jetter, *Geschichte*, p. 202.

56 O'Donaghue, p. 317. A system for boarding the insane in private homes in Gheel, Belgium, and having them work in the community predated Willis by centuries and persists to this day.

57 Ibid., p. 318.

58 George III, it was recently discovered, actually suffered from a rare hereditary disease, porphyria, only one of whose symptoms is mental disorder. Cf. Ida Macalpine and Richard Hunter, *Porphyria—a Royal Malady*, British Medical Association, 1968.

59 Tuke, *Retreat*, p. 147.

60 See above, p. 53. "Viewing these things . . . day after day, and often reflecting upon them, and with a deep impression, partly derived from the perusal, again and again . . . of the excellent 'Description of the Retreat near York' . . . I was not long before I determined, that whatever difficulties there might be to encounter, no mechanical restraint should be permitted in the Hanwell Asylum" (Conolly, Introduction to *Lunatic Asylums*, p. 23).

61 Ibid., Introduction, p. 25.

62 Then or now, but now the restraints are pharmaceutical.

63 Conolly remarks that if an institution is planned for the actual number of lunatics in a county, within ten years it will have laid in such a backlog of incurables that to take fresh cases it will have to be enlarged (pp. 10–11).

64 The noise from the insane disturbed the seriously ill on the upper floors. The seriously ill infected the insane. Yet when a second wing was added 40 years later, the arrangements were repeated. At the New York Hospital the insane were placed in the basement, in scattered cells among the other patients, and in the newly added upper stories (1791–1803). In 1808 New York Hospital was the first to undertake a separate asylum for the insane (fig. 108; Jetter, "Anfänge der Irrenfürsorge," pp. 218–21).

65 Kirkbride, *On the Construction, Organization, and General Arrangements of Hospitals for the Insane*, 2nd ed., Philadelphia: Lippincott, 1880, p. 51.

CHAPTER 4

1 *Lazarettos*, p. 58; *Prisons*, p. 122.

2 "The Entrances should be Grand, the Rooms Noble and Spacious, and should be contiguous to each other, without the Interruption of Passages or Staircases. . . . [A] Vista through the Middle of the Building should be always had . . . and the Doors of one Room, in a Range of Rooms should be dispos'd to answer each other in a Line, to preserve a Grandeur proportion'd to the Magnitude of the Building" (Robert Morris, *Lectures*, 1730–35, quoted in Emil Kaufmann, *Architecture in the Age of Reason*, New York: Dover, 1955, pp. 23–24).

3 Jetter, *Geschichte*, p. 66.

4 Ulrich Craemer, *Das Hospital als Beautyp des Mittelalters*, p. 93.

5 Cf. Banister Fletcher, *A History of Architecture on the Comparative Method*, pp. 667, 694. "The Italian 'piano nobile' was adopted for many country houses with basement, not necessarily below ground, for cellarage and kitchen offices, while the principal rooms are approached either by a great external staircase with a portico, or by an internal stair from the basement" (pp. 964–67).

6 Vallery-Radot, *Paris d'autrefois, ses vieux hôpitaux*, p. 154.

7 Talbot Hamlin, *Architecture Through the Ages*, p. 329.

8 Palladio, paraphrased by Kaufmann, *Architecture in the Age of Reason*, p. 11.

9 Thomas R. Forbes, *Chronicle from Aldgate*, p. 177.

10 Ibid., p. 183.

11 Benjamin Golding, *An Historical Account of St. Thomas's Hospital, Southwark*, pp. 113–14. Subsequent page numbers refer to this volume.

12 E. M. McInnes, *St. Thomas' Hospital*, p. 61.

13 Hujohn A. Ripman, *Guy's Hospital 1725–1948*, London: Guy's Hospital, 1951, p. 114.

14 Text of 1765, quoted under a reproduction of Thomas Bowles's print on the walls of the present Guy's Hospital.

15 This particular bill, says Dr. Nellie Kerling, Archivist of Bart's, who showed it to us and permitted it to be photographed, was for servicing one of the houses in the neighborhood belonging to the hospital. In 1893 Burdett remarked that "the value of excrement from the point of view of manure must not be left out of sight, when 400 patients yield an annual value in this way of 240–300 pounds" (*Hospitals and Asylums of the World*, 2: 149).

16 Ripman, *Guy's Hospital*, p. 14.

17 Ibid., p. 138.

18 Marcus Faulkner, *An Historical and Descriptive Account of the Royal Hospital . . . at Chelsea*, London: T. Faulkner, 1805, p. 46.

19 *Essai sur l'architecture*, Paris: Duschesne, 1755, pp. 169–70.

20 John Summerson, *Architecture in Britain: 1530–1830*, Baltimore: Penguin, 1963, p. 196.

21 Andrea Palladio, *The Four Books of Architecture*, 2: 51.

22 O'Donel T. D. Browne, *The Rotunda Hospital 1745–1945*, pp. 30–31.

23 *The History and Statutes of the Royal Infirmary of Edinburgh*, frontispiece.

24 The difficulties faced by physicians doing their best to learn from the clinical research made possible by hospitals are well described in Richard H. Shryock, *The Development of Modern Medicine*, pp. 45–56.

25 *History and Statutes*, p. 16.

26 "Clarendon House was among the first great classical homes to be built in London and easily the most striking of them. It was imitated far and wide, both closely and loosely" (Summerson, *Architecture in Britain*, pp. 87–88).

27 Cf. above, chap. 3, n. 64.

28 *History and Statutes*, p. 85.

29 *A History of Public Health*, New York: M. D. Publications, 1958, pp. 117, 147.

30 Thomas G. Morton, *The History of the Pennsylvania Hospital 1751–1895*, Philadelphia: Times Printing House 1897, pp. 36–39.

31 *Benjamin Franklin's Memoirs*, Berkeley: University of California Press, 1949, p. 310.

32 *The Papers of Benjamin Franklin*, ed. Leonard W. Labaree and Whitfield J. Bell, Jr., New Haven: Yale University Press, 1962, 5: 312.

33 Ibid., p. 326.

34 Morton, *Pennsylvania Hospital*, p. 40.

35 James William Beekman, *Centenary Address delivered before the Society of the New York Hospital*, published by the Society, 1871, pp. 11–12.

36 *An Account of the New-York Hospital*, pp. 11–12.

37 Beekman, *Centenary Address*, p. 13.

38 Ibid., p. 37.

39 It is hard to decide where to list Charity Hospital of New Orleans in the order of precedence. Endowed by a sailor's bequest in 1736 as St. John's Hospital, destroyed by hurricane in 1779, rebuilt for 24 poor and needy on the same site but destroyed by fire, renamed Charity Hospital and moved to a new building site on Canal Street, it had 120 patients in six wards and ten years later a 500-bed hospital was built on the present site. Charity Hospital now has 3,500 beds (Mary Risley, *The House of Healing*, pp. 217–18).

40 Cf. N. I. Bowditch, *A History of the Massachusetts General Hospital*, n. on pp. 3–9 for the full text of this argument.

41 Ibid., p. 207.

42 Figures 112 and 113 were supplied by Martin Bander, public relations officer of the hospital.

43 Frederic A. Washburn, *The Massachusetts General Hospital*, p. 648.

44 Grace Whiting Myers, *History of the Massachusetts General Hospital*, Boston: Griffith–Stillings Press, 1929, p. 23.
45 Washburn, *Massachusetts General*, p. 547.
46 Ibid., p. 549.
47 Ibid., p. 550.
48 S. B. Clough and C. W. Cole, *Economic History of Europe*, Boston: D. C. Heath & Co., 1946, p. 202.
49 *Prisons*, Appendix, p. 80.

50 Edvard Gotfredsen, *Det Kongelige Frederiks Hospital*, p. 14.
51 Christopher Lloyd and Jack L. S. Coulter, *Medicine and the Navy*, Edinburgh: Livingstone, 1961, 3: 253.
52 As an example of the most appetizing food we have run across in an eighteenth-century hospital, here is the menu John Howard found hanging in a ward of Frederiks Hospital (*Prisons*, Appendix, pp. 80–81):

FULL DIET.

DINNER *at One.*

		SUPPER *at Seven.*
Sunday.	Soup with forced meat balls; veal cutlets; lamb or beef fteaks; paftry or pud-*N.B. Bread and beer or ale every day.*	Hafty pudding with butter; bread and butter with eggs; beer. *N.B. Bread and butter and beer every night.*
Monday.	Bouillon-foup with pearl barley; veal or lamb fricafee.	Water-gruel with raifins, and toafted bread.
Tuefday.	Broth with toafted wheaten bread and meat; ¹fh roafted or boiled.	Hafty pudding with butter.
Wednefday.	Bouillon-foup with rice; boiled veal, lamb or beef, with fpinach, four krout, cauliflower or carrots.	Soup of bread and beer.
Thurfday.	Soup with bread dumplins, or green cole; broiled meat.	Wine foup, with rice or Scotch barley.
Friday.	Soup with greens, eggs and toafted bread; beef and horfe-radifh.	As on Monday.
Saturday.	Rice milk; fifh or fteaks.	Cherry-foup with toafted bread.

COMMON DIET.

DINNER *at Eleven.*

		SUPPER *at Six.*
Sunday.	Soup, three pints, with beef four ounces, or lamb five ounces with rice; rye bread half a pound; beer a pint. *Bread and beer or ale every day.*	Thick barley boiled in water with grits, a pint, and butter, quarter of an ounce; rye bread half a pound, with butter half an ounce; beer a pint. *Bread and butter and beer every night.*
Monday.	Soup and meat, with Scotch barley.	Water-gruel, with wheaten bread, vinegar and fugar; or cherry foup with wheaten bread and fugar.
Tuefday.	Soup and meat, with oat grits.	Thick boiled barley with butter.
Wednefday.	Soup and meat, with rice.	Water-gruel with wheaten bread, vinegar and fugar.
Thurfday.	Broth, with toafted bread and meat.	As on Tuefday.
Friday.	As on Monday.	Barley-foup with vinegar and fugar.
Saturday.	As on Tuefday.	Rye flour and water hafty pudding, or, as on Tuefday.

Each patient has for breakfast two biscuits and a pint of milk; and weekly one ounce of congou tea, and half a pound of white sugar.—The soup shall be well supplied with vegetables according to the season.

For such patients as are confined to particular diet, the physician or surgeon, instead of the usual food, *orders*, veal-soup, barley-soup, sorrel, spinnach, asparagus, codlins, french plums, and wheaten bread.—Broth and water-gruel is always ready for use.

Frederick's Hospital, 1st July, 1774.

This may be compared with French cuisine at the Hospital Notre-Dame des Fontenilles, Tonnerre, in the fourteenth and fifteenth centuries, as abstracted from hospital records by Dr. Jean Fromageot:

Lamb, beef, veal for soups; pork; fish from the pools and the river. Garlic, onions and beans often mentioned, with "kinds of mustard." Many good cheeses, honey, grapes, fruits and even figs. Wine. Certain specialties seemingly reserved for exceptional circumstances: simnels [a bun or bread of fine wheat flour, says *Webster's Seventh New Collegiate Dictionary*]; cheeses to make "*flancs*" for Easter—probably *flans*, custard tarts; Parisian spices; river birds, hens for the sick, venison paté, beef snouts; cherry "bousillonées;" truffles and baby chicks, generally reserved for "personnages de distinction" [most likely the Tonnerre equivalent of the rich patients who rated private rooms at the Hôpital St. Louis, Paris, cf. below p. 146 and fig. 150]. Milk was always an *aliment distingué*, and among the drugs were listed items that may well have been confections for the patients: violet sugar, rose sugar, assorted syrups, barley water, *lactuères*, and something called *graines de Paradis*.

53 Page 14. As we pinch our noses let us remind ourselves that in some of *our* lakes neither toads nor leeches nor fish nor eels can survive.

54 On Struensee cf. W. G. Petersen in *Annals of Medical History,* New Series 4 (1932): 364–76.

55 *History and Statutes,* p. 9.

56 Henry C. Burdett, Hospitals and Asylums of the World, 5: 43.

57 Wellcome Library, London.

58 Vallery-Radot, *Nos hôpitaux Parisiens,* p. 70, n.

59 S. Gill Wylie, *Hospitals: Their History, Organization, and Construction,* p. 202. Wylie adds, "At the time of our visit, not a window in it was open, and we considered it a receptacle for foul air."

60 *Manuel d'archéologie française,* p. 93.

61 Victor-L. Tapié, *The Age of Grandeur,* New York: Praeger, 1966, p. 208.

62 The controversy is reviewed in Erna Lesky, "Das Wiener Allgemeine Krankenhaus, Seine Gründung und Wirkung auf deutsche Spitäler," pp. 23–37. We thank Professor Lesky for supplying, patiently, enthusiastically, indefatigably, the most useful materials dealing with this hospital.

63 Ibid., pp. 28–29.

64 Ibid., p. 27.

65 Johann Georg Krünitz, *Oekonomisch-technologische Encyklopädie,* pp. 448–49. It is sad to remember that in this hospital Semmelweis tracked down the source of a persistent puerperal fever in the maternity wards and attributed it to the medical staff's habit of going straight from dissection room to delivery room without washing their hands—and that he was ostracized by his colleagues for calling the matter to their attention. Even as early as 1802, it was noted that "in a period of twelve years, more doctors have become victims of contagious hospital fever in the Allgemeines Krankenhaus of Vienna than would normally be the case in five hospitals of the same size" (Erna Lesky, Introduction to *Nachricht an das Publikum über die Einrichtung des Hauptspitals in Wien,* p. 10.)

66 Krünitz, *Encyklopädie,* p. 447.

67 Dr. Egill Snorrason informs us that in the eighteenth century women murdered their children because before being beheaded for the crime the mothers were given absolution by the priest and would go straight to heaven. Otherwise they would remain in purgatory for some years. A woman might also be executed by drowning or by being buried alive, but hanging was considered too demeaning for a wife. A thief might be hung, but very seldom.

68 Lesky, Introduction to *Nachricht,* pp. 19–20.

69 Lesky, "Das Wiener Allgemeine Krankenhaus," p. 30.

70 Ibid., p. 31.

71 Jetter, *Geschichte,* p. 145. For centuries, to prevent their being abandoned in the streets, babies had been admitted to hospitals via the *ruota,* a baby-sized receptacle operating on the principle of a revolving door (or, in some cases, a mailbox), behind which waited a representative of the maternity service. Such an arrangement existed at the Ospedale Maggiore. The mother (or whoever) might deposit the baby, tug the bell, and run.

72 Krünitz, *Encyklopädie,* p. 449.

73 *Nachricht,* p. 11.

74 *Lazarettos,* p. 68.

75 *Nachricht,* p. 6.

76 Ibid., pp. 39–41.

77 Eberhard Hempel, *Baroque Art and Architecture in Central Europe,* Baltimore: Penguin, 1965, p. 10.

78 Jetter, *Geschichte,* p. 158.

79 Ibid., pp. 151, 154.

80 An interesting application of the Milan privy principle can be found at the Holy Infirmary of Valetta, Malta, which was built by the Knights of St. John between 1662 and 1666. The series of doors between beds still runs down the courtyard side of the great hall. Today these doors lead into a corridor with miscellaneous small rooms and—every now and then—a toilet.

CHAPTER 5

1 A critique of recent American medical practice may be found in Eli Ginzberg and Miriam Ostow, *Men, Money and Medicine.*

2 *L'Hôtel-Dieu de Paris au Moyen Age,* 1: 155–59.

3 Vallery-Radot, *Paris d'autrefois, ses vieux hôpitaux,* p. 47.

4 Coyecque, *L'Hôtel-Dieu,* pp. 104–07.

5 Marcel Fosseyeux, *L'Hôtel-Dieu de Paris au XVIIe et au XVIIIe siècle,* p. 273.

6 M. Tenon, *Mémoires sur les hôpitaux de Paris,* p. 140. Our thanks to Professor George Rosen for an extended loan of his personal copy of this book.

7 Quoted in Mary Risley, *The House of Healing,* p. 138.

8 Fosseyeux, *L'Hôtel-Dieu,* p. 274.

9 Phyllis Richmond, "The Hôtel-Dieu of Paris on the Eve of the Revolution," p. 343.

10 *Cours d'architecture,* Paris: Desaint, 1773, 2: 337.

11 "Frankreichs Bemühen um bessere Hospitäler," pp. 147–69.

12 J. Fleming, H. Honour, and N. Pevsner, *The Penguin Dictionary of Architecture,* Baltimore: Penguin, 1967, pp. 166–67.

13 Reginald Blomfield, *A History of French Architecture,* London: G. Bell, 1921, pp. 198–99. Professor Dieter Jetter first called the influence of the palace of Marly to our attention.

14 Jean and Alfred Marie, *Marly,* Paris: Editions "Tel," 1947, p. 7.

15 Ibid., p. 13.

16 Eberhard Hempel, *Baroque Art and Architecture in Central Europe,* Baltimore: Penguin, 1965, pp. 181, 184, 224.

17 As early as 1749, Carré is supposed to have suggested adding many parallel structures to the two wings of the Hôtel-Dieu (Jetter, "Frankreichs Bemühen," p. 152).

18 Tenon, *Mémoires,* p. 440.

19 Ibid., pp. 436–37. Tenon always acknowledged that his ideas on planning were assembled from other hospitals he had seen; the floor plan for the smallpox wards was taken from the Smallpox Hospital and the Inoculation Hospital in London. While it is extremely difficult to put one's finger upon the first instance of any arrangement, it may be possible to indicate an early example of its general use.

20 "Pavilions for the patients' convenience and the sisters', for the wood supply, and the cleaning room and the linen changing; a single one is common to two wards" (*Mémoires,* p. 372).

21 *Oeuvres de Lavoisier,* 3: 696, n.

22 Ibid., p. 705, item E of the key.

23 Ibid., p. 695.

24 Ibid., pp. 698–99.

25 Ibid., pp. 699–700.

26 Antoine Depage, P. Vandervelde, and Victor Cheval, *La construction des hôpitaux,* p. 101.

27 Ibid., pp. 102–03.

28 François Guérard, *L'hôpital de Lariboisière,* Paris, 1888, p. 13.

29 Albert J. Ochsner and Meyer J. Sturm, *The Organization, Construction and Management of Hospitals,* p. 465.

30 Depage, Vandervelde, and Cheval, *La construction,* p. 102.

31 Christopher Lloyd and Jack L. S. Coulter, *Medicine and the Navy,* Edinburgh: Livingstone, 1961, 3: 275.

32 Ibid., p. 265.

33 *Prisons,* p. 389.

34 Lloyd and Coulter, *Medicine and the Navy,* p. 275.

35 *Oeuvres de Lavoisier,* 3: 682.

36 Lloyd and Coulter, p. 268.
37 *Oeuvres de Lavoisier*, pp. 684–85.
38 Lloyd and Coulter, pp. 268, 279.
39 Howard, *Prisons*, p. 389.
40 *Oeuvres de Lavoisier*, p. 700.
51 At Charenton (fig. 64) they did use pavilions for the insane, but only for certain categories of insane. The violent remained in single cells.
42 "Erwägungen beim Bau französischer Pesthauser," p. 252.
43 Ibid., p. 255. Full keys to the plan and elevation may be found in Tenon, *Mémoires*, pp. 60–70.
44 Jetter, "Erwägungen," p. 43. The best of plans needs human cooperation, and can rot in 175 years. In 1784 John Howard named St. Louis and the Hôtel-Dieu of Paris as the two worst hospitals he ever visited. "These two hospitals are a disgrace to Paris" (*Prisons*, p. 177).
45 Tenon, *Mémoires*, p. 64.
46 Norman Moore, *The History of St. Bartholomew's Hospital*, London: Pearson, 1918, p. 20.
47 Professor Jetter brought this plan to our attention. Cf. Victor Fürst, *The Architecture of Sir Christopher Wren*, London: Lund Humphries, 1956, pp. 86–95. Fürst plausibly interprets the two versions of the elevation as Wren's proffered alternatives.
48 Charles Edward-Amory Winslow, *The Conquest of Epidemic Disease*, pp. 177, 182.
49 As paraphrased by B. W. Richardson, *Snow on Cholera*, New York: The Commonwealth Fund, 1936, p. xxxix.
50 *Hospital and Jayl-Fevers*, pp. 4–5. This is not the John Pringle who in 1722 produced *A Rational Enquiry into the Nature of the Plague*, London: J. Peele, a volume arriving at a similar conclusion: "The Air bears the greatest Share in the producing, or communicating the Plague" (p. 7).
51 James Tilton, *Economical Observations on Military Hospitals*, p. 29.
52 *Observations on the Diseases of the Army*, pp. 91–92.
53 *Plain Concise Practical Remarks on the Treatment of Wounds and Fractures*, Appendix, p. 18.
54 *Economical Observations*, p. 48.
55 Ibid., pp. 49–50.
56 The account of Renkioi is taken from Isambard Brunel, *The Life of Isambard Kingdom Brunel*, pp. 461–73.
57 F. J. Stone, "Elements of the Hospital: 1300–1900," *Architectural Review* 137 (June 1965): 415.
58 Cecil Woodham-Smith, *Florence Nightingale*, p. 135.
59 *Eminent Victorians*, New York: Capricorn, 1963, p. 189.
60 *Notes on Hospitals*, p. 23.
61 Ibid., p. 14.
62 *Selected Writings of Florence Nightingale*, ed. Lucy Seymer, p. 119.
63 Winslow, *Conquest of Epidemic Disease*, p. 266.
64 Woodham-Smith, *Florence Nightingale*, p. 227.
65 Ochsner and Sturm, *Organization, Construction and Management*, p. 471.
66 Robert Furneaux Jordan, *Victorian Architecture*, Baltimore: Penguin, 1966, p. 76.
67 Talbot Hamlin, *Architecture Through the Ages*, pp. 578–79.
68 One recalls Cluny, St. Louis, and the project of Le Roy and Viel.
69 Henry C. Burdett, *Hospitals and Asylums of the World*, 4: 137, 156–57.

CHAPTER 6

1 U.S. Sanitary Commission no. 23, *Report on Hospitals in Washington and Vicinity*, p. 2.
2 W. Gill Wylie, *Hospitals, their History, Organization, and Construction*, p. 49.

3 Russell V. Bowers, "A Confederate General Hospital," *The Scarab*, Medical College of Virginia, 2, no. 4 (Nov. 1962): 1–2.
4 Lawrence Wodehouse, "John McArthur, Jr. (1823–1890)," *Journal of the Society of Architectural Historians* 28, no. 4 (Dec. 1969): 271–83.
5 *Hospital Plans: Five Essays*, pp. 17–18.
6 Ibid., pp. xv, xvii.
7 *Description of the Johns Hopkins Hospital*, p. 30.
8 *Hospital Plans*, p. xvii.
9 Ibid., p. xv.
10 Alan M. Chesney, *The Johns Hopkins Hospital and the Johns Hopkins University School of Medicine*, Baltimore: Johns Hopkins Press, 1943, 1: 20–21.
11 *Hospital Plans*, p. xi.
12 Figures 211 and 212. Folsom suggested a rectangular building, high central corridor, and clerestory lighting and ventilation, with 16 single rooms to either side of it, each ventilated by a fireplace; to which two 2-bed rooms were added, plus three large singles with perforated floor for extraordinary ventilation.
13 Siegfried Giedion, *Space, Time, and Architecture*, Cambridge: Harvard University Press, 1962, pp. 206–09.
14 Morris does not always cite sources, and perhaps certain notions hung in the air. In 1867 John Simon wrote, "The Question, what infecting powers are prevalent in given atmospheres, should never be regarded as a mere question of stink. It is of the utmost practical importance to recognize in regard of Filth, that agents which destroy its stink may yet leave all its main powers of disease-production undiminished" (quoted in Winslow, *The Conquest of Epidemic Disease*, p. 20). It may update the problems wrestled with by an earlier generation to quote from an Associated Press release of recent date (*New Haven Register*, Oct. 6, 1971, p. 1):

The problem of hospital cross-infection—or nosocomial infection, as it is called—is major, if not critical, in the view of medical authorities. . . . No one really knows how many such infections occur or how many people die as a result—there might be 100,000 deaths a year. . . . Conservative estimates of the incidence of hospital infections range from 2 to 5 per cent of all admissions. . . . This represents an annual cost of $48 million. . . . Diagnosis and therapy of these infections probably add at least one-third of a billion dollars annually to the cost of hospitalization for the patients who acquire them. It is widely accepted that if hospital personnel would wash their hands more religiously, more carefully and more frequently between patient contacts, hospital infection would be reduced. The two best disinfectants for use in a hospital . . . are soap and elbow grease. Chemical disinfectants do not work if there are too many bacteria present.

15 Billings, *Description*, p. 31.
16 Chesney, *Johns Hopkins*, 1: 61, 69–73.
17 Billings, *Description*, p. 87.
18 Ibid., pp. 88–90.
19 Ibid., pp. 92–94. Cf. figure 112.
20 This arrangement was explained to us by the Assistant Director of Architectural Planning of Johns Hopkins Hospital, William E. Severtsen.
21 In the Frue Kirk, Copenhagen, where, elevated behind the altar, it is reduced to size by its architectural setting. In niches along both long sides of the church are similar-size statues of the twelve apostles.
22 *Address at the Opening of the Hospital, May 7, 1889*, Baltimore: Johns Hopkins Hospital, 1889, p. 67.

23 *Hospital Plans,* p. xvii.

24 Ibid., pp. 43–44.

25 George Rosen, "Louis, P. C. A.," in *International Encyclopedia of the Social Sciences,* New York: Macmillan and Free Press, 1968. 9: 478–79.

26 *The Development of Modern Medicine,* p. 160.

27 Ibid., pp. 161, 176.

28 Malcolm T. MacEachern, *Hospital Organization and Management,* Chicago: Physicians' Record Co., 1957, p. 20.

29 A brief list with dates and discoverers may be found in Erwin H. Ackerknecht, *A Short History of Medicine,* New York: Ronald Press, 1955, pp. 167–68.

30 George Rosen, "The Hospital," in *The Hospital in Modern Society,* ed. Eliot Friedson, p. 28.

31 E. L. H. Corwin, *The American Hospital,* New York: Commonwealth Fund, 1946, pp. 183–84.

32 Ochsner and Sturm, *The Organization, Construction and Management of Hospitals,* pp. 117–19.

33 *Architecture Through the Ages,* p. 601.

34 Ibid., p. 628.

35 *The Big Money,* p. 24, in *U.S.A.,* New York: Modern Library, 1939.

36 "Efficiency in Nursing," *Journal of the American Medical Association* 61, no. 24 (Dec. 13, 1913): 2146–49.

37 "A Plan for the Construction of Ward Buildings in Crowded Cities," *Transactions of the American Hospital Association* 12 (1911): 178–79.

38 Ibid., p. 183.

39 *On Hospitals,* pp. 226, 228.

40 Ibid., p. 240.

41 The description of Beaujon is taken from Vallery-Radot, *Nos hôpitaux Parisiens,* pp. 173–80.

42 John Langdon-Davies, *Westminster Hospital,* pp. 233–35.

CHAPTER 7

This material was published in somewhat different form in *Episteme,* March 1970, pp. 37–76.

1 *Hospitals,* May 1, 1963, p. 41.

2 *Notes on Hospitals,* p. 17.

3 Ibid., p. 102.

4 *Selected Writings of Florence Nightingale,* ed. Lucy Seymer, p. 166.

5 *Notes on Hospitals,* p. 18.

6 Ibid., pp. 6–7.

7 *Hospitals and Asylums,* 4: 59.

8 *The Hospitals, 1800–1948,* p. 137.

9 Ibid., pp. 141–42.

10 Ibid., p. 148.

11 *Pay Hospitals and Paying Wards Throughout the World,* pp. 78–79.

12 Billings, *Description of the Johns Hopkins Hospital,* p. 85.

13 Ibid., p. 96.

14 Goldwater, *On Hospitals,* pp. 270–72.

15 *Transactions of the American Hospital Association* 12 (1911): 171.

16 Ibid., pp. 173–75.

17 Asa S. Bacon, "Efficient Hospitals," *Journal of the American Medical Association* (Jan. 10, 1920): 123–26.

18 John D. Thompson and Robert B. Fetter, "Economics of Occupancy with Varying Mixes of Private and other Patient Accommodations: A Simulation," *Health Services Research* (Spring 1969): 42–52; see chap. 7 below.

19 Folsom, in his plan of 1875 for Johns Hopkins Hospital, considered the advisability of having a water closet and bathroom attached to each private room. "It would add much to the convenience and elegance of the ward. But comfort does not require it, as movable bath-tubs and commodes can be supplied for such as need them" (*Hospital Plans,* p. 91).

20 " 'Efficient Hospitals': Success of Private Room Plan at Temple, Texas," *Journal of the American Medical Association* 74, no. 7 (Feb. 14, 1920): 479.

21 "The Individual Room Hospital—the hospital of the future," *The Modern Hospital* 17 (Dec. 1921): 475–79.

22 *On Hospitals,* pp. 286–90. This chapter, a collaboration with E. M. Bluestone, was written in 1922–25.

23 Goldwater, quoted in Arthur C. Bachmeyer and Gerhard Hartman, *Hospital Trends and Developments,* New York: Commonwealth Fund, 1948, p. 545.

24 *On Hospitals,* p. 290.

25 Goldwater, in Bachmeyer and Hartman, *Hospital Trends and Developments,* p. 545.

26 "The Ward of the Future," *British Hospital Journal and Social Service Review* (hereafter *BHJSSR*) (Dec. 31, 1965): 2466.

27 *On Hospitals,* p. 288.

28 "The Open Ward vs. Single Rooms," *The Modern Hospital* (hereafter *MH*) 18 (March 1922): 233–34.

29 "Bedpandemonium, or, the Two-Bed Room Shouldn't Happen to a Dog!" *MH* 77 (Oct. 1951): 54–57.

30 "Today's Most Talked-about Hospital," *Architectural Forum* 101 (July 1954): 108–15.

31 "Seaside Hospital Has Residential Atmosphere," *Hospitals* 42 (Dec. 1968): 20.

32 "Clustered Patient Rooms Save Space on Nursing Unit," *Hospitals* 42 (Dec. 1968): 20.

33 *Hospitals—Integrated Design,* p. 58.

34 "Integrated Communication through Construction," *Hospital Progress* (Aug. 1960): 64–67.

35 Sanford, "Bedpandemonium," p. 57.

36 "There Can Be Privacy in 'Shared Accommodations,' " *MH* 77 (Oct. 1951): 55.

37 *Architectural Record* 138 (Sept. 1965): 220.

38 M. L. Bobrow, "Design Innovations for Single-Bed Rooms," *Hospitals* 42 (May 16, 1968): 56.

39 "A Trustee Views Hospital Service from the Bed of a Patient," *Hospital Management,* May 1929 (author's reprint, no pagination).

40 "Corner Bunks or Island Beds? A Plea for Comfort and Efficiency," *MH* 34, no.1 (Jan. 1930) 75.

41 O'Connor, "The Corner Bed Location," p. 35.

42 "Patients Want Privacy If They Can Pay for It," *MH* 93 (Oct. 1959): 89–94.

43 "Circular Nursing Division Runs Rings around Rectangle," *MH* 91 (Nov. 1958): 71–73.

44 "Something New in Hospital Circles," *MH* 89 (March 1957): 74–79.

45 "The Minimal Room Offers Privacy At a Price the Patient Can Pay," *MH* 77 (Sept. 1951): 51–55.

46 Carl Walters, "Progressive Care Calls for a Progressive Design," *MH* 92 (March 1959): 79–80.

47 "Why Not Build Patient Room as a Special Care Unit?" *MH* 110 (March 1968): 92–93.

48 "All Rooms Are Private in This Compact Nursing Plan," *Hospitals* 37 (Oct. 1, 1963): 35–41.

49 *Yale Studies of Hospital Function and Design,* U.S. Public Health Service, 1959, p. P21 and chart 4.

50 John D. Thompson, "Patients Like These Four-Bed Wards," *MH* 85 (Dec. 1955): 84–86.

51 M. F. Angell and G. L. Spaeth, "Multibed Rooms Improve Morale, Patient Survey Shows," *Hospitals* 42 (Nov. 1, 1968): 57–58.

52 "Progressive Care Calls for a Progressive Design," p. 80.

53 "A Psychological Study of the Hospital–Patient Relationship," *MH* 83 (Dec. 1954): 72–73.

54 "Nursing Sisters' Revolutionary Plan. The Automated Hospital—with a Room for Every Patient," *Nursing Mirror*, Feb. 24, 1967, pp. 498–99. When last we checked on this project, it was still slated for all single rooms, but the British National Health Service having refused to approve the plan, it was to be opened as a pay hospital. The remark has been made that it does seem odd that in this day and age, nuns should see it as their mission to provide an all-single-room hospital for private patients for profit.

CHAPTER 8

1 Christoph Ludwig Hoffmann, *Bestättigung der Nothwendigkeit, einum jeden Kranken in einem Hospitale sein eigenes Zimmer zu geben* (Mainz, 1788). We thank Professor Erna Lesky for generously responding to our request with the xeroxed text and Dr. Sela Nelson for preparing a summary translation. All quotations can be found within the 204 pages of the text more or less in the order presented. Direct quotes are placed within quotation marks. Other dialogue is paraphrased.

CHAPTER 9

1 A term that came into use with the National Health Service. An amenity patient never paid full cost of maintenance as a private patient and the transaction did not involve a private consultant.

2 *House of Lords Official Report*, April 14, 1970, column 427 "The patient of course realizes why he is screened or moved in this way—a clumsy method of informing him, though difficult to avoid" (Hugh Gainsborough and John Gainsborough, *Principles of Hospital Design*, p. 35, hereafter Gainsborough and Gainsborough 1964. Hugh is a doctor, John an architect).

3 "Ward Complexes—A Modern Approach," *BHJSSR* (Jan. 13, 1967): 55.

4 *The Falkirk Ward*, vol. 4, *Hospital Design in Use*, p. 42.

5 Robert Vaughan Hudson, "The Conversion of General Wards into Private Wards," *Lancet* (July 9, 1960): 90; Gainsborough and Gainsborough 1964, p. 21; Hugh Gainsborough, "Audiovisuality in Hospital Ward Design," *Architects' Journal* 133 (May 18, 1961): 732.

6 Audrey Partington, "From Nightingale to Partitioned PPC Ward," *Nursing Times* (Jan. 26, 1968): 129.

7 Hudson, "Conversion of General Wards," n. 4.

8 "Prefabricated Hospital Wards Designed for Privacy," *Hospital Management* (Sept. 1965): 112.

9 Miles C. Hardie, "Islands of Change," pp. 21–22.

10 Nuffield Provincial Hospitals Trust, *Studies in the Functions and Design of Hospitals*, pp. 14, 15, 22.

11 Gainsborough and Gainsborough 1964, p. 141.

12 Hardie, "Islands of Change," p. 22.

13 "Ward Design," *Nursing Times* (April 10, 1964): 472.

14 *The Evaluation of a Deep Ward Plan*, p. 6 (hereafter *Wycombe Evaluation*).

15 Ibid., p. 2.

16 "Hospital Ward Block," *Architects' Journal Information Library* (April 17, 1968): 827; *Wycombe Evaluation*, p. 41.

17 *Wycombe Evaluation*, p. 19.

18 Ibid., p. 14; George F. Ellis, "Ward Design" (unpublished lecture delivered to ward sisters at the Royal College of Nursing, Sept. 1962), p. 11.

19 *Deep Plan (Race-Track) Ward Units*, Ministry of Health Hospital Building note no. 17, May 1963, p. 10; *Wycombe Evaluation*, p. 51.

20 "Double Corridor Wards and All That," *Hospital Management* (Aug. 1965): 615; "Principles of Hospital Design,"

BHJSSR (July 16, 1965): 1351; *Deep Plan (Race-Track) Ward Units*, p. 2; *BHJSSR* (Aug. 21, 1970): 1637; *Wycombe Evaluation*, p. 50; Hardie, "Islands of Change," p. 27.

21 *The Falkirk Ward*, p. 4.

22 "Principles of Hospital Design," p. 1351; *Deep Plan (Race-Track) Ward Units*, p. 1; *The Falkirk Ward*, p. 52; "Hospital Ward Block," p. 833.

23 Gainsborough and Gainsborough 1964, p. 80; "Principles of Hospital Design," p. 1351; *Ward Units*, Department of Health and Social Security, Oct. 1968, p. 3.

24 Gainsborough and Gainsborough 1964, pp. 59, 121.

25 Phyllis M. Rountree et al., "Staphylococcal Sepsis in a New Surgical Ward," *British Medical Journal* (Jan. 21, 1967): 134–35.

26 "Principles of Hospital Design," p. 1351.

27 Gainsborough and Gainsborough 1964, pp. 61, 77, 109, 143, 167.

28 "Ward Complexes—A Modern Approach," p. 60.

29 *The Falkirk Ward*, pp. 50–51.

30 "Design for Planning," *BHJSSR* (Feb. 17, 1967): 302.

31 *Greenwich District Hospital*, Ministry of Health, Feb. 1968, pp. 8, 10–11.

32 Ibid., pp. 25–26.

33 Plus a lower ground floor and a plant room on top.

34 "The New St. Thomas' Hospital," *Hospital, London*, Sept. 1966, pp. 429–41.

35 Slough Hospital, *British Hospitals Home and Overseas*, London: Trafalgar Press, 1965, p. 63.

36 *New District General Hospitals at Bury St. Edmunds and Frimley*, Ministry of Health, March 1968, p. 7; Nigel Thompson, "Structure in Hospitals," *British Hospitals Home and Overseas* (1968): 12–13. This seems almost a return to a medieval concept of the partitioning of open space (cf. the quotation from Enlart, chap. 3, n. 1 above).

37 *Bury and Frimley*, p. 23.

38 "The Ward of the Future," p. 2465 (see chap. 7, n. 26).

39 "Principles of Hospital Design," p. 1351; *An Evaluation of New Guy's House*, London: King Edward's Hospital Fund, 1963, p. 5 and *passim*; Gainsborough and Gainsborough 1964, p. 37.

40 "Planning," *BHJSSR* (July 25, 1969): 1391.

41 *Hansard Paliamentary Debates, House of Lords Official Report*, April 14, 1970, cols. 421–36.

42 "Audio-visuality in Hospital Ward Design," *Architects' Journal* 133 (May 18, 1961): 732–33).

43 Myre Sim, "Edgbaston Nursing Home: A Development in Private Practice," *British Medical Journal* (Dec. 11, 1965): 1422.

44 "Ward Complexes—A Modern Approach," p. 56.

45 Gainsborough and Gainsborough 1964, p. 34.

46 To nurses of this ilk, a monitoring device was recently demonstrated that, in the event of there being no one in the ward at night, causes a light to flash on in the nearby night sister's office when a certain sound level is reached. "The idea of the installation of this incredible device was greeted by complete silence on the part of the sisters. . . ." "Geriatric Units," *Nursing Times* (Nov. 6, 1964): 1479.

CHAPTER 10

1 "Building on Past Experience," *Hospitals* 26 (Oct. 1952): 49–52.

2 *Design and Construction of General Hospitals*, Chicago: Modern Hospital Publishing Co., n.d. (c. 1947).

3 Poisson distribution is explained later on in this chapter.

4 See below, chap. 18, n. 1.

5 John D. Thompson, "How Many Oxygen Outlets Are Enough?" *MH* 92 (Jan. 1959): 116–19.

6 This was mathematically ascertained in a study on the relationship of births at the Yale–New Haven Hospital to the phases of the moon, which was undertaken to satisfy our own curiosity. It was never published.

7 *Poisson's Exponential Binomial Limit,* New York: Van Nostrand, 1947.

8 John Young, *A Queuing Theory Approach to the Control of Hospital Inpatient Census,* Baltimore: Operations Research Division, Johns Hopkins Hospital, 1962.

CHAPTER 11

The original research for this chapter was done in conjunction with Jane Hartman and Robert J. Pelletier.

1 Elizabeth A. Greener, "The Purchase, Preparation, and Service of Food Supplies," *MH* 2 (May 1914): 291.

2 "Hospital Planning, Fifteen Years After," *MH* 31 (Sept. 1928): 55–60.

3 Elva J. Kahrs, "We Need a New Perspective on Hospital Food Service," *MH* 70 (March 1948): 110.

4 A Study of Food Temperatures, *MH* 31 (July 1928): 142–44.

5 "Certain Factors in Hospital Food Service Affecting the Acceptability of Food to the Patient," 0.0. diss., University of Chicago, 1933.

6 "Desirable Food Temperatures in Hospital Food Service and the Cooling Rates in Various Types of Containers," M.S. diss., Ohio State University, 1954.

7 This may explain the higher temperature criteria of May and Stanton [cf. E. N. May, *Economics of Hospital Food Service,* Wilmington, Del.: Charitable Research Foundation, p. 91; Mark Stanton, "The Cafeteria Comes to the Patient," *MH* 84 (May 1955): 118. See also Evelyn Theresa Farnsworth, "Coffee Temperature Study," M.A. diss., Yale University, 1955, pp. 6, 10].

8 Bessie Brooks West and Levelle Wood, *Food Service in Institutions,* New York: Wiley, 1955, p. 296.

CHAPTER 12

1 P. A. Jewett, *Semi-Centennial History of the General Hospital of Connecticut,* New Haven, Conn.: Tuttle, Morehouse and Taylor, 1876, p. 15.

2 *A Century of Growth,* Pamphlet no. 2 on the New Haven Hospital, c. 1933, pp. 17–20.

3 Ibid., pp. 59–60.

4 Hasbrouck Wallace, album on the history of the New Haven Hospital, Medical Library, Yale University.

CHAPTER 13

1 A comparable study for Great Britain is Winifred Raphael, *Patients and Their Hospitals,* King Edward's Hospital Fund for London, 1969.

2 Private rooms at Genesee Hospital are discussed above, pp. 219–21.

3 "A Psychological Study of the Hospital–Patient Relationship," *MH* 83 (Nov. 1954): 61.

4 John Francis O'Connor, *"The Corner Bed Location,"* M.A. diss., Yale University, p. 38.

5 August B. Hollingshead and Frederick C. Redlich, *Social Class and Mental Illness,* p. 67 and chap. 4.

6 Tables and charts may be found in J. D. Thompson and Doris Johnson, "How Hot is Hot Enough?" *Hospitals* 37 (Sept. 1, 1963): 61–68.

CHAPTER 14

1 Three early studies on mechanical aids to supervision are E. A. Jacobs, "Two Way Audible Communication," *Hospitals* 21 (Oct. 1947): 44; "Call System Conserves Nurses'

Time," *Hospital Management* 77 (Feb. 1954): 62; F. L. George and D. Popovitch, "What about a Voice Intercom System? *Hospitals* 28 (Feb. 1954): 80. Cf. chap. 8 for recent experiences in Britain with smaller rooms that involve the reluctant adoption of mechanical aids as a substitute for direct nurse supervision. At the new Greenwich Hospital, however, a feature of staff-to-staff communication is built into the system: the patient–nurse audio system includes a facility for the nurse to call to adjoining wards if she is on her own and needs help (*Greenwich District Hospital,* Ministry of Health, Feb. 1968, p. 32).

CHAPTER 15

1 At the time of the study, there was a shortage of professional nurses at the hospital. But the auxiliary nursing help (aides and ward secretaries) had been trained by the nursing department and had been in service for a number of years. At this hospital *properly trained* nurses' aides are allowed to perform about 80 percent of the basic nursing services anyway (81 percent when measured by frequency). Licensed practical nurses may perform about 96 percent of all services for patients. The additional 4 percent of services have to do with the administration of medication, either orally or by hypodermic syringe; this can be done only by a professional nurse. Since, quantitatively speaking, her exclusive share of the job was so small, our conclusions about traffic flow are not much affected by the number of professional nurses, practical nurses, and nurses' aides on the floor during the different periods.

2 Some difference inevitably shows up and would have been seen in this study too because we were studying units contrasting drastically in this respect, if it were not that in the private units so many private nurses were being used. Private nurses travel less; they seldom visit other patient rooms in the ordinary course of their duties, and their presence on the private units of the Yale–New Haven tended to conceal what would otherwise be an inevitable consequence of patient segregation.

3 This has been substantiated, to a degree, by the report of Richard Dudek and Dorothy M. Gailani ["Frequency of Nursing Procedures Performed at the Bedside," *Nursing Research* 9, no. 1 (Winter 1960): 43], who found in hospitals in different sections of this country no distinct differences in the top ten nursing procedures—though it did make some difference whether the hospital was a teaching hospital when it came to ranking the frequency with which those nursing procedures were performed.

4 John D. Thompson and Robert J. Pelletier, "Privacy vs. Efficiency in the Inpatient Unit," *Hospitals* 36 (Aug. 16, 1962): 56.

CHAPTER 16

The original research for this chapter was done in conjunction with Robert B. Fetter.

1 First assumed by C. H. Hamilton in 1947 to be four times the square root of the average daily census ((*Hospital Care in the United States,* New York: The Commonwealth Fund, p. 279).

2 The development and validation of this simulation model were reported on in J. D. Thompson and R. B. Fetter, "Predicting Requirements for Maternity Facilities," *Hospitals* 37 (Feb. 16, 1963): 45–49, 132.

3 These occupancies run counter to the theme of this paper and experience elsewhere in the state. The higher occupancy of the smaller unit can be explained by the pattern of medi-

cal practice in the city. Whereas some obstetricians admit only to the smaller hospital and others only to the larger, one group can admit to both depending on the availability of a bed. Thus the smaller unit does not have to be large enough to care for every possible patient requiring admission. Because of these double staff appointments, overflow beds are available for some patients in the larger hospital.

CHAPTER 17

The original research for this chapter was done in conjunction with Robert B. Fetter.

1 Cf. chaps. 7 and 9 and instances throughout history listed in the index under "privacy."
2 New York: Harper and Row, 1968, pp. 36–37, 294.
3 Goldwater, *On Hospitals,* pp. 287–90. See above pp. 214–15.
4 John D. Thompson, "How Many Oxygen Outlets Are Enough?" *MH* 92 (Jan. 1959): 116–22.
5 Hollingshead and Redlich, *Social Class and Mental Illness,* pp. 66–135; see above p. 224.
6 Increased costs are minimized when the small private room (19'9" × 9'9") is employed.
7 "All Private Room Units: They May Be an Unexpected Bargain," *MH* 110 (March 1968): 100, 103.
8 The inpatient unit simulator was written in MAD by Harry David of the Department of Administrative Sciences, Yale University. Computations were done at the Yale Computer Center.
9 Charles Wagner, *Planning the Patient Care Unit in the General Hospital,* Washington D.C., Public Health Service Publication no. 930-D-1, 1962, p. 10.
10 R. B. Fetter and J. D. Thompson, "The Simulation of Hospital Systems," *Operations Research* 13, No. 5 (1965): 697.
11 Donald Wilkinson, "A Study of Patient Transfers in the Memorial Unit of Yale–New Haven Hospital," M.A. diss., Yale University, 1970, pp. 46–50.

12 C. T. Lotreck, "Patients Want Privacy If They Can Pay for It," *MH* 93 (Oct. 1959): 89.
13 J. D. Thompson and R. J. Pelletier, "Privacy vs. Efficiency in the Inpatient Unit," *Hospitals* 36 (Aug. 16, 1962): 57.
14 See above, p. 277.
15 J. F. O'Connor, "The Corner Bed Location," pp. 37–38, and see above, pp. 219–20.

CHAPTER 18

1 Michael L. Bobrow, "Evolution of Nursing Space," pp. 151–54.
2 Robert J. O'Connor et al., "Effective Use of Nursing Resources: A Research Report," *Hospitals* 35 (May 1, 1961): 30–39; Robert J. O'Connor, "A Work Sampling Study of Variations in Nursing Work Load," *Hospitals* 35 (May 1, 1961): 40–41; M. A. Rockwell, *A Summary of Coronary-Care-Unit Literature,* Santa Monica, Calif.: RAND Corp., 1969.
3 *Elements of Progressive Patient Care,* Sept. 1962, p. 2.
4 C. D. Flagle et al., *Estimating Bed Needs in a Progressive Patient Care Hospital,* U.S. Public Health Service (n.d.).
5 R. B. Fetter and J. D. Thompson, "A Decision Model for the Design and Operation of a Progressive Patient Care Hospital," *Medical Care* 7 (Nov.–Dec. 1969): 450–62.

CHAPTER 19

1 *Hospital Guide Issue* (Aug. 1, 1971): 480.
2 M. A. Rockwell, *A Summary of Coronary-Care-Unit Literature,* Santa Monica, Calif.: RAND Corp., 1969, p. 4.
3 *Group Practice and Prepayment of Medical Care,* Washington, D.C.: Public Affairs Press, 1966, pp. 206–07.
4 "Reflections on Violence," *New York Review of Books* (Feb. 27, 1969): 24.

Bibliography

For the convenience of at least two groups of readers, the bibliography comes in two sections. The first contains books and shorter pieces having to do with the historic hospital, the second material on the modern hospital. Both are arranged alphabetically. Roughly, the dividing line between the two, on the basis of subject matter and not date of publication, is 1900. A few items belong in both bibliographies but since repetition was avoided, they will have to be sought first in one, then in the other.

There are selective bibliographies. In the one dealing with the modern hospital, inclusion of an item does not necessarily mean it was referred to in the text but does imply the authors' personal recommendation.

Books on the Historic Hospital

Abel-Smith, Brian. *The Hospitals, 1800–1848.* London: Heinemann, 1964.

An Account of the New-York Hospital. New York: Collins, 1811.

Ackerknecht, Erwin H. *Medicine at the Paris Hospital.* Baltimore: Johns Hopkins Press, 1967.

Austin, Anne L. *History of Nursing Source Book.* New York: Putnam: 1957.

Bentham, Jeremy. *Management of the Poor.* Dublin: James Moore, 1796.

————. *Panopticon; or, The Inspection House.* Dublin; reprinted London, 1791.

Billings, John S. *Description of the Johns Hopkins Hospital.* Baltimore, 1890.

Bonenfant, Paul. "Hôpitaux et bienfaisance publique dans les anciens Pays-Bas, des origines à la fin du XVIIIe siècle." *Annales de la Societé Belge d'Histoire des Hôpitaux* 3, 1965.

Bowditch, N. I. *A History of the Massachusetts General Hospital.* Boston: Houghton Mifflin, 1939.

Browne, O'Donel T. D. *The Rotunda Hospital 1745–1945.* Edinburgh: Livingstone, 1947.

Bru, Paul. *Histoire de Bicêtre.* Paris, 1890.

Brunel, Isambard. *The Life of Isambard Kingdom Brunel: Civil Engineer.* London: Longsmans Green, 1870.

Burdett, Henry C. *Hospitals and Asylums of the World.* 5 Vols. (one of plans) London: Churchill, 1891.

————. *Pay Hospitals and Paying Wards Throughout the World.* Philadelphia: P. Blakiston, 1880.

Conant, Kenneth J. *Carolingian and Romanesque Architecture 800 to 1200.* Baltimore: Penguin, 1959; 3rd ed., 1974; 1st paperback ed. 1974.

————. *Cluny, les églises et la maison du chef d'ordre.* Cambridge, Mass.: Medieval Academy of America, 1968.

Conolly, John. *The Construction and Government of Lunatic Asylums* (first published 1847). Edited by Richard Hunter and Ida Macalpine. London: Dawson's, 1968.

Coyecque, E. *L'Hôtel-Dieu de Paris au Moyen Age.* Paris: Champion, 1891.

Craemer, Ulrich. *Das Hospital als Beautyp des Mittelalters.* Köln: W. Kohlhammer, 1963.

Depage, Antoine; Vandervelde, P.; and Cheval, Victor. *La construction des hôpitaux.* Brussels: Misch & Thron, 1909.

Edelstein, Emma J., and Edelstein, Ludwig. *Asclepius.* Baltimore: Johns Hopkins Press, 1945.

Enlart, Camille. *Manuel d'archéologie française.* Vol. 1. Paris: Picard, 1929.

Esquirol, J. E. D. *Mental Maladies, a Treatise on Insanity.* A fascimile of the English edition of 1845. New York: Hafner, 1965.

Fletcher, Banister. *A History of Architecture on the Comparative Method.* New York: Scribner, 1963.

Forbes, Thomas Rogers. *Chronicle from Aldgate, Life and Death in Shakespeare's London.* New Haven: Yale University Press, 1971.

Fosseyeux, Marcel. *L'Hôtel-Dieu de Paris au XVIIe et au XVIIIe siècle.* Paris: Berger-Levrault, 1912.

Foucault, Michel. *Madness and Civilization.* New York: Random House, 1965.

Gabriel, Albert. *La Cité de Rhodes.* 2 Vols. Paris: Boccard, 1921. Volume 1, chapter 3 deals with the hospital.

Goldin, Grace. "A Walk through a Ward of the Eighteenth Century." *Journal of the History of Medicine and Allied Sciences* 22, no. 2 (1967): 121–38.

Golding, Benjamin. *Historical Account of St. Thomas's Hospital, Southwark.* London: Longman, 1819.

Gotfredsen, Edvard. *Det Kongelige Frederiks Hospital.* Copenhagen, 1957.

Grassi, Liliana. *La Ca' Granda.* University of Milan, 1957–58.

Guérard, François. *L'Hôpital de Lariboisière*. Paris, 1888.

Hamlin, Talbot. *Architecture Through the Ages*. New York: Putnam, 1953.

Henry, Marthe. *La Salpêtrière sous l'Ancien Régime*. Paris: Librairie le François, 1922.

The History and Statutes of the Royal Infirmary of Edinburgh. Edinburgh: Balfour and Smellie, 1778.

Horn, Walter. "La Maquette d'après le plan de St. Gall." *Charlemagne, oeuvre, rayonnement et survivances*, 10e Exposition sous les auspices de conseil de l'Europe, ed. Wolfgang Braunfels, Aix-la-Chapelle, 1965, pp. 391–400.

———. "On the Author of the Plan of St. Gall and the Relation of the Plan to the Monastic Reform Movement." In *Studien zum St. Galler Klosterplan*, ed. Johannes Duff, 1962, pp. 103–27.

———. "On the Origins of the Medieval Bay System." *Journal of the Society of Architectural Historians* 17 (summer 1958): 2–23.

Hospital Plans: Five Essays. New York: William Wood, 1875.

Howard, John. *An Account of the Principal Lazarettos in Europe*. London, 1791.

———. *The State of the Prisons in England and Wales*. London: Warrington, 1784.

Husson, Armand. *Etude sur les hôpitaux*. Paris: Paul Dupont, 1862.

Jeanselme, E., and Oeconomos, L. *Les oeuvres d'assistance et les hôpitaux Byzantins au siècle des Comnènes*. Anvers, 1921.

Jetter, Dieter. "Die Anfange der Irrenfursorge in den Vereinigten Staaten von Amerika." *Confinia Psychiatrica* 2 (1968): 210–24.

———. "Die Psychiatrischen Krankenhäuser als Anstalten besonderer Art." *Confinia Psychiatrica* 9 (1966): 198–222.

———. "Erwägungen beim Bau französischer Pesthauser." *Archives internationales d'histoire des sciences* 76 (Sept. 1966): 247–62.

———. "Frankreichs Bemühen um bessere Hospitäler." *Sudhoffs Archiv fuer Geschichte der Medizine und der Naturwissenschaften* 49 (1965): 147–69.

———. *Geschichte des Hospitals*. Vol. 1. Wiesbaden, 1966.

Jones, John. *Plain Concise Practical Remarks on the Treatment of Wounds and Fractures*. New York: Holt, 1775.

Krunitz, Johann Georg. *Oekonomisch-technologische Encyklopädie* 47 (1789): 444–70.

Langdon-Davies, John. *Westminster Hospital*. London: John Murray, 1952.

Laugier, Marc Antoine. *Essai sur l'architecture*. Paris: Duchesne, 1755.

Lavoisier, Antoine. *Oeuvres de Lavoisier*. Vol. 3. Paris: Imprimerie Impériale, 1865, pp. 603–704.

Leistikow, Dankwart. *Ten Centuries of European Hospital Architecture*. Ingelheim am Rhein: C. H. Boehringer, 1967.

Lesky, Erna. "Das Wiener Allgemeine Krankenhaus, Seine Grundung und Wirkung auf deutsche Spitäler." *Clio Medica* 2 (1967): 23–37.

McInnes, E. M. *St. Thomas's Hospital*. London: Allen & Unwin, 1963.

Manzoni, Alessandro. *The Betrothed* (original publication 1827). Translated by Archibald Colquhoun. London: Everyman's, 1968.

Meyer-Steineg, Theodore. *Kranken-anstalten im griechisch-romischen Altertum*. Jena: Gustav Fisher, 1912.

Møller-Christensen, Vilh. *Bogen om Æbelholt Kloster*. Copenhagen: Dansk Videnskabs Forlag, 1958, pp. 17–73.

Nachricht an das Publikum über die Einrichtung des Hauptspitals in Wien. Original publication 1784; facsimile by the Wiener Bibliophilangesellschaft, Vienna, 1960, with an introduction by Erna Lesky.

Nightingale, Florence. *Notes on Hospitals*. London: John W. Parker & Son, 1859.

———. *Selected Writings of Florence Nightingale*. Edited by Lucy Seymer. New York: Macmillan, 1954.

O Donaghue, Edward G. *The Story of Bethlehem Hospital*. London: Unwin, 1914.

Palladio, Andrea. *The Four Books of Architecture*. New York: Dover, 1965.

Pinel, Philippe. *A Treatise on Insanity*. Original publication 1802. Translated by D. D. Davis. New York: Hafner, 1962.

Pringle, John. *Observations on the Diseases of the Army*. Originally published 1752. Edited by Benjamin Rush. Philadelphia: Finley, 1812.

———. *Observations on the Nature and Cure of Hospital and Jayl-Fevers*. London: Millar, 1750.

Richmond, Phyllis. "The Hôtel-Dieu of Paris on the Eve of the Revolution." *Journal of the History of Medicine and Allied Sciences* 16 (Oct. 1961): 335–53.

Risley, Mary. *The House of Healing*. New York: Doubleday, 1961.

Rosen, George. "The Hospital." In *The Hospital in Modern Society*, edited by Eliot Friedsen. Glencoe (Ill.): Free Press, 1965.

———. *Madness in Society*. New York: Harper and Row, 1968.

Sand, René. *The Advance to Social Medicine*. London: Staples, 1952.

Schaumann, Gustav. *Das Heiligen-geist-Hospital*. Lübeck, 1906.

Shryock, Richard H. *The Development of Modern Medicine*. New York: Knopf, 1947.

Sigerist, Henry E. *Medicine and Human Welfare.* New Haven: Yale University Press, 1941.

Snow, John. *Snow on Cholera.* Edited by B. W. Richardson. New York: The Commonwealth Fund, 1936.

Spencer, John R., ed. *Filarete's Treatise on Architecture.* New Haven: Yale University Press, 1965; vol. 1, pp. 137–46; vol. 2, 81r–82v.

Spinelli, Salvatore. *La Ca' Granda.* Milan, 1958.

Studien zum St. Galler Klosterplan. St. Gall, Switzerland: Fehr'sche Buchhandlung, 1962.

Tchalenko, Georges. *Villages antiques de la Syrie du nord.* 2 Vols. Paris: Guethner, 1963.

Tenon, M. *Mémoires sur les hôpitaux de Paris.* Paris: Ph.-D. Pierres, 1788.

Tilton, James. *Economical Observations on Military Hospitals and the Prevention and Cure of Diseases Incident to an Army.* Wilmington, Del.: J. Wilson, 1813.

Tollet, Casamir. *De l'Assistance Publique et des Hôpitaux jusqu'au XIXe siècle.* Paris, 1889.

———. *Les edifices hospitaliers depuis leur origine jusqu'à nos jours.* Paris, 1892.

Tuke, Samuel. *Description of the Retreat.* First published 1813. Edited by Richard Hunter and Ida Macalpine, London: Dawson's, 1964.

U.S. Sanitary Commission, no. 23. *Report on Hospitals in Washington and Vicinity.* July 31, 1861.

Van Puyvelde, L. *Un hôpital du moyen age et une abbaye y annexée.* Paris: Champion, 1925.

Vallery-Radot, Pierre. *Nos hôpitaux Parisiens, un siècle d'histoire hospitalière de Louis-Philippe jusqu'à nos jours (1837–1949).* Paris: Éditions Paul Dupont, 1948.

———. *Paris d'autrefois, ses vieux hôpitaux. Deux siècles d'histoire hospitalière de Henri IV à Louis-Philippe (1602–1836).* Paris: Éditions Paul Dupont, 1947.

Viollet-le-Duc, E. *Dictionnaire raisonné de l'architecture française.* Vol. 6. *Hôtel-Dieu.* Paris: Morel, 1875, pp. 99–120.

Washburn, Frederic A. *The Massachusetts General Hospital.* Boston: Houghton Mifflin, 1939.

Willis, Robert. "Description of the Ancient Plan of the Monastery of St. Gall." *The Archaeological Journal* 5 (1848): 85–116.

———. *The Conventual Buildings of the Monastery of Christ Church in Canterbury.* London: Kent Architectural Society, 1869.

Winslow, Charles-Edward Amory. *The Conquest of Epidemic Disease.* New York: Hafner, 1967.

Woodham-Smith, Cecil. *Florence Nightingale.* New York: McGraw-Hill, 1951.

Wright, Lawrence. *Clean and Decent.* New York: Viking, 1960.

Wylie, S. Gill. *Hospitals: Their History, Organization, and Construction.* New York: Appleton, 1877.

Books on the Modern Hospital

Bachmeyer, Arthur C., and Hartman, Gerhard. *The Hospital in Modern Society.* New York: The Commonwealth Fund, 1943.

Bacon, Asa S. "Efficient Hospitals." *Journal of the American Medical Association* (January 10, 1920): 123–26.

Becker, Harry, ed. *Prepayment and the Community.* Vol. 2. *Financing Hospital Care in the United States.* New York: McGraw-Hill, 1955.

Bobrow, Michael L. "The Evolution of Nursing Space Planning for Efficient Operation." *Architectural Record* (September 1971): 151–54.

Design and Construction of General Hospitals. Chicago: Modern Hospital Publishing, n.d. Originally appeared in *The Modern Hospital,* March 1947.

Dichter, Ernest. "The Hospital–Patient Relationship." *The Modern Hospital* 83, 1954, Sept., p. 51 +; Oct., p. 56 +; Nov., p. 61 +; Dec., 69 +; Jan. 1955, p. 74+.

The Economics of Health and Medical Care. Ann Arbor: University of Michigan Press, 1964.

Elements of Progressive Patient Care. U.S. Department of Health, Education and Welfare, Sept. 1962.

The Evaluation of a Deep Ward Plan. Oxford Regional Hospital Board, August 1970.

The Falkirk Ward. Vol. 4. *Hospital Design in Use.* Edinburgh: Scottish Home and Health Department, 1969.

Faxon, Nathaniel W. *The Hospital in Contemporary Life.* Cambridge, Mass.: Harvard University Press, 1949.

Flexner, Abraham. *Medical Education in the United States and Canada.* Carnegie Foundation, Bulletin no. 4, 1910. Reproduced in 1960 by William F. Fell Co.

Gainsborough, Hugh, and Gainsborough, John. *Principles of Hospital Design.* London: Architectural Press, 1964.

Ginzberg, Eli, and Ostow, Miriam. *Men, Money and Medicine.* New York: Columbia University Press, 1969.

Goldwater, S. S. "A Plan for the Construction of Ward Buildings in Crowded Cities." *Transactions of the American Hospital Association* 12 (1911): 178–85.

———. *On Hospitals.* New York: Macmillan, 1949.

Hardie, Miles C. "Islands of Change." *Hospital Administration* (summer 1969): 7–40.

Hill-Burton Publications. An Annotated Bibliography. Rev. ed. 1963. United States Department of Health, Education and Welfare, Public Health Service Publication no. 930-G-3.

Hollingshead, August B., and Redlich, Frederick C.

Social Class and Mental Illness: A Community Study. New York: Wiley, 1958.

Hudenburg, Roy. *Planning the Community Hospital.* New York: McGraw-Hill, 1967.

An Investigation of the Relation Between Nursing Activity and Patient Welfare. State University of Iowa, 1960.

Lave, Judith R. "A Review of the Methods Used to Study Hospital Costs." *Inquiry* (May 1966): 57–81.

MacColl, William A. *Group Practice and Prepayment of Medical Care.* Washington, D.C.: Public Affairs Press, 1966.

McGibony, John R. *Principles of Hospital Administration.* New York: Putnam, 1952.

McNerney, Walter J. *Hospital and Medical Economics.* 2 Vols. Chicago: Hospital Research and Educational Trust, 1962.

Manual on Obstetrical Practice in Hospitals. Chicago: American Hospital Association, 1936.

Medical Care for the American People. The Final Report of the Committee on the Costs of Medical Care. First printing, University of Chicago Press, October 1932. Reprint. United States Department of Health, Education and Welfare, 1970.

Molina, E. C. *Poisson's Exponential Binomial Limit.* New York: Van Nostrand, 1947.

Nuffield Provincial Hospitals Trust. *Children in Hospital.* London: Oxford University Press, 1963.

Nuffield Provincial Hospitals Trust. *Studies in the Functions and Design of Hospitals.* London: Oxford University Press, 1955.

Ochsner, Albert J., and Sturm, Meyer J. *The Organization, Construction and Management of Hospitals.* Chicago: Cleveland Press, 1907.

O'Connor, John Francis. "The Corner Bed Location." M.A. thesis, Yale University, 1959.

Rosenfield, Isadore. *Hospitals—Integrated Design.* New York: Reinhold, 1947.

Sloan, Raymond P. *This Hospital Business of Ours.* New York: Putnam, 1952.

Smalley, Harold E., and Freeman, John R. *Hospital Industrial Engineering.* New York: Reinhold, 1966.

Somers, Herman M., and Somers, Anne R. *Medicare and the Hospitals, Issues and Prospects.* Washington D.C.: Brookings Institution, 1967.

Thompson, John D., and Fetter, Robert B. "Economics of Occupancy with Varying Mixes of Private and Other Patient Accommodations: A Simulation." *Health Services Research* (Spring 1969): 42–52.

Thompson, W. Gilman. "Efficiency in Nursing." *Journal of the American Medical Association* 61, no. 24 (Dec. 13, 1913): 2146–49.

Weeks, Lewis E., and Griffeth, John R., eds. *Progressive Patient Care, an Anthology.* Ann Arbor: University of Michigan Press, 1964.

Wheeler, E. Todd. *Hospital Design and Function.* New York: McGraw-Hill, 1964.

Wright, Marion J. *Improvement of Patient Care, a Study at Harper Hospital.* New York: Putnam, 1954.

ADDENDUM

Received too late for inclusion in text or notes: Louis S. Greenbaum, " 'Measure of Civilization': The Hospital Thought of Jacques Tenon on the Eve of the French Revolution." *Bulletin of the History of Medicine* 49 (Spring, 1975): 43–56.

> The physical stature of man was basic. From it could be determined the proper size of a hospital bed. . . . Man's oxygen requirements, derived from Lavoisier's 1785 respiration experiments, determined the height of ceilings, governed the number of patients per ward and hence its size. . . . Man's water requirements for health and cleanliness . . . directly determined the planning of kitchens and wards and the location of reservoirs, toilets, baths, laundries, kitchens, pharmacies, taps and sewers. The sick man's gait determined the design and construction of staircases. The variety of human ailment governed the location of wards within the hospitals. (pp. 48–49)

Index